FIRST AID FOR THE USMLE STEP 1

A STUDENT TO STUDENT GUIDE

UPDATED FOR 98

VIKAS BHUSHAN, MD
University of California, San Francisco, Class of 1991
Diagnostic Radiologist

TAO LE, MD
University of California, San Francisco, Class of 1996
Yale–New Haven Hospital, Resident in Internal Medicine

CHIRAG AMIN, MD
University of Miami, Class of 1996
Orlando Regional Medical Center, Resident in Orthopaedic Surgery

VIPAL SONI
1998 Student Editor
University of California, Los Angeles, Class of 1999

HOANG NGUYEN
1998 Student Editor
Northwestern University, Class of 1999

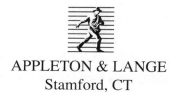

APPLETON & LANGE
Stamford, CT

S0-BYC-484

Copyright © 1998 by Appleton & Lange
A Simon & Schuster Company
Copyright © 1997, 1996, 1995, 1994, 1993, 1992, 1991 by Appleton & Lange
First edition copyright © 1990, 1989 by Vikas Bhushan, Jeffrey Hansen, and Edward Hon

Information from the following titles was incorporated into Section II: Database of High-Yield Facts, and was used with permission: Stobo, *The Principles and Practice of Medicine,* 23rd ed., Appleton & Lange, 1996; McPhee, *Pathophysiology of Disease,* 2nd ed., Appleton & Lange, 1997; Paulsen, *Basic Histology,* 3rd ed., Appleton & Lange, 1996; Katzung BG (editor), *Basic & Clinical Pharmacology,* 7th ed., Appleton & Lange, 1997; Goldman HH, *Review of General Psychiatry,* 5th ed., Appleton & Lange, 1992; Ganong WF, *Review of Medical Physiology,* 18th ed., Appleton & Lange, 1996; Levinson W, *Medical Microbiology and Immunology: Examination and Board Review,* 4th ed., Appleton & Lange, 1996; Chandrasoma P, *Concise Pathology,* 3rd ed., Appleton & Lange, 1997; Costanzo L, *BRS Physiology,* 1st ed., Williams & Wilkins, 1995. The diagram on p. 179 was adapted from *Curr Opin Infect Dis* 1992; **5:**214. Portions of the material in Section I are copyright © 1997 by The Federation of State Medical Boards of the United States, Inc., and the National Board of Medical Examiners®.

98 99 00 01 / 10 9 8 7 6 5 4 3 2 1

Prentice Hall International (UK) Limited, *London*
Prentice Hall of Australia Pty. Limited, *Sydney*
Prentice Hall of Canada, Inc., *Toronto*
Prentice Hall Hispanoamericana, S.A., *Mexico*
Prentice Hall of India Private Limited, *New Delhi*
Prentice Hall of Japan, Inc., *Tokyo*
Simon & Schuster Asia Pte. Ltd., *Singapore*
Editora Prentice Hall do Brasil Ltda., *Rio de Janeiro*
Prentice Hall, *Upper Saddle River, New Jersey*

ISBN 0-8385-2603-9

90000

9 780838 526033

Acquisitions Editor: Marinita Timban
Production: Rainbow Graphics, Inc.
Editorial Consultant: Andrea Fellows

PRINTED IN THE UNITED STATES OF AMERICA

To the contributors to this and future editions, who took
time to share their knowledge, insight, and
humor for the benefit of students.

&

To our families, friends and loved ones, who endured
and assisted in the task of assembling this guide.

1998 Contributors

ANTHONY GLASER, MD, PhD
Contributing Author, IMG Section
Medical University of South Carolina, Resident

RICK KULKARNI
Contributing Author, Website
University of California, San Francisco, Class of 1998

JENNIFER STEINFELDT
Contributing Author, Review Resources
University of California, Los Angeles, Class of 1999

ANTONIO WONG
Contributing Author, Website
University of California, San Francisco, Class of 1998

1998 Associate Contributors

VISHAL BANTHIA
University of California, San Francisco, Class of 1999

JOSÉ FIERRO, MD
Toluca, Mexico

1998 Faculty Reviewers

WILLIAM GANONG, MD
Lange Professor of Physiology Emeritus
University of California, San Francisco

BERTRAM KATZUNG, MD, PhD
Professor of Pharmacology
University of California, San Francisco

WARREN LEVINSON, MD, PhD
Professor of Microbiology and Immunology
University of California, San Francisco

HENRY SANCHEZ, MD
Assistant Clinical Professor of Pathology
University of California, San Francisco

Contents

Preface to the 1998 Edition

With the 1998 edition of *First Aid for the USMLE Step 1,* we continue our commitment to providing students with the most useful and up-to-date preparation guide for the USMLE Step 1. The 1998 edition represents a thorough revision in many ways and includes:

- Revisions and new material based on student experience with the June 1997 administration of the USMLE Step 1.
- A revised and updated guide to efficient exam preparation, including new Step 1 statistics, new study and test-taking strategies for clinical vignettes, and the latest information on the upcoming **computerized adaptive USMLE Step 1.**
- A new section on **high-yield clinical vignettes** for each discipline.
- Revised USMLE advice geared toward international medical graduates and osteopathic medical students.
- More than 850 frequently tested facts and useful mnemonics, including **more than 100 new or expanded entries with over 50 new diagrams and illustrations.**
- An updated listing of more than 250 high-yield study topics that highlight key areas of basic science and clinical material recently emphasized on the USMLE Step 1.
- A **completely revised, in-depth guide** to over 200 basic science review and sample examination books, based on a random survey of thousands of third-year medical students across the country. Includes **more than 40 new books and software titles.**

The 1998 edition would not have been possible without the help of the hundreds of students and faculty members who contributed their feedback and suggestions. We invite students and faculty to continue sharing their thoughts and ideas to help us improve *First Aid for the USMLE Step 1.* (*See* How to Contribute, p. xv, and User Survey, p. xxiii.)

Los Angeles	Vikas Bhushan
New Haven	Tao Le
Orlando	Chirag Amin
Los Angeles	Vipal Soni
Chicago	Hoang Nguyen

November 1997

Foreword

The purpose of *First Aid for the USMLE Step 1: A Student-to-Student Guide* is to help medical students and foreign medical graduates review the basic medical sciences and prepare for the United States Medical Licensing Examination, Step 1 (USMLE Step 1). Preparing for this examination can be a stressful, difficult, and costly task. This book helps students make the most of their limited time, money, and energy. As is often the case in medical school, we found that the best advice a student can receive is from other medical students. We also recognized that certain basic science topics and details are "popular" and appear frequently on examinations. With this in mind, *First Aid for the USMLE Step 1* was started in 1989.

As we studied for the NBME Part I, we examined and evaluated scores of review books and thousands of sample questions. We kept track of useful study strategies, frequently tested facts, and helpful mnemonics through a simple computer database. The printed database was first distributed to the medical school class of 1992 at the University of California, San Francisco (UCSF). The next year, a revised edition was self-published under the name *High-Yield Basic Science Boards Review: A Student-to-Student Guide.* This guide was distributed to the UCSF class of 1993 and to numerous faculty and medical students at various institutions.

The title reflects the potential value of this book as the "first" one to get before buying others, and the fact that boards examinations are stressful and unpleasant experiences that students may "aid" each other in overcoming. We feel that this study guide provides a unique and pragmatic approach to the USMLE Step 1 and that it contains useful components not found in current boards review material. *First Aid for the USMLE Step 1* has three major sections:

Section I: Guide to Efficient Exam Preparation is a compilation of general student advice and study strategies for taking the USMLE Step 1.

Section II: Database of High-Yield Facts contains short descriptions of frequently tested facts and concepts as well as mnemonics and diagrams to facilitate learning. It includes a unique summary of subject-by-subject examination emphases as estimated by students who have recently taken the examination.

Section III: Database of Basic Science Review Books is designed to save students time and money by identifying high-quality, reasonably priced review and sample examination books and software. The comments and ratings are based on our analyses and on a nationwide random sampling of third-year medical students.

First Aid for the USMLE Step 1 is not designed to be a comprehensive text or the sole study source for the USMLE Step 1; it is meant as a **guide** to one's preparation for the USMLE Step 1. The material in this book has been written to strengthen one's familiarity with a large number of topics in a short, fact-based review. The authors do not advocate blindly memorizing the lists of facts, and we hope medical students realize that memorization cannot replace an understanding of the concepts that underlie these key points.

Entries in *First Aid for the USMLE Step 1* originated from hundreds of students, international medical graduates, and faculty members, who synthesized the facts, notes, and mnemonics from a variety of textbooks, review books, lecture notes, and personal notes. We regret the inability to reference each individual fact or mnemonic owing to the diverse and often anecdotal sources. Although the material has been reviewed by faculty members and medical students, errors and omissions are inevitable. We urge readers to identify errors and suggest improvements. We regret that some students may find certain mnemonics trivializing or offensive. The mnemonics are meant solely as optional devices for learning.

The authors and Appleton & Lange intend to continue updating *First Aid for the USMLE Step 1* so that the book grows in quality and scope and continues to reflect the material covered on the USMLE Step 1. If you have any study strategies, high-yield facts with mnemonics, or book reviews for the next edition, please use the forms included to submit your contributions. (*See* How to Contribute, p. xv.) Any student or faculty member who submits material subsequently used in the next edition of *First Aid for the USMLE Step 1* will receive personal acknowledgment in the next edition and one $10 coupon per complete entry, good toward the future purchase of any Appleton & Lange medical book.

Good luck in your studies!

Acknowledgments

This has been a collaborative project from the start. We gratefully acknowledge the thoughtful comments, corrections, and advice of the many hundreds of medical students, international medical graduates, and faculty who have supported the authors in the continuing development of *First Aid for the USMLE Step 1*.

For submitting major contributions to the 1998 edition, often including dozens of new entries, book reviews, or entire annotated books, we give special thanks to Tamseel Awan, Jackie Faircloth, Michael Friedman, Laurie Hickey, Sundar Jayaraman, Warren Krackov, James Moak, Riva Rahl, James Smith, and Mark Tanaka.

Thanks to Jan Lewis (Director of Administration, NBOME), Sunil Singhania, Grace Torres, and Chad Friel for reviewing and contributing to the Section I Supplement. For helping us obtain information concerning review books, we thank Milberry Union Bookstore (UCSF), Discount Medical Books (San Francisco), Reiter's Scientific & Professional Books (Washington, DC), and UCLA Health Sciences Bookstore. Thanks to Noam Maitless for the original book design, Evenson Design Group and Ashley Pound for design revisions, and Design Group Cook for the cover design.

For support and encouragement throughout the process, we are grateful to Sameer Bhushan, Dr. Sana Khan, Dr. Eric Schulze, Dr. Daniela Drake, Jonathan Kirsch, Esq., and the UCSF Office of Medical Student Affairs.

Thanks to our publisher, Appleton & Lange, for offering a coupon for each new contribution used in future editions of this book, and for the valuable assistance of their staff. For enthusiasm, support, and commitment for this ongoing and ever-challenging project, thanks to our tireless editor, Marinita Timban. For personal and last-minute production support, thanks to our able administrative assistant, Gianni Le Nguyen, our personal copyeditor, Andrea Fellows, Jimmy and Bennie Sauls (Rainbow Graphics), and John Williams, Deborah King, Lisa Guidone, and Frank Del Vecchio (Appleton & Lange).

For submitting contributions, corrections, and book surveys for the 1998 edition, we thank J. Abdou, Apul Abramson, David Adelman, Arman Afagh, Avinash Agarwal, Neera Agarwal, Naseez Ahmad, Chris Aiken, Jerry Ainsworth, Lee Akst, Brannon Alberty, Amarin Alexander, Laura Andrews, Sonia Angell, Karen Ashton, Ghassan Atiyeh, Sujatha Ayyagari, Amy Badberg, Sujay Banerjere, Laurie Bankston, Peter Bartz, Manuel Benavides, Adam Bennett, William Bennet, Joshua Berlin, Michael Bertram, Jonelle Bingham, Doug Blackmon, Robyn Blair, Lauren Bliss, Aminah Bliss, Julia Bolding, Sudip Bose, Brandy Box, Peter Bray, Vanessa Brennan, Rebecca Brightly, Joshua Broder, Julianne Brown, Heather Burton, Consuelo Cagande, Douglas Calhoun, Henry Capps, C. Caraang, Yah Cason, Dean Cauley, Alicia Chang, Teresa Chang, Tess Chapman, W.Y.C. Cheathan, Julie Cheek, Lindsay Cheng, Daniel Chertow, Doris Chih, Arnold Chin, Ericka Choi, Madhu Chopra, Laura Chyung, Lauren Cianciaruso, Heather Coert, Abigail Collins, Doug Collins, Corinna Corbin, Laura Coulson, Alison Crager, Julia Cron, Timothy Cruz, Will Davenport, Ramona de Jesus, Corey Dean, Elizabeth DeBacts, Evan Dellon, Frank Demery, Shawn Dhupar, Rayner Dickey, Jimmy Doan, Aaron Donnell, Chandler Dora, Ian Doten, Katherine Dragisic, Lisa Driscoll, William Eck, Susan Ehrlich, Elly Falzarano, Jesse Flaxenburg, Priscilla Fowler, Bart Francis, John Franson, Chad Friel, Melinda Fung, Sean Garcia, Ravi Ghanta, Karol Gieszczykiewicz, Kanwal Gill, Raymond Golish, Chengxin Gong, Brad Gordan, Helen Gorlitsky, Kristi Griffin, Jadie Guo, Arun Gupta, Jennifer Hager, Daniel Hall, Stuart Hall, Greg Hallert, Joni Hamilton, David Hanauer, Clovene Hanchard, Maria Hansberry, Teresa Harper, Diana Harris, Mary Hartman, Nader Hebela, Amanda Heidemann, Kazu Hernandez, Jason Hester, Mark Hiatt, James Hitchcock,

Tuan Ho, Ronald Homer, Kim Hood, Rachel Hotard, Anthony Hou, Daniel Hrad, Mark Huber, Joshua Hurwitz, Michael Hutchen, Serge Iliver, Justin Indyk, Jennifer Ireland, Kiera Irvin, Kristen Jacobs, Jason James, Yarub Jamiel, Jason Johnson, Romaine Johnson, David Jones, Nnemdi Kamanu, James Kao, Anne Kasmar, Brian Katt, Matt Keefer, Travis Keller, Zachary Kerwin, Mohammed Khan, Edward Kim, Eugene Kim, Rich Kim, John King, Octavia Kingcaid, Paul Klekotka, Anita Kohli, Lawrence Kohn, Cyrus Komer, Mary Kona, Liping Kong, Meredith Kosann, Katherine Kougias, Mark Krivopal, Ellen Kwan, Eleanor Lai, Christopher Lansford, Daphne Lashbrook, David Lasko, Mimi Le, Gus Leotta, Dan Lee, Soo Lee, Alfred Lee, Abe Lee, Caroline Lee, Jordan Leonard, Yuk-Yuen Leung, Joseph Lim, Andy Lin, Joann Lin, Wei Lin, Juliann Lipps, Mike Liu, James Livermore, Christine Loo, Glenda Lovell, Ben Lowenstein, Patricia Lugar, Yvonne Lui, Jonathan MacCabe, Michael Margolin, Kim Mark, Junnie Mark, Kenneth Mautner, Bryan Maxwell, Alissa McClure, Craig McCotter, Heidi McElhaney, Brandy McKelvy, Rohit Mehta, Michal Melamed, Sudeep Menachery, Travis Miller, Lumil Mitrev, Laleh Moazen, M. Moharrami, Allan Moore, Zeyad Morcos, Anne Mullet, Yoon Myung, Richard Navitsky, Sarah Newell, Song Nguyen, Brett Niblack, Deanna Nobleza, John Nolen, Garey Noritz, Karen Nork, Essie Ocamp-Marapao, Jon Oda, April Odom, Clifton Otto, Abby Patchan, Birju Patel, Falguni Patel, Abhijit Patel, Michele Pauporte, Ryan Peters, Dan Peters, Janelle Peterson, Tan Pham, Jennifer Phan, David Pinkstaff, Jessica Pinzon, Bobby Pittman, Rob Poirier, Adebowale Popoola, David Presser, Jose Prince, Simona Prochazka, Stephen Przynosch, Rodolfo Quintero, Dina Ragheb, Francis Ramos, Shoaib Rashid, Kesari Reddy, Rachan Reddy, Alejandro Rey, Martin Richman, Eric Risovi, Jason Rosenberg, Claudia Roussos, Mitzi Rubin, Anne Rutledge, Kenneth Sable, Ahmad Sadat, Ibrahim Saeed, Dana Salomy, David Sanders, Nisha Saran, Minna Saslaw, S. Scanlon, John Schilling, Jennifer Schutzman, Hamilton Schwartz, Sam Sered, Andrew Shea, Heather Shenteman, Helen Shigemitsu, David Shih, Shira Shiloah, Margaret Shnorhavonar, Andrew Shpall, Andrea Silver, Rebecca Slaunwhite, Matt Slavin, Maria Smith, Lucia Sobrin, John Spencer, Malini Srinivasan, Rachel St. John, William Stacey, Lucy Stapleton, Kristan Staudenmayer, Jason Stein, Paul Sterman, John Stoutenburg, Sara Sukalich, Khoji Suzuki, Jakub Svoboda, Moshe Szlechter, James Takayesu, Ursina Teitelbaum, Smita Thamban, Pitchar Theerathorn, Eliza Thomasson, Toya Tillis, Jenna Timm, Binh Tran, Kevin Tran, Thomas Trybucek, Patricia Tsai, Peter Tucker, Lawrence Uzochukwy, Jason Van Ittersum, Sonya Vieira, Joseph Villacis, Bolivar Villacis, Todd Villines, Salvatore Viscomi, Arati Wagh, Bryan Wahl, Billy Wang, Tammy Watkins, Joanne Watson, Andrew Weiss, Cacia Welch, Christopher Wen, Jeffrey Westpheling, Todd Whitenhurst, Bryan Wilcox, Billie Wilkerson, Tonya Williams, Brian Williams, Penny Williams, Timothy Williams, Scott Wilson, Zev Wimpfheimer, Sony Wiriosuparto, James Wise, Todd Witte, Lee Wolfe, Chris Wright, Jinoos Yazdany, Helen Yeni-Komshian, Suzanne Yoon, Dana Zappetti, M.M. Ziebert, Eli Ziv, and Edwin Zong. Our apologies if we missed you.

Finally, thanks to Ted Hon, one of the founding authors of this book, for his vision in developing this guide on the computer. Eddie Chu and Jeffrey Hansen were also among the founding authors of this book. For major contributions to previous editions, we thank Hatem Abou-Sayed, Taejoon Ahn, Shaun Anand, Alireza Atri, Lisa Backus, Ross Berkeley, John Bethea, Jr., Stephen Gomperts, Robert Hosseini, Freddy Huang, Kassem Kahlil, Ketan Kapadia, Shin Kim, Kambiz Kosari, Thong Le, Ross Levine, Kathleen Liu, Kieu Nguyen, Christine Pham, Thao Pham, Michael Rizen, Radhika Sekhri-Breaden, Judy Shih, Yi Chieh Shiuey, David Steensma, Dax Swanson, Gary Ulaner, Matthew Voorsanger, and Ziqiang Wu.

Los Angeles   Vikas Bhushan
New Haven   Tao Le
Orlando   Chirag Amin
Los Angeles   Vipal Soni
Chicago   Hoang Nguyen

How to Contribute

This version of *First Aid for the USMLE Step 1* incorporates hundreds of contributions and changes suggested by faculty and student reviewers. We invite you to participate in this process.

Please send us your suggestions for:

- New facts, mnemonics, diagrams, or strategies
- High-yield topics that may reappear on future Step 1 exams
- Personal ratings and comments on review books that you have examined

For each entry incorporated into the next edition, you will receive one $10 coupon per entry good toward the purchase of any Appleton & Lange medical book, as well as personal acknowledgment in the next edition. Diagrams, tables, partial entries, updates, corrections, and study hints are also appreciated, and significant contributions will be compensated at the discretion of the publisher. Also let us know about material in this edition that you feel is low yield and should be deleted.

The **preferred** way to submit entries, suggestions, or corrections is via electronic mail, addressed to the authors:

vbhushan@aol.com
taotle@aol.com
chiragamin@aol.com

The preferred way to contact the publisher is via electronic mail, addressed to:

marinita_timban@prenhall.com

For *First Aid for the USMLE Step 1* updates and corrections, visit our Internet website at:

http://www.s2smed.com

Otherwise, please send entries, neatly written or typed or on disk (Microsoft Word), to: First Aid for the USMLE Step 1, 720 Orange St. #2, New Haven, CT 06511–9046, Attention: Contributions. Please use the contribution and survey forms on the following pages. Each form constitutes an entry. (Attach additional pages as needed.)

Another option is to send in your entire annotated book. We will look through your additions and notes and will send you Appleton & Lange coupons based on the quantity and quality of any additions that we incorporate into the 1998 edition. Books will be returned upon request. Contributions received by July 15, 1998, receive priority consideration for the 1999 edition of *First Aid for the USMLE Step 1.*

Note to Contributors

All entries are subject to editing and reviewing. Please verify all data and spellings carefully. In the event that similar or duplicate entries are received, only the first entry received will be used. Include a reference to a standard textbook to facilitate verification of the fact. Please follow the style, punctuation, and format of this edition if possible.

Contribution Form I

For entries, mnemonics, facts, strategies, corrections, diagrams, etc.

Contributor Name: ____________________

School/Affiliation: ____________________

Address: ____________________

____

Telephone: ____________________

E-mail: ____________________

Topic:

Subject/Subsection:
Page number in '98 ed.:

Fact and Description:

Notes, Diagrams, and Mnemonics:

Reference:

Please return by July 15, 1998. You will receive personal acknowledgment and a $10 coupon toward selected Appleton & Lange books for each entry that we use in future editions.

Please seal with tape only.
No staples or paper clips.

- (fold here) -

NO POSTAGE
NECESSARY
IF MAILED
IN THE
UNITED STATES

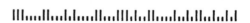

- (fold here) -

Contribution Form II

For high-yield vignettes for
Section II Supplement

Contributor Name: _____

School/Affiliation: _____

Address: _____

_____

Telephone: _____

E-mail: _____

Please place the subject heading (e.g., Anatomy) on the first line and the high-yield vignette or topic on the following two lines.

1. Subject: _____
   Vignette: _____
   _____

2. Subject: _____
   Vignette: _____
   _____

3. Subject: _____
   Vignette: _____
   _____

4. Subject: _____
   Vignette: _____
   _____

5. Subject: _____
   Vignette: _____
   _____

6. Subject: _____
   Vignette: _____
   _____

7. Subject: _____
   Vignette: _____
   _____

8. Subject: _____
   Vignette: _____
   _____

9. Subject: _____
   Vignette: _____
   _____

10. Subject: _____
    Vignette: _____
    _____

Please return by July 15, 1998. You will receive personal acknowledgment and a $10 coupon toward selected Appleton & Lange books for each entry that is used in future editions.

Please seal with tape only.
No staples or paper clips.

- (fold here) -

BUSINESS REPLY MAIL
FIRST-CLASS MAIL PERMIT NO. 596 NEW HAVEN CT

POSTAGE WILL BE PAID BY ADDRESSEE

FIRST AID FOR THE USMLE STEP 1
720 ORANGE ST #2
NEW HAVEN CT 06511-9046

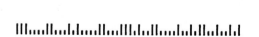

- (fold here) -

Contribution Form III

For review resource ratings
for Section III

Contributor Name: _____

School/Affiliation: _____

Address: _____

_____

Telephone: _____

E-mail: _____

We welcome additional comments on review resources rated in Section III as well as reviews of resources not rated in Section III. Please fill out each review entry as completely as possible. Please do not leave "Comments" blank. Rate texts using the letter grading scale provided on p. 308, taking into consideration current ratings of other books on that subject.

1. ***Title/Author:*** _____ Days needed to read: _____

   Publisher/Series: _____ ISBN Number: _____

   Rating: _____ ***Comments:*** _____

   _____

   _____

2. ***Title/Author:*** _____ Days needed to read: _____

   Publisher/Series: _____ ISBN Number: _____

   Rating: _____ ***Comments:*** _____

   _____

   _____

3. ***Title/Author:*** _____ Days needed to read: _____

   Publisher/Series: _____ ISBN Number: _____

   Rating: _____ ***Comments:*** _____

   _____

   _____

   _____

4. ***Title/Author:*** _____ Days needed to read: _____

   Publisher/Series: _____ ISBN Number: _____

   Rating: _____ ***Comments:*** _____

   _____

   _____

5. ***Title/Author:*** _____ Days needed to read: _____

   Publisher/Series: _____ ISBN Number: _____

   Rating: _____ ***Comments:*** _____

   _____

   _____

Please seal with tape only.
No staples or paper clips.

- (fold here) -

BUSINESS REPLY MAIL
FIRST-CLASS MAIL PERMIT NO. 596 NEW HAVEN CT

POSTAGE WILL BE PAID BY ADDRESSEE

FIRST AID FOR THE USMLE STEP 1
720 ORANGE ST #2
NEW HAVEN CT 06511-9046

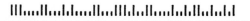

- (fold here) -

User Survey

Contributor Name: _____

School/Affiliation: _____

Address: _____

_____

Telephone: _____

E-mail: _____

What student-to-student advice would you give someone preparing for the USMLE Step 1?

Are you aware of any commercial review courses not listed in Section I: Guide to Efficient Exam Preparation? If so, which ones? What commercial courses have you been enrolled in, and what were your overall assessments of the courses?

What would you change about the study and test-taking strategies listed in Section I: Guide to Efficient Exam Preparation?

Were there any high-yield facts, topics, or vignettes in Section II that you think were inaccurate or should be deleted? Which ones and why? What would you change or add?

What review resources for the USMLE Step 1 are not covered in Section III? Would you change the rating of any of the review resources in Section III? If so, which one(s) and why?

What other suggestions do you have for improving *First Aid for the USMLE Step 1*? Any other comments or suggestions? What did you like most about the book?

Please seal with tape only.
No staples or paper clips.

- (fold here) -

BUSINESS REPLY MAIL
FIRST-CLASS MAIL PERMIT NO. 596 NEW HAVEN CT

POSTAGE WILL BE PAID BY ADDRESSEE

FIRST AID FOR THE USMLE STEP 1
720 ORANGE ST #2
NEW HAVEN CT 06511-9046

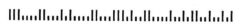

- (fold here) -

How to Use This Book

Medical students who have used previous editions of this guide have given us feedback on how best to make use of the book.

It is recommended that you begin using this book as early as possible when learning the basic medical sciences. You can use Section III to select first-year course review books and then use those books for review while taking your medical school classes.

Use different parts of the book at different stages in your preparation for the USMLE Step 1. Before you begin to study for the USMLE Step 1, we suggest that you read Section I: Guide to Efficient Exam Preparation and Section III: Database of Science Review Books. **If you are an international medical graduate student, an osteopathic medical student, a podiatry student, or a student with a disability,** refer to the appropriate Section I supplement for additional advice. Devise a study plan and decide what resources to buy. We strongly recommend that you invest in at least one or two top-rated review books in each subject. *First Aid* is not a comprehensive review book, and it is not a panacea for not studying during the first two years of medical school. Scanning Section II will give you an initial idea of the diverse range of topics covered on the USMLE Step 1.

As you study each discipline, **use the corresponding high-yield fact section in *First Aid for the USMLE Step 1* as a way of consolidating the material and testing yourself** to see if you have covered some of the frequently tested items. Work with the book to integrate important facts into your fund of knowledge. Using *First Aid for the USMLE Step 1* as a review can serve as both a self-test of your knowledge and a repetition of important facts to learn. High-yield topics and vignettes are abstracted from recent exams to help guide your preparation.

Return to Section II frequently during your preparation and fill your short-term memory with remaining high-yield facts a few days before the USMLE Step 1. The book can serve as a useful way of retaining key associations and high-yield facts fresh in your memory just prior to the examination. Some students choose to skim the book between the two exam days.

Reviewing the book immediately after the exam is probably the best way to **help us improve the book in the next edition.** Decide what was truly high and low yield and **send in the contribution forms or your entire annotated book.**

Guide to Efficient Exam Preparation

INTRODUCTION

Relax.

This section is intended to make your exam preparation easier, not harder. Our goal is to reduce your stress and help you make the most of your study effort by helping you understand more about the United States Medical Licensing Examination, Step 1 (USMLE Step 1). As a medical student, you are no doubt familiar with taking standardized examinations and absorbing large amounts of material. However, in confronting the USMLE Step 1, it is easy to become sidetracked and not achieve your goal of studying with maximum effectiveness. Common mistakes that students make when studying for the boards include the following:

- "Stressing out" due to an inadequate understanding of the test
- Not understanding how scoring is performed and what your score means
- Starting *First Aid* too late
- Starting to study too late
- Using inefficient or inappropriate study methods
- Buying the wrong books or buying more books than you can ever use
- Buying only one publisher's review series for all subjects
- Buying too many review books too late
- Not using practice examinations for maximum benefit
- Not using review books along with your classes
- Not analyzing and improving your test-taking strategies
- Getting bogged down by reviewing difficult topics excessively
- Studying material that is rarely tested on the USMLE Step 1
- Failing to master certain high-yield subjects due to overconfidence
- Using this book as your sole study resource

In this section, we offer advice to help you avoid these pitfalls and be more productive in your studies. First, it is important to understand what the examination involves.

USMLE STEP 1—THE BASICS

The purpose of the USMLE Step 1 is to test your understanding and application of important concepts in basic biomedical sciences. [2]

A degree of concern about your performance on the USMLE Step 1 examination is expected and appropriate. However, medical students all too often become unnecessarily anxious about the examination. It is important to take a moment to understand what it involves. As you become more familiar with the USMLE Step 1, you can translate your anxiety into more efficient preparation.

The USMLE Step 1 is the first of three examinations that you must pass in order to become a licensed physician in the United States.[1] The USMLE is a joint endeavor of the National Board of Medical Examiners (NBME) and the Federation of State Medical Boards (FSMB). In previous years, the examination was strictly organized around seven traditional disciplines: anatomy, behavioral science, biochemistry, microbiology, pathology, pharmacology, and physiology. In June 1991, the NBME began administering the "new" NBME Part I examination, which offers a more integrated and multidisciplinary format and more **clinically** oriented questions.

In 1992, the USMLE replaced both the Federation Licensing Examination (FLEX) and the certifying examinations of the NBME.[3] The USMLE now serves as the **single** examination system for United States medical students and international medical graduates seeking medical licensure in the United States.

Many students report that Step 1 is looking more and more like Step 2.

Format

The USMLE Step 1 is a multiple-choice examination administered over a two-day period (Fig. 1). It consists of four booklets, each containing approximately 180 items. On each day of the examination, one booklet is administered in the morning and one is administered in the afternoon. You are allotted three hours to complete each test booklet. A sample answer sheet is provided within each

FIGURE 1. Schematic of the 1997 USMLE Step 1 Examination

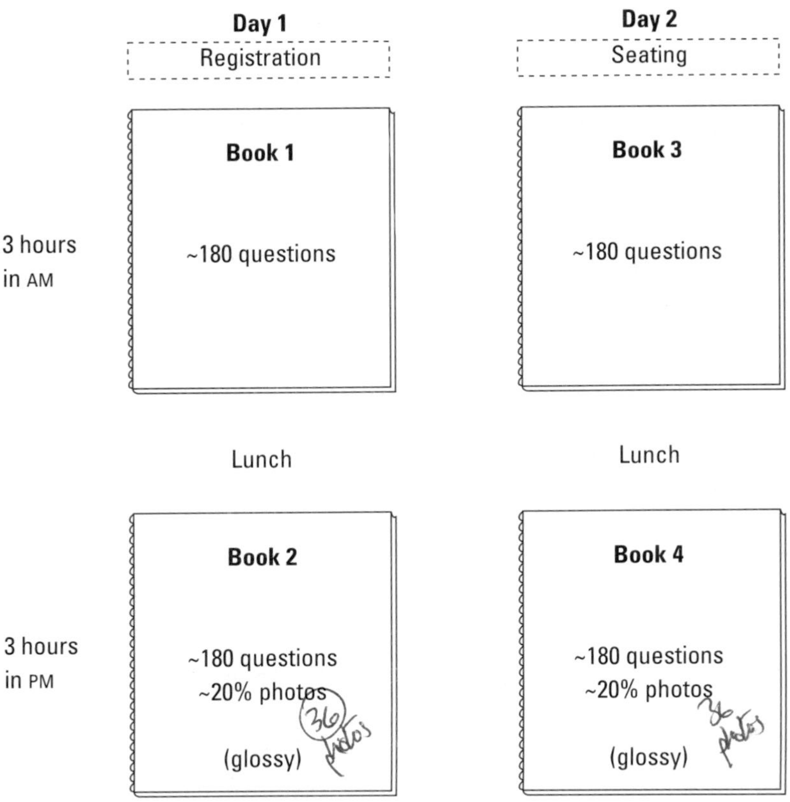

Glossy booklet photographs include:

- *Gross photos*
- *Histology slides*
- *Radiographs*
- *EMs*
- *Line drawings*

booklet and is shown in the *USMLE Step 1 General Instructions, Content Outline, and Sample Items.*[4]

Figure 1 should give you a mental image of the exam structure. Note that:

- Booklets vary in overall difficulty. Unlike the SAT, there does not seem to be a pattern of increasing or decreasing difficulty as you proceed through the exam.
- Subject areas vary randomly from question to question. Many questions incorporate multiple basic science and medical concepts.
- The morning booklets are printed on plain paper. They may contain line drawings but do not contain photographs.
- The afternoon booklets are usually printed on high-quality glossy paper and include a number of photographs. In 1997, students reported a black-and-white glossy booklet during the afternoon of one of the days and a color glossy booklet during the afternoon of the other day.
- The exam is scored if all four booklets are opened.[5] Otherwise, a notation on the USMLE transcript is made that the examination was incomplete.

Test booklets vary in difficulty, so do not become discouraged early in the exam.

Nearly two-thirds of the 1997 Step 1 questions began with a description of a patient.[6]

Question Types

One-best-answer items are the most commonly used multiple-choice format. They usually consist of a clinical scenario or direct question followed by a list of five or more options. You are required to select the one best answer among the options. A number of options may be partially correct, in which case you must select the option that best answers the question or completes the statement. A variation of this format employs **negatively phrased questions** that include negative words such as EXCEPT, LEAST, and NOT.

Matching sets consist of a list of approximately 4 to 26 items from which you choose the one best answer that corresponds to each of the numbered items or questions located below the list. Once again, a number of options may be partially correct, in which case you must select the option that best answers the question or completes the statement.

Student experience from the June 1997 administration indicates that questions in each booklet are organized by type, starting with the one-best-answer items, followed by negatively phrased one-best-answer items, and ending with matching sets. Although the numerical proportions of question types vary with each booklet, students recall that the **one-best-answer** items constituted approximately 95% of all questions, while **negatively phrased one-best-answer** items constituted about 3% and **matching sets** made up roughly 2% of the questions (Fig. 2). Many students recommend quickly flipping through each booklet at the beginning to assess the question mix. Don't count on much of a time cushion at the end given the relatively few (or no) matching-set questions.

FIGURE 2. Question Type and Order

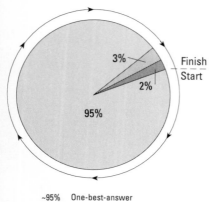

3%
2%
Finish
Start
95%

~95% One-best-answer
~3% Negatively phrased one-best-answer
~2% Matching and extended matching

FIGURE 3A. Simulated Score Report—Front Page

Doe, John I.
000 Main St.
Any Town, CA 12345

USMLE ID: 0-123-456-7
Test Date: June 1997

The USMLE is a single examination program for all applicants for medical licensure in the United States; it replaces the Federation Licensing Examination (FLEX) and the certifying examinations of the National Board of Medical Examiners (NBME Parts I, II, and III). The program consists of three Steps designed to assess an examinee's understanding of and ability to apply concepts and principles that are important in health and disease and that constitute the basis of safe and effective patient care. Step 1 is designed to assess whether an examinee understands and can apply key concepts of the basic biomedical sciences, with an emphasis on principles and mechanisms of health, disease, and modes of therapy. The inclusion of **Step 1** in the USMLE sequence is intended to ensure mastery of not only the basic medical sciences undergirding the safe and competent practice of medicine in the present, but also the scientific principles required for maintenance of competence through lifelong learning. Results of the examination are reported to medical licensing authorities in the United States and its territories for use in granting an initial license to practice medicine. The two numeric scores shown below are equivalent; each state or territory may use either score in making licensing decisions. These scores represent your results for the administration of Step 1 on the test date shown above.

PASS	The result is based on the minimum passing score set by USMLE for Step 1. Individual licensing authorities may accept the USMLE-recommended pass/fail result or may establish a different passing score for their own jurisdictions.

200	This score is determined by your overall performance on Step 1. For recent administrations, the mean and standard deviation for first-time examinees from U.S. medical schools are approximately 205 and 20, respectively, with most scores falling between 165 and 245. A score of 176 is set by USMLE to pass Step 1. The standard error of measurement (SEM)* for this scale is four points.

82	This score is also determined by your overall performance on the examination. A score of 82 on this scale is equivalent to a score of 200 on the scale described above. A score of 75 on this scale, which is equivalent to a score of 176 on the scale described above, is set by USMLE to pass Step 1. The SEM* for this scale is one point.

* Your score is influenced by both your general understanding of basic biomedical sciences and the specific set of items selected for this Step 1 examination. The SEM provides an estimate of the range within which your scores might be expected to vary by chance if you were tested repeatedly using similar tests.

Scoring and Failure Rates

Each Step 1 examinee receives a score report that has the examinee's pass/fail status, two test scores, and a graphic depiction of the examinee's performance by discipline and organ system or subject area (Figs. 3A and 3B). The actual organ system profiles reported may depend on the statistical characteristics of a given administration of the examination.

FIGURE 3B. Simulated Score Report—Back Page

INFORMATION PROVIDED FOR EXAMINEE USE ONLY

The Performance Profile below is provided solely for the benefit of the examinee.
The USMLE will not provide or verify the Performance Profile for any other person, organization,
or agency.

USMLE STEP 1 PERFORMANCE PROFILE

	Lower Performance	Borderline Performance	Higher Performance
Behavioral Sciences			xxxxxxxxxxx
Biochemistry			xxxxxxxxx
Cardiovascular System			xxxxxxxxxxxxx
Gastrointestinal System			xxxxxxxxxxxxx
General Principles of Health & Disease			xxxxxxx
Gross Anatomy & Embryology		xxxxxxxxxxxxx	
Hematopoietic & Lymphoreticular Systems			xxxxxxxxxxxxxx
Histology & Cell Biology		xxxxxxxxxxxxx	
Microbiology & Immunology			xxxxxxxxx
Musculoskeletal, Skin, & Connective Tissue			xxxxxxxxxxxxxxx
Nervous System/Special Senses			xxxxxxxxx
Pathology			xxxx*
Pharmacology			xxxxxxx
Physiology		xxxxxxx	
Renal/Urinary Systems			xxxxxxxxxxxxx
Reproductive & Endocrine Systems			xxxxxxxxxxx
Respiratory System			xxxxxxxxxx*

The above Performance Profile is provided to aid in self-assessment. The shaded area defines a borderline level of performance for each content area; borderline performance is comparable to a HIGH FAIL/LOW PASS on the total test.

Performance bands indicate areas of relative strength and weakness. Some bands are wider than others. The width of a performance band reflects the precision of measurement; narrower bands indicate greater precision. The band width for a given content area is the same for all examinees. An asterisk indicates that your performance band extends beyond the displayed portion of the scale.

This profile should not be compared to those from other Step 1 administrations.

Additional information concerning the topics covered in each content area can be found in the *USMLE Step 1 General Instructions, Content Description, and Sample Items.*

FIGURE 4. Scoring Scales for the USMLE Step 1: Approximate 1994 Equivalencies

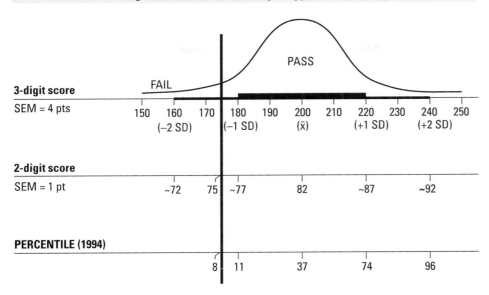

FIGURE 5. Score to Percentile Conversion[7]

Three-Digit Score	95/96 Norms* (% ile)
248	99
244	97
240	94
235	90
230	83
225	75
220	67
215	58
210	48
205	40
200	31
195	24
190	19
185	14
180	10
176	**7**
170	5
165	3
160	2
156	2
154	1

* 1995/1996 US and Canadian 1st-time takers

For 1996, USMLE provided two overall test scores based on the total number of items answered correctly on the examination. The first score, the three-digit score, was reported as a scaled score, in which the mean was 208 and the standard deviation was 20. This means that a score of 208 roughly corresponded to the 50th percentile, while a score of 225 roughly corresponded to the 85th percentile.[8] The June 1996 USMLE score report for students did not include any percentile score equivalents. Percentile performance norms for 1994 were provided to medical schools and have been summarized in Figure 5. The second score scale, the two-digit score, defines 75 as the minimum passing score (equivalent to a score of 176 on the first scale). A score of 82 is equivalent to a score of 200 on the first score scale (Fig. 4). To avoid confusion, we refer to scores using the three-digit scale with a mean of 208 and a standard deviation of 20.

In 1997, a score of 176 or higher was required to pass Step 1. The pass/fail standard for Step 1 is predominantly "content-based." The passing mark is determined by reviewing test items and defining a mastery level of performance.[9] In 1996, 93% of all first-time test takers passed the June administration of the USMLE Step 1, and the failure rate appears to have stabilized (Figs. 6 and 7). An unofficial estimate of the mean score for first-time test takers in the United States was 213 for the June 1997 Step 1 exam. It is estimated that passing Step 1 corresponds to answering between 55% and 65% of the questions correctly.

The mean Step 1 score for US medical students rose from 200 in 1991 to 208 in 1995.

Passing Step 1 is estimated to correspond to answering 55–65% of the questions correctly.

FIGURE 6. Passing Rates for 1996 USMLE Step 1[10]

	June 1996		October 1996		Total 1996	
	No. Tested	Passing (%)	No. Tested	Passing (%)	No. Tested	Passing (%)
NBME-Registered Examinees						
First-Time Takers	15,884	93	1,132	82	17,016	93
Repeaters	916	48	1,343	57	2,259	53
NBME Total	**16,800**	**91**	**2,475**	**69**	**19,275**	**88**
ECFMG*-Registered Examinees						
First-Time Takers	7,865	58	9,004	52	16,869	55
Repeaters	6,474	32	6,592	30	13,066	30
ECFMG Total	**14,339**	**46**	**15,596**	**42**	**29,935**	**44**

* Educational Commission for Foreign Medical Graduates.

According to the USMLE, medical schools receive a listing of total scores and pass/fail results plus group summaries by discipline and organ systems. Students can withhold their scores from their medical school if they wish. Official USMLE transcripts, which can be sent on request to residency programs, include only total scores, not performance profiles.

The preceding information is based on students' experience with the June 1996 and June 1997 administrations of the USMLE Step 1 and information published by the NBME (refer to the NBME publications listed in Section III). The format and the scoring of the examination are subject to change, and it is best to consult the latest NBME publications and your medical school for the most current and accurate information regarding the examination.

NBME/USMLE Publications

We strongly encourage students to use the free materials provided by the testing agencies (see p. 35), to study in detail the following NBME publications, and to retain them for future reference:

■ *USMLE Step 1 General Instructions, Content Outline, and Sample Items* (information given free to all examinees)

FIGURE 7. Trends in Performance on USMLE Step 1[11]

	Percent Failing (< 176)	Percent > 225
1991	11	10
1992	9	11
1993	7	14
1994	8	11
1995	8	15
1996	7	—

(NBME-registered first-time test takers only)

■ *USMLE Bulletin of Information* (information given free to all examinees)
■ *USMLE Special Bulletin on Computer-based Testing*

The *USMLE Step 1 General Instructions, Content Outline, and Sample Items* booklet contains approximately 180 questions that are similar (but not identical) in format and content to the questions on the actual USMLE Step 1. This practice test is one of the better methods for assessing your boards test-taking skills. However, it does not contain enough questions to simulate the full length of the examination, and its content is a very limited sample of the possible basic science material covered. Also, most students felt that the 1997 exam was more difficult than these questions. Some students report encountering a few near-duplicates of these questions on the actual Step 1. Presumably, these are "experimental" questions, but who knows!

The extremely detailed 25-page Step I Content Outline provided by the USMLE has not proved useful for students studying for the exam. The USMLE even states that "the content outline is not intended as a guide for curriculum development or as a study guide."[12] We concur with this assessment.

The *USMLE Bulletin of Information* booklet accompanies application materials for the USMLE. This publication has detailed procedural and policy information regarding the USMLE, including descriptions of all three Steps, scoring of the exams, reporting of scores to medical schools and residency programs, procedures for score rechecks and other inquiries, policies for irregular behavior, and test dates.

The now-out-of-print *Retired NBME Basic Medical Sciences (Part I) Test Items* contains nearly 1000 "retired" questions, the content of which still may reappear on the new USMLE Step 1. This publication allows you to assess your performance on basic science topics and to identify areas of weakness. The retired test items include old NBME Part I questions of the K (multiple true/false) and C (A/B/both/neither) variety, neither of which appears on the USMLE Step 1. Although these question **types** are not found on the current version of the boards, the **content** of these questions is still relevant.

Another out-of-print NBME publication useful to students in preparing for the USMLE Step 1 is the *Self-Test in the Part I Basic Medical Sciences,* with 630 questions drawn from the old NBME Part I item pool. It can be used in the same way as the *Retired NBME Basic Sciences (Part I) Test Items.* There is some overlap in content between the two publications. Unfortunately, these question booklets are **no longer available from the NBME,** and the NBME does not grant permission to reprint these publications to individuals, medical schools, or organizations.[13] Some medical schools, however, still have old copies of these booklets available for their students. Ideally, a copy should be placed on reserve in the medical library. Another source would be third- and fourth-year students who have saved their copies.

The original questions are becoming more difficult to find every year. However, explanatory answers to all 1623 questions in the *Retired* and *Self-Test* booklets are available as an independent publication titled *Underground Step 1 Answers to the NBME Retired and Self-Test Questions.* This book is designed to be read alone or as a study guide to the NBME questions. This publication is by the same authors as *First Aid for the USMLE Step 1* and is available for $22.95 plus shipping and handling at (800) 247-6553 (see p. 313 for a review and the inside back cover of this book for more information).

Although the NBME Self-Test and Retired Test Items *are both out of print, they remain a decent source of practice content for the USMLE Step 1.*

The most productive way to use these study aids is to take the practice examinations and to identify carefully the questions that were missed or that were answered correctly by guessing. Try some questions early to assess your strengths and weaknesses; save some questions for the few weeks before the exam to evaluate your progress. Students often find that many missed questions originate from a limited number of seemingly trivial topics (e.g., congenital diseases involving sphingolipid synthesis). It is worthwhile to study these subjects thoroughly, because student experience has shown that the topics covered in these retired questions (trivial or not) remain predictors of many topics tested on the new USMLE Step 1, even though the old NBME publications no longer approximate the style of questions appearing on the current USMLE Step 1 examinations. Thus, we suggest that you study these questions only if you are able to easily find them and only if you have the time.

DEFINING YOUR GOAL

It is useful to define your own personal performance goal when approaching the USMLE Step 1. Your style and intensity of preparation can then be matched to your goal. Your goal may depend on your school's requirements, your specialty choice, your grades to date, and your personal assessment of test importance.

Comfortably Pass

As mentioned earlier, the USMLE Step 1 is the first of three standardized examinations that you must pass to become a licensed physician in the United States. For many medical schools, passing the USMLE Step 1 is also required before you can continue with your clinical training. The NBME, however, feels that medical schools should not use Step 1 as the sole determinant of being advanced to the third year.[14] If you are headed for a "noncompetitive" residency program and you have consulted advisers and fourth-year medical students in your area of interest, you may feel comfortable with this approach. Obviously, aiming for a 176 is a risky way to "comfortably pass" the exam.

Beat the Mean

Although the NBME warns against the misuse of examination scores to evaluate student qualifications for residency positions, some residency program directors continue to use Step 1 scores to screen applicants (Fig. 8).[15] Thus, many students feel it is important to score higher than the national average.

Internship and residency programs vary greatly in their requests for scores. Some simply request your pass/fail status, whereas others request your total score. Some programs have been known to request a photocopy of your score report to determine how well you performed on the individual sections; however, this is unusual. It is unclear how the continuing changes in the USMLE Step 1 examination and score reporting will affect the application process for residency programs. The best sources of bottom-line information are fourth-year medical students who have recently completed the residency application process.

Fourth-year medical students have the best feel for how Step 1 scores factor into residency applications.

Several years ago, *First Aid for the USMLE Step 1* conducted a small informal post-match survey of fourth-year medical students at several US medical schools regarding the use of Step 1 scores. The results are summarized in Figure 9. Use this information only as a rough guide for goal setting. Trends in certain specialties are evolving rapidly (see also Le, Bhushan, Amin: *First Aid for the Match,* and Iserson: *Getting into Residency*).

FIGURE 8. Academic Factors Important to Residency Directors

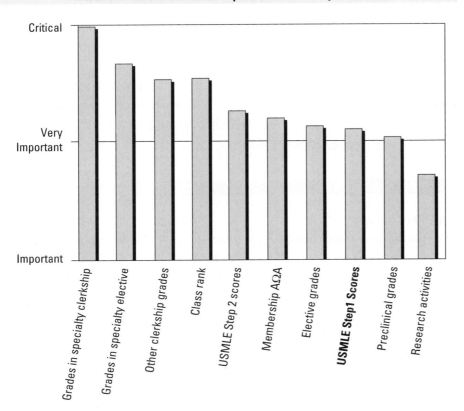

FIGURE 9. Informal Post-Match Survey: Step 1 Goals*

Comfortably Pass	Beat the Mean	Ace the Exam
Pediatrics →	Emergency Medicine	Dermatology
Family Practice →	OB/GYN	ENT
Internal Medicine →	←Radiology	Orthopedics
Anesthesiology	General Surgery	←Ophthalmology
Psychiatry		

* Based on the 1995 results of 110 respondents to an informal survey distributed to US fourth-year medical students at UCSF, UCLA, the University of Louisville, and the University of Miami. Arrows indicate perceived trends from 1996: → = increasing; ← = decreasing score.

Some medical students may wish to "beat the mean" for their own personal satisfaction. For these students, there may be a psychological advantage to scoring higher than the national average.

Some competitive residency programs use Step 1 scores in their selection process.

Ace the Exam

Certain highly competitive residency programs, such as those in otolaryngology and orthopedic surgery, have acknowledged the use of Step 1 scores in the selection process. In such residency programs, greater emphasis may be placed on attaining a high score, so students who wish to enter these programs may want to consider aiming for a very high score on the USMLE Step 1. However, use of the USMLE scores for residency selection has been criticized because neither Step 1 nor Step 2 was designed for this purpose.[16] In addition, only a subset of the basic science facts and concepts that are tested is important to functioning well on the wards. Alternatively, some students may wish to score well in order to feel a sense of mastery. High scores are particularly important for IMGs appyling in all specialties.

TIMELINE FOR STUDY

There are three basic study patterns:

- *the compulsive (months—ace exam)*
- *the crammer (weeks—just pass)*
- *the IMG (months—variable)*

Make a Schedule

After you have defined your goals, map out a study schedule consistent with your objectives, your vacation time, and the difficulty of your ongoing coursework (Fig. 10). Determine whether you want to spread out your study time or concentrate it into 14-hour study days in the final weeks. Factor in your own history in preparing for standardized examinations (e.g., SAT, MCAT), but remember that the USMLE Step 1 is longer and covers far more material than other tests you may have taken.

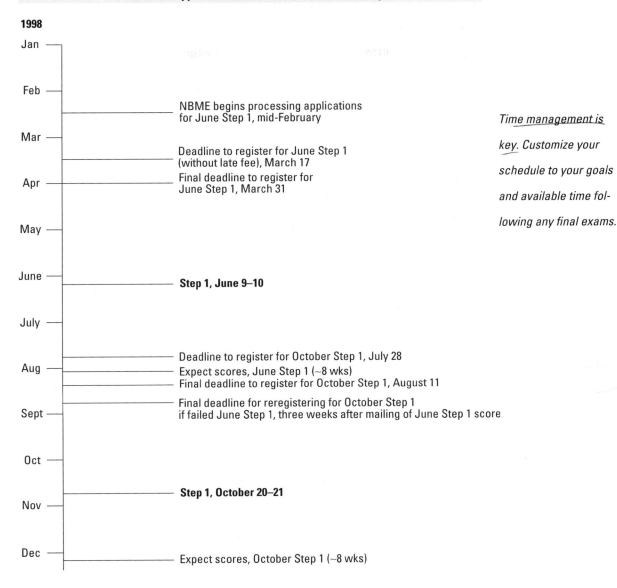

FIGURE 10. Approximate Timeline for 1998 USMLE Step 1

1998

Jan

Feb

Mar — NBME begins processing applications for June Step 1, mid-February

Apr — Deadline to register for June Step 1 (without late fee), March 17
Final deadline to register for June Step 1, March 31

May

June — **Step 1, June 9–10**

July

Aug — Deadline to register for October Step 1, July 28
Expect scores, June Step 1 (~8 wks)
Final deadline to register for October Step 1, August 11

Sept — Final deadline for reregistering for October Step 1 if failed June Step 1, three weeks after mailing of June Step 1 score

Oct

Nov — **Step 1, October 20–21**

Dec — Expect scores, October Step 1 (~8 wks)

Time management is key. Customize your schedule to your goals and available time following any final exams.

Another important consideration is when you will study each subject. Some subjects lend themselves to cramming, whereas others demand a substantial long-term commitment. The "crammable" subjects for Step 1 are those for which concise yet relatively complete review books are available. (See Section III for highly rated review and sample examination books.) Behavioral science and physiology are two subjects with concise review books. Three subjects with longer but quite complete review books are microbiology, pharmacology, and biochemistry. Thus, these subjects could be covered toward the end of your schedule, whereas other subjects (anatomy and pathology) require a longer time commitment and could be studied earlier. An increasing minority of students report using a "systems-based" approach (e.g., GI, renal, CV) toward boards review.

"Crammable" subjects should be covered later and less "crammable" subjects earlier.

Practically speaking, spending a given amount of time on a crammable or high-yield subject (particularly in the waning days before the test) generally produces more correct answers on the examination than spending the same amount of time on a low-yield subject. Student opinion indicates that knowing the crammable subjects extremely well probably results in a higher overall score than knowing all the subjects moderately well.

Allow time in your study schedule for getting sidetracked by personal emergencies.

If you are having difficulty deciding when to start your test preparation, you may find the reverse-calendar approach helpful. Start with the day of the test and plan backward, setting deadlines for objectives to be met. Where the planning ends on your calendar defines a possible starting point.

Make your schedule realistic, with achievable goals. Many students make the mistake of studying at a level of detail that requires too much time for a comprehensive review—reading *Gray's Anatomy* in a couple of days is not a realistic goal! Revise your schedule regularly based on your actual progress. Be careful not to lose focus. Beware of feelings of inadequacy when comparing study schedules and progress with your peers. Avoid students who stress you out. Focus on a few top-rated books that suit your learning style—not on some obscure books your friends may have unearthed. Do not set yourself up for frustration. Accept the fact that you cannot learn it all. Maintain your sanity throughout the process.

Avoid burnout. Maintain proper diet, exercise, and sleep habits. You need to reach and maintain peak concentration on exam day.

You will need time for uninterrupted and focused study. Some students recommend a study schedule that mirrors the exam (e.g., three hours in the morning, lunch break, three hours in the afternoon). Plan your personal affairs to minimize crisis situations near the date of the test. Allot an adequate number of breaks in your study schedule to avoid burnout. Maintain a healthy lifestyle, with proper diet, exercise, and sleep. Getting sick before or during the test will not help your cause.

Year(s) Prior

Buy review books early (first year) and use while studying for courses.

USMLE asserts that the best preparation for the USMLE Step 1 is "broadly based learning that establishes a strong general foundation of understanding of concepts and principles in basic sciences."[17] We agree. Although you may be tempted to rely solely on "cramming" in the weeks and months before the test in order to pass, you should not have to. The knowledge gained during your first two years of medical school and even during your undergraduate years provides the groundwork on which to base your test preparation. The majority of your boards preparation should involve resurrecting dormant information stored away during the basic science years.

Ways to help resurrect and integrate this information include:

- Tutoring first-year students during your second year.
- Reviewing related first-year material in your second year. For example, review first-year cardiac physiology and histology while learning second-year cardiac pathology.
- At the end of each medical school course, compiling and organizing key tables, charts, and mnemonics into a "Step 1" binder. Then, when it comes time to study, you will have a head start with familiar high-yield material.
- Attending all "Introduction to Clinical Medicine" and "problem-based learning" classes and reviews to gain experience with clinical vignettes.

We recommend that you buy highly rated review books early in your first year of medical school and use them as you study throughout the two years. When Step 1 comes along, the books will be more familiar and will be personalized to the way in which you learn. It is risky to buy unfamiliar review books in the final two or three weeks.

Review first-year material in parallel with related second-year topics.

Talk to third- and fourth-year medical students to familiarize yourself with strengths and weaknesses in your school's curriculum. Identify subject areas in which you excel or with which you have difficulty. If you have any doubts concerning your reading speed, consider a speed-reading course. Content typically learned in the second year receives more coverage on Step 1 than do first-year topics due to the emphasis placed on integration of basic science information across many courses.[18] Be aware of your school's testing format and determine whether you have adequate exposure to multiple-choice and matching questions in the form of clinical vignettes.

Month(s) Prior
Review test dates and the application procedure. In 1998, the dates of the USMLE Step 1 are June 9–10 and October 20–21 (Fig. 11). Choose the most appropriate testing site for optimal performance. Many US students simply take the exam at the closest site with all their classmates. A few students report traveling to more distant sites for privacy. Judge for yourself whether you find familiarity reassuring or stressful. If you have any disabilities or "special circumstances," contact the NBME as early as possible to discuss test accommodations (see p. 56, First Aid for the Student with a Disability).

Simulate the USMLE Step 1 under "real" conditions before beginning your studies.

Before you begin to study earnestly, simulate the USMLE Step 1 under "real" conditions to pinpoint strengths and weaknesses in knowledge and test-taking skills. Be sure that you are well informed about the examination and have planned your strategy for studying. Consider what study methods you will use, the study materials you will need, and how you will obtain your materials. Some review books may not be available at your local bookstore, and you may have to order ahead of time to get copies (see list of publisher contacts at the end of Section III). Plan ahead. Get advice from third- and fourth-year medical students who have recently taken

FIGURE 11. Test Dates for the USMLE Step 1, Step 2, and Step 3

	Step 1	Step 2	Step 3
1998	June 9–10 October 20–21	March 3–4 August 25–26	May 12–13 December 1–2*
1999	June 8–9* October 12–13*	March 2–3 August 24–25*	May 11–12* December 7–8*
2000	June 13–14* October 10–11*	March 7–8* August 29–30*	May 9–10* December 5–6*

1999 and 2000 test dates are tentative.

*Indicates exam planned for computer-based administration. Dates with asterisks may not be used for paper-and-pencil testing if computer-based testing is implemented on current timeline.

A major shift to a computer-based Step 1 exam is planned beginning June 1999.

the USMLE Step 1. There might be strengths and weaknesses in your school's curriculum that you should take into account in deciding where to focus your efforts. You might choose to share books, notes, and study hints with classmates. That is how this book began.

Three Weeks Prior

Two to four weeks before the examination is a good time to resimulate the USMLE Step 1. You may want to do this earlier depending on the progress of your review, but do not do it later, when there will be little time to remedy defects in your knowledge or test-taking skills. Make use of remaining good-quality sample USMLE test questions, and try to simulate the test conditions so that you gain a fair assessment of your test performance. Realize that time pressure is increasing as more and more questions are framed as clinical vignettes. Most sample exam questions are shorter than the real thing. Focus on reviewing the high-yield facts, your own notes, picture books, and very short review books.

In the final two weeks, focus on review and endurance. Avoid unfamiliar material.

One Week Prior

Make sure you have your admission ticket and items necessary for the day of the examination, including five or six #2 pencils, a nonbeeping digital timer, and non-smudge erasers. Review the site location and test time. Work out how you will get to the test site and what parking and traffic problems you might encounter. Visit the testing site (if possible) to get a better idea of the testing conditions. Determine what you will do for lunch. Make sure you have everything you need to ensure that you will be comfortable and alert at the test site (e.g., seat cushions, your favorite talismans). Some students recommend loose earplugs to muffle distracting noises, with the caveat that you must be able to hear the directions. Assess your pre-exam living and sleeping arrangements. Do you have an inconsiderate roommate or a loud neighbor who could possibly disrupt your sleep or concentration several days before the exam? Politely announce your upcoming exam to people in your environment in order to avoid confrontations the night before the test. Take aggressive measures to ensure an environment fit for concentration and sufficient sleep. If you really need absolute quiet and have the money, reserve a hotel room for the night(s) before the exam. If you must travel a long distance to the test site, consider arriving the day before and staying overnight with a friend or at a nearby hotel (make early hotel reservations).

One Day Prior

Try your best to relax and rest the night before the test. Double-check your admissions and test-taking materials as well as comfort measures as discussed earlier so you do not have to deal with such details the morning of the exam. Do not study any new material. If you feel compelled to study, then quickly review short-term-memory material (e.g., Section II: Database of High-Yield Facts) before going to sleep (the brain does a lot of information processing at night). However, do not quiz yourself, as you may risk becoming flustered and confused. Do not underestimate your abilities. Remember that regardless of how hard you studied, you cannot know everything. There will be things on the exam that you have never even seen before, so do not panic.

Ensure that you will be comfortable and alert. You must be able to think, not just regurgitate.

Many students report difficulty sleeping the night prior to the exam. This is often exacerbated by going to bed much earlier than usual. Do whatever it takes to ensure a good night's sleep (e.g., massage, exercise, warm milk). Do not change much about your daily routine prior to the exam. Exam day is not the day for a caffeine-withdrawal headache.

Morning of the Exam

Wake up at your regular time and eat a normal breakfast. Drink coffee, tea, or soda in moderation, or you may end up wasting exam time on bathroom breaks. Make sure you have your admission ticket, test-taking materials, and comfort measures as discussed earlier. Wear loose, comfortable clothing. Plan for a variable temperature in the testing center. Remember that you will arrive early in the morning, when it may be cool, and you will not leave until late in the afternoon, when it may be warmer. Arrive at the test site a few minutes before the time designated on the admission ticket; however, do not come too early, as this may increase anxiety. Seating will be assigned, but ask to be reseated if necessary. You need to be seated in an area that will allow you to remain comfortable and to concentrate. Some students find that sitting in the very front or the very back of the room is the least distracting. Listen to your proctors regarding any changes in instructions or testing procedures specific to your test site.

No notes, books, calculators, pagers, recording devices, or alarm timers are allowed. If you must leave, you will be escorted and will not receive extra time.

Remember that it is natural (and even beneficial) to be a little nervous. Focus on being mentally clear and alert. Avoid panic. Avoid panic. Avoid panic. When asked to begin each booklet, catch your breath, read the directions carefully, rapidly skim the entire booklet, and then begin. Remember your time budget. If time and the testing center permit, take breaks to stretch and relax.

Plan bathroom breaks so you do not lose valuable testing time.

Certain "theme" topics
tend to recur throughout
the exam and across
both days.

The lunch break is an excellent opportunity to relax, reorganize your thoughts, and regain composure if you are feeling overly stressed or panicked. Some students use the break to discuss questions with classmates or to look up information. Some students also recommend reviewing theme topics during lunch and between days one and two. However, do what feels comfortable. If you decide to review the morning session, do not dwell on perceived mistakes. Remain focused and briefly review topics that you feel are likely to reappear.

Between the First and Second Days

Try your best to relax. You need the rest to avoid fatigue on the second day. Maintain a positive attitude and do not be discouraged. If you feel absolutely compelled, you can lightly review short-term memory material or "theme" topics heavily tested on the first day. Many students report topics being repeated on the second day. Opinions vary as to the value of looking up topics from the first day. Pros: The topic may be repeated and you may be better prepared. Cons: You may increase your stress and anxiety over questions you believe you have already answered incorrectly.

Relax between test days.
Consider exercise,
massage, or whatever it
takes to stay clear-
headed.

Do a quick analysis of your test-taking technique and how you might modify it for the second day. Assess whether your pace of answering questions was too slow, too fast, or just right. Again, do whatever it takes to ensure a good night's sleep.

After the Test

Have fun and relax regardless of the outcome. Taking the test is an achievement in itself. Enjoy the free time you have before your clerkships. Expect to experience some "reentry" phenomena as you try to regain a real life. Some students report transient feelings of emptiness and anticlimax after it's all over. Once you have recovered sufficiently from the test (or from partying), we invite you to send us your feedback, corrections, and suggestions for entries, facts, mnemonics, strategies, book ratings, and so on (*see* How to Contribute, p. xv). Sharing your experience benefits fellow medical students and international medical graduates.

If you pass Step 1, you
are not allowed to re-
take the exam in an at-
tempt to raise your
score.

IF YOU THINK YOU FAILED

After the test, many examinees feel that they have failed, and most are at least unsure of their pass/fail status. Many students find the whole experience to be miserable and disillusioning. There are several sensible steps you can take to plan for the future if you do not achieve a passing score. First, save and organize all your study materials, including review books, practice tests, and notes.

If you studied from borrowed materials, make sure that you have immediate access to them. Review your school's policy regarding requirements for graduation and promotion to the third year. About one-half of the medical schools accredited by the Liaison Committee on Medical Education require passing Step 1 for promotion to the third year, and two-thirds require passing Step 1 as a requirement for graduation.[19] Even if passing Step 1 is not necessary for promotion to the third year, it is probably best to retake the exam at the next available administration. Weigh your options carefully. Finally, familiarize yourself with reapplication procedures for Step 1, including application deadlines and upcoming test dates.

USMLE Step 1 results usually arrive in the mail about six weeks after the test administration. In 1997, scores for the June administration were delayed due to reports of irregular behavior. If you do not achieve a passing score on the June administration of Step 1, then you have about eight weeks to prepare for the October Step 1. The deadline for the October administration is generally extended two weeks past the June Step 1 score mailings for examinees who fail and wish to repeat the exam.[20]

If you believe that your scores were incorrectly determined, you may request that your answer sheets be rechecked by hand. The resulting scores will be honored. The request must be submitted in writing with a fee to the test administration entity that registered you for the Step 1.

The performance profiles on the back of the USMLE Step 1 score report provide valuable feedback concerning your relative strengths and weaknesses (see Fig. 3B). Study the performance profiles closely. Set up a study timeline to repair defects in knowledge as well as to maintain and improve what you already know (see Timeline for Study, p. 12). Do not neglect high-yield subjects. Finally, it is normal to feel somewhat anxious about retaking the test. However, if anxiety becomes a problem, seek appropriate counseling.

Sixty-three percent of the NBME-registered first-time takers who failed the June 1996 Step 1 repeated the exam in October. The overall pass rate for that group in October was 71% (up from 57% in 1995). However, pass rates varied widely depending on previous performance on the June 1996 administration (Fig. 12).

Although the NBME allows an unlimited number of attempts to pass the Step 1, both the NBME and the FSMB recommend that licensing authorities allow a minimum of three and a maximum of six attempts for each Step examination.[22] Again, review your school's policy regarding retakes.

FIGURE 12. Pass Rates for USMLE Step 1 Repeaters 1995–96[21]

Score in June	% Pass Oct. 95	% Pass Oct. 96
173–175	82	94
170–172	76	89
165–169	57	79
160–164	29	59
150–159	11	35
<150	0	14
Overall	**57**	**71**

IF YOU FAILED

Even if you came out of the exam room feeling that you failed, seeing that failing grade in cold print can be traumatic, and it is natural to feel upset. Different people react in different ways: For some it is a stimulus to buckle down and study harder; for some it "takes the wind out of their sails" for a few days; and for some it may lead to a reassessment of their goals and abilities. For a few, however, failure may trigger weeks or months of sadness, feelings of hopelessness, social withdrawal, and inability to concentrate—in other words, a true clinical depression.

If you are depressed, seek help. As you know from your studies, depression is a common, potentially disabling, and at times even fatal illness. Depression is also very treatable, and you must use the same resources that you plan to offer your patients. In other words, you must seek treatment, whether from a school counselor, psychiatrist, or psychologist. Do not "treat" yourself with alcohol, illegal drugs, or anything else—you need the same skilled help that anyone else with this problem needs.

Even if your reaction is not so intense, ask yourself the following questions:

- Who says I should never fail? To never experience failure is to be perfect, and it is absurd to expect anyone to be perfect.
- Is failing a true catastrophe? Certainly it would be better if you had not failed. Failing does not mean that you will never reach your goal of becoming a US licensed physician.

Near the failure threshold, each three-digit scale point is equivalent to about three questions answered correctly.[23]

As Figure 12 shows, the majority of people who fail Step 1 the first time will pass on their second attempt, especially if they were near the failure threshold. But be realistic: If you obtained a very low mark or have already failed several times before, you need to reevaluate not only your study methods but also your goals. Although there are some people who are merely "bad test takers" with the potential to become good physicians, you need to ask yourself if it is really in your best interests to pursue a career that is giving you such a hard time. Remember that you will never run out of exams to take: after Step 1 come Step 2 and Step 3, in-service exams as a resident, specialty board exams at the end of residency, and then possible recertification exams in your specialty every few years.

STUDY METHODS

It is important to have a set of study methods for preparing for the USMLE Step 1. There is too much material to study by random reading and memorization. Experiment with different ways of studying. You do not know how effective something might be until you try it. This is best done months before the test in order to determine what works and what you enjoy. Possible study options include:

- Studying review material in groups
- Creating personal mnemonics, diagrams, and tables
- Using *First Aid* as a framework on which to add notes
- Taking practice tests alone or in groups
- Attending faculty review sessions
- Making or sharing flashcards
- Reviewing old syllabi and notes
- Making cassette tapes of review material to study during commuting time
- Playing Trivial Pursuit–style games with facts and questions
- Getting away from home for an extended period to avoid distractions and to immerse yourself in studying

Study Groups

A good study group has many advantages. It can relieve stress, organize your time, and allow people with different strengths to exchange information. Study groups also allow you to pool resources and spend less money on review books and sample tests.

Balance individual and group study.

There are, however, potential problems with study groups. It is difficult to study with people who have different goals and study paces. Avoid large, unwieldly groups. Otherwise, studying can be inefficient and time-consuming. Some study groups also tend to socialize more than study.

If you choose not to belong to a study group, it may be a good idea to find a support group or study partner simply to keep pace with and share study ideas. It is good to get different perspectives from other students in evaluating what is and is not important to learn. Do not become intimidated or discouraged by interactions with a few overly compulsive students; everyone studies and learns differently.

Mnemonics and Memorizing

Cramming is a viable way of memorizing short-term information just before a test, but after one or two days you will find that much of that knowledge has dissipated. For that reason, cramming and memorization by repetition ("brute force") in the weeks before the exam are not ideal techniques for long-term memorization of the overwhelming body of information covered by Step 1. Mnemonics are memory aids that work by linking isolated facts or abstract ideas to acronyms, pictures, patterns, rhymes, and stories—information that the mind tends to store well.[24] The best mnemonics are your own, and develop-

Developing good mnemonics takes time and work.

Quiz yourself periodically. Do not simply reread highlighted material.

ing them takes work. The first step to creating a mnemonic is understanding the information to be memorized. Play around with the information and look for unique features that help you remember it. In addition, make the mnemonic as colorful, humorous, or outlandish as you can; such mnemonics are the most memorable. Effective mnemonics should link the topic with the facts in as specific and unambiguous a manner as possible. In memorizing the mnemonic, engage as many senses as possible by repeating the fact aloud or by writing or acting it out. Keep the information fresh by quizzing yourself periodically with flashcards, in study groups, and so on. Do not make the common mistake of simply rereading highlighted review material. The material may start to look familiar, but that does not mean you will be able to remember it in another context during the exam.

Review Sessions

Faculty review sessions can be helpful. Review sessions that are geared specifically toward the USMLE Step 1 tend to be more helpful than general review sessions. Open "question and answer" sessions tend to be inefficient and not worth the time. Focus on reviews given by faculty who are knowledgeable in the content and testing format of the USMLE Step 1.

Commercial Courses

Commercial preparation courses can be helpful for some students, but they are expensive and require significant time commitment. They are often effective in organizing study material for students who feel overwhelmed by the volume of material. Note that the multiweek courses may be quite intense and may thus leave limited time for independent study. Note also that some commercial courses are designed for first-time test takers and that others focus on students who are repeating the examination. Some courses focus on international medical graduates who must take all three Steps in a limited amount of time. See page 359 for summarized data and excerpted information from several commercial review courses.

STUDY MATERIALS

Quality and Cost Considerations

Although there is an ever-increasing number of board review books and software on the market, the quality of the material is highly variable. Some common problems:

- Certain review books are too detailed for review in a reasonable amount of time or cover subtopics not emphasized on the exam (e.g., a 400-page histology book).

- Many sample question books were originally written years ago and have not been updated adequately to reflect trends on the revised USMLE Step 1.
- Many sample question books use poorly written questions or contain factual errors in the explanations.
- Explanations for sample questions range from nonexistent to overly detailed.
- Software for boards review is of highly variable quality, may be difficult to install, and may be fraught with bugs.

In 1997, students felt that even the top-rated sample exams did not accurately reflect the clinical focus of the actual exam.

Basic Science Review Books

Most review books are the products of considerable effort by experienced educators. There are many, and you must choose which ones to buy based on their relative merits. Although recommendations from other medical students are useful, many students simply recommend whatever books they used without having compared them to other books on the same subject. Do not waste time with very outdated "hand-me-down" review books. Some students blindly advocate one publisher's series without considering the broad range of quality encountered within most series. Weigh different opinions against each other, read the reviews and ratings in Section III of this guide, examine the books closely in the bookstore, and choose review books very carefully. You are investing not only money but also your limited study time. Do not worry about finding the "perfect" book, as many subjects simply do not have one, and different students prefer different styles.

If a given review book is not working for you, stop using it, no matter how highly rated it may be.

There are two types of review books: books that are stand-alone titles and books that are part of a series. The books in a series generally have the same style, and you must decide if that style is helpful for you. However, a given style is not optimal for every subject. For example, charts and diagrams may be the best approach for physiology and biochemistry, whereas tables and outlines may be better for microbiology.

Find out which books are up to date. Some new editions represent major improvements, whereas others contain only cursory changes. You should take into consideration how a book reflects the format of the USMLE Step 1. Note that some of the books reviewed in Section III have not been updated adequately to reflect the clinical emphasis and question format of the current USMLE Step 1. Books that emphasize obscure facts and minute details tend to be less helpful for the USMLE Step 1, because there are now fewer "picky" questions and more problem-solving questions.

Many students regret not using the same books for medical school exam review and Step 1 review.

Clinical Review Books

Keep your eye out for early purchase and review of more clinically oriented review books. A number of students are turning to Step 2 books, pathophysiology books, and case-based reviews in order to prepare for the clinical vignettes.

Examples of such books (not yet rated) include:

- *NMS Medicine* (Williams & Wilkins)
- *PreTest Physical Diagnosis* (McGraw-Hill)
- *Washington Manual* (Little, Brown)
- *Laboratory Medicine Case Book* (Appleton & Lange)
- Various USMLE Step 2 review books

Texts, Syllabi, and Notes

Limit your use of texts and syllabi for Step 1 review. Many textbooks are too detailed for high-yield boards review and include material that is generally not tested on the USMLE Step 1 (e.g., drug dosages, complex chemical structures). Syllabi, although familiar, are inconsistent and often reflect the emphasis of the faculty, which often does not correspond to the emphasis of the boards. Syllabi also tend to be less organized and to contain fewer diagrams and study questions than the top-rated review books. In our opinion, they are often a waste of time for the faculty to write and suboptimal for the student to read (when compared with the best review books). Make sure that your instructors are aware of the best books, and supplement your classes with case-based problem-solving curricula that reflect the current exam format. Old class notes have the advantage of presenting material in the way you learned it but suffer from the same disadvantages as syllabi.

When using texts or notes, engage in **active learning** by making tables, diagrams, new mnemonics, and conceptual associations whenever possible. Supplement incomplete or unclear material with reference to other appropriate textbooks. Keep a good medical dictionary at hand to sort out definitions.

Practice Tests

Most practice exams are shorter and less clinical than the real thing.

Taking practice tests provides valuable information about strengths and weaknesses in your fund of knowledge and test-taking skills. Some students use practice examinations simply as a means of breaking up the monotony of studying and adding variety to their study schedule. Other students study almost solely from practice tests. There is a wide range of quality in available practice material, and it is easy to become frustrated by low-quality sample questions or questions without explanations. Students report that many current practice exam books have questions that are, on average, shorter and less clinically oriented than the current USMLE Step 1. Many Step 1 questions demand fast reading skills and application of basic science facts in a problem-solving format. Approach sample examinations critically, and do not waste time with low-quality questions until you have exhausted better sources.

Use practice tests to identify concepts and areas of weakness, not just facts that you missed.

After taking a practice test, try to identify concepts and areas of weakness, not just the facts that you missed. Do not panic if you miss a lot of questions on a practice examination. Use the experience to motivate your study and prioritize what areas need the most work.

Use quality practice examinations to improve your test-taking skills. Analyze your ability to pace yourself so that you have enough time to complete each test booklet comfortably. Practice examinations are also a good means of training yourself to concentrate for long periods of time under appropriate time pressure. Consider taking practice tests with a friend or in a small group to increase motivation while simulating more accurately the format and schedule of the real examination. Analyze the pattern of your responses to questions to determine if you have made systematic errors in answering questions. Common mistakes are reading too much into the question, second-guessing your initial impression, and misinterpreting the question.

GENERAL STUDY STRATEGIES

The USMLE Step 1 was created according to an integrated outline that organizes basic science material in a multidisciplinary approach. Broad-based knowledge is more important than in prior years. The exam is designed to test basic science material and its application to clinical situations. A little over half of the questions include clinical situations, although some are brief.

In spite of the change in the organization of the subject matter, the detailed Step 1 content outline provided by the USMLE has not proved useful for students. We feel that it is still best to approach the material along the lines of the seven traditional disciplines. In Section II, we provide suggestions on how to approach the material within each subject.

Practice questions that include case histories or descriptive vignettes are critical in preparing yourself for the clinical slant of the USMLE Step 1. It is not necessary to memorize all normal laboratory values, because they are printed on the insides of both the front and back covers of all test booklets. However, it's worth knowing the commonly encountered normals so that you can answer questions faster. For this purpose, we have highlighted the high-yield normal values on duplicates of the tables provided within the exam booklet (see Fig. 13).

Familiarize yourself with the commonly tested normal laboratory values.

TEST-TAKING STRATEGIES

Your test performance is influenced by both your fund of knowledge and your test-taking skills. You can increase your performance by considering each of these factors. Test-taking skills and strategies should be developed and per-

Practice and perfect test-taking skills and strategies well before the test date.

FIGURE 13. USMLE Step 1 Laboratory Values

* = Included in the Biochemical Profile (SMA-12)

BLOOD, PLASMA, SERUM	REFERENCE RANGE	SI REFERENCE INTERVALS
* Alanine aminotransferase (ALT, GPT at 30°C)	8–20 U/L	8–20 U/L
Amylase, serum	25–125 U/L	25–125 U/L
* Aspartate aminotransferase (AST, GOT at 30°C)	8–20 U/L	8–20 U/L
Bilirubin, serum (adult)		
Total // Direct	0.1–1.0 mg/dL // 0.0–0.3 mg/dL	2–17 µmol/L // 0–5 µmol/L
* Calcium, serum (Total)	8.4–10.2 mg/dL	2.1–2.8 mmol/L
* Cholesterol, serum	140–250 mg/dL	3.6–6.5 mmol/L
Cortisol, serum	0800 h: 5–23 µg/dL // 1600 h: 3–15 µg/dL	138–635 nmol/L // 82–413 nmol/L
	2000 h: ≤ 50% of 0800 h	Fraction of 0800 h: ≤ 0.50
Creatine kinase, serum (at 30°C) ambulatory	Male: 25–90 U/L	25–90 U/L
	Female: 10–70 U/L	10–70 U/L
* Creatinine, serum	0.6–1.2 mg/dL	53–106 µmol/L
Electrolytes, serum		
Sodium	135–147 mEq/L	135–147 mmol/L
Chloride	95–105 mEq/L	95–105 mmol/L
* Potassium	3.5–5.0 mEq/L	3.5–5.0 mmol/L
Bicarbonate	22–28 mEq/L	22–28 mmol/L
Estriol (E_3) total, serum (in pregnancy)		
24–28 wks // 32–36 wks	30–170 ng/mL // 60–280 ng/mL	104–590 // 208–970 nmol/L
28–32 wks // 36–40 wks	40–220 ng/mL // 80–350 ng/mL	140–760 // 280–1210 nmol/L
Ferritin, serum	Male: 15–200 ng/mL	15–200 µg/L
	Female: 12–150 ng/mL	12–150 µg/L
Follicle-stimulating hormone, serum/plasma	Male: 4–25 mIU/mL	4–25 U/L
	Female: premenopause 4–30 mIU/mL	4–30 U/L
	midcycle peak 10–90 mIU/mL	10–90 U/L
	postmenopause 40–250 mIU/mL	40–250 U/L
Gases, arterial blood (room air)		
P_{O_2}	75–105 mm Hg	10.0–14.0 kPa
P_{CO_2}	33–44 mm Hg	4.4–5.9 kPa
pH	7.35–7.45	[H^+] 36–44 nmol/L
* Glucose, serum	Fasting: 70–110 mg/dL	3.8–6.1 mmol/L
	2-h postprandial: < 120 mg/dL	< 6.6 mmol/L
Growth hormone - arginine stimulation	Fasting: < 5 ng/mL	< 5 µg/L
	provocative stimuli: > 7 ng/mL	> 7 µg/L
Immunoglobulins, serum		
IgA	76–390 mg/dL	0.76–3.90 g/L
IgE	0–380 IU/mL	0–380 kIU/mL
IgG	650–1500 mg/dL	6.5–15 g/L
IgM	40–345 mg/dL	0.4–3.45 g/L
Iron	50–170 µg/dL	9–30 µmol/L
Lactate dehydrogenase (L → P, 30ºC)	45–90 U/L	45–90 U/L

FIGURE 13. USMLE Step 1 Laboratory Values (continued)

BLOOD, PLASMA, SERUM	REFERENCE RANGE	SI REFERENCE INTERVALS
Luteinizing hormone, serum/plasma	Male: 6–23 mIU/mL	6–23 U/L
	Female: follicular phase 5–30 mIU/mL	5–30 U/L
	midcycle 75–150 mIU/mL	75–150 U/L
	postmenopause 30–200 mIU/mL	30–200 U/L
Osmolality, serum	275–295 mOsmol/kg	275–295 mOsmol/kg
Parathyroid hormone, serum, N-terminal	230–630 pg/mL	230–630 ng/L
* Phosphatase (alkaline), serum (p-NPP at 30°C)	20–70 U/L	20–70 U/L
* Phosphorus (inorganic), serum	3.0–4.5 mg/dL	1.0–1.5 mmol/L
Prolactin, serum (hPRL)	< 20 ng/mL	< 20 µg/L
* Proteins, serum		
Total (recumbent)	6.0–7.8 g/dL	60–78 g/L
Albumin	3.5–5.5 g/dL	35–55 g/L
Globulins	2.3–3.5 g/dL	23–35 g/L
Thyroid-stimulating hormone, serum or plasma	0.5–5.0 µU/mL	0.5–5.0 mU/L
Thyroidal iodine (^{123}I) uptake	8–30% of administered dose/24 h	0.08–0.30/24 h
Thyroxine (T_4), serum	5–12 µg/dL	64–155 nmol/L
Triglycerides, serum	35–160 mg/dL	0.4–1.81 mmol/L
Triiodothyronine (T_3), serum (RIA)	115–190 ng/dL	1.8–2.9 nmol/L
Triiodothyronine (T_3) resin uptake	25–35%	0.25–0.35
* Urea nitrogen, serum (BUN)	7–18 mg/dL	1.2–3.0 mmol urea/L
* Uric acid, serum	3.0–8.2 mg/dL	0.18–0.48 mmol/L
CEREBROSPINAL FLUID		
Cell count	0–5 cells/mm^3	0–5 × 10^6/L
Chloride	118–132 mmol/L	118–132 mmol/L
Gamma globulin	3–12% total proteins	0.03–0.12
Glucose	40–70 mg/dL	2.2–3.9 mmol/L
Pressure	70–180 mm H_2O	70–180 mm H_2O
Proteins, total	< 40 mg/dL	< 0.40 g/L
HEMATOLOGIC		
Bleeding time (template)	2–7 minutes	2–7 minutes
Erythrocyte count	Male: 4.3–5.9 million/mm^3	4.3–5.9 × 10^{12}/L
	Female: 3.5–5.5 million/mm^3	3.5–5.5 × 10^{12}/L
Hematocrit	Male: 41–53%	0.41–0.53
	Female: 36–46%	0.36–0.46
Hemoglobin, blood	Male: 13.5–17.5 g/dL	2.09–2.71 mmol/L
	Female: 12.0–16.0 g/dL	1.86–2.48 mmol/L
Hemoglobin, plasma	1–4 mg/dL	0.16–0.62 µmol/L
Leukocyte count and differential		
Leukocyte count	4500–11,000/mm^3	4.5–11.0 × 10^9/L
Segmented neutrophils	54–62%	0.54–0.62
Band forms	3–5%	0.03–0.05
Eosinophils	1–3%	0.01–0.03
Basophils	0–0.75%	0–0.0075
Lymphocytes	25–33%	0.25–0.33
Monocytes	3–7%	0.03–0.07

FIGURE 13. USMLE Step 1 Laboratory Values (continued)

HEMATOLOGIC (cont.)	REFERENCE RANGE	SI REFERENCE INTERVALS
Mean corpuscular hemoglobin	25.4–34.6 pg/cell	0.39–0.54 fmol/cell
Mean corpuscular hemoglobin concentration	31–36% Hb/cell	4.81–5.58 mmol Hb/L
Mean corpuscular volume	80–100 µm³	80–100 fl
Partial thromboplastin time (nonactivated)	60–85 seconds	60–85 seconds
Platelet count	150,000–400,000/mm³	150–400 × 10⁹/L
Prothrombin time	11–15 seconds	11–15 seconds
Reticulocyte count	0.5–1.5% of red cells	0.005–0.015
Sedimentation rate, erythrocyte (Westergren)	Male: 0–15 mm/h	0–15 mm/h
	Female: 0–20 mm/h	0–20 mm/h
Thrombin time	< 2 seconds deviation from control	< 2 seconds deviation from control
Volume		
Plasma	Male: 25–43 mL/kg	0.025–0.043 L/kg
	Female: 28–45 mL/kg	0.028–0.045 L/kg
Red cell	Male: 20–36 mL/kg	0.020–0.036 L/kg
	Female: 19–31 mL/kg	0.019–0.031 L/kg
SWEAT		
Chloride	0–35 mmol/L	0–35 mmol/L
URINE		
Calcium	100–300 mg/24 h	2.5–7.5 mmol/24 h
Chloride	Varies with intake	Varies with intake
Creatinine clearance	Male: 97–137 mL/min	
	Female: 88–128 mL/min	
Estriol, total (in pregnancy)		
30 wks	6–18 mg/24 h	21–62 µmol/24 h
35 wks	9–28 mg/24 h	31–97 µmol/24 h
40 wks	13–42 mg/24 h	45–146 µmol/24 h
17-Hydroxycorticosteroids	Male: 3.0–10.0 mg/24 h	8.2–27.6 µmol/24 h
	Female: 2.0–8.0 mg/24 h	5.5–22.0 µmol/24 h
17-Ketosteroids, total	Male: 8–20 mg/24 h	28–70 µmol/24 h
	Female: 6–15 mg/24 h	21–52 µmol/24 h
Osmolality	50–1400 mOsmol/kg	
Oxalate	8–40 µg/mL	90–445 µmol/L
Potassium	Varies with diet	Varies with diet
Proteins, total	< 150 mg/24 h	< 0.15 g/24 h
Sodium	Varies with diet	Varies with diet
Uric acid	Varies with diet	Varies with diet

fected well in advance of the test date so you can concentrate on the test itself. We suggest you try the following strategies to see if they might work for you.

Pacing

You have 180 minutes to complete approximately 180 questions (down from 185). This works out to 60 questions per hour and about 60 seconds per question. Most students report having at most a few minutes at the end of the examination to verify answers and to go over any particularly difficult questions that they may have guessed or skipped. Most students prefer to mark a temporary answer on all skipped questions in case they do not have time to return. You may find that some question types (e.g., extended matching) may require less time to process than others. Dealing with such question types first may prevent you from leaving quickly answerable questions unanswered.

An old NBME analysis of previous board examinations revealed that some students left a few items unanswered in the first examination book of the first morning.[25] This indicates that pacing yourself may be especially important when working on the first booklet. Make the necessary pacing adjustments as you work on each booklet. Pacing errors leading to unanswered questions have been known to occur even among students who were considered to be very well prepared.

Dealing with Each Question

There are several established techniques for efficiently approaching multiple-choice questions. See what works for you. All questions can be identified as easy, workable, or impossible. Your goal should be to answer all easy questions, to work out all workable questions in a reasonable amount of time, and to make quick and intelligent guesses on all impossible questions. Most students read the stem, think of the answer, and turn immediately to the choices. A second technique is to first skim the answer choices and the last sentence of the question. Then read through the passage quickly, extracting only relevant information to answer the question. Try a variety of techniques on practice exams and see what works best for you.

In 1997, students have reported feeling quite rushed and often unable to return to skipped questions.

In general, when you eliminate an incorrect choice on a question, mark it out to avoid rereading it unnecessarily. If you are unsure about a choice, place a question mark by it. When you think you have determined the best answer, circle it and mark your answer sheet accordingly.

Difficult Questions

Questions on the USMLE Step 1 require varying amounts of time to answer. Some problem-solving questions take longer than simple, fact-recall questions. Because of the exam's clinical emphasis, you may find that many of the questions appear workable but take more time than is available. It can be tempting to dwell on these types of questions for an excessive amount of time because you feel you are on the verge of "figuring it out." Resist this temptation and budget your time. Answer the question with your best guess, make a mark signifying "tentative" on your booklet or answer sheet, and come back to the

Do not dwell excessively on questions that you are on the verge of "figuring out." Make your best guess and move on.

question after you have completed the rest of the booklet. This keeps you from inadvertently leaving any blank questions in your efforts to beat the clock. Remember to save a few minutes at the end to remove all stray marks from the answer sheet and to make sure that all questions have been answered.

Inevitably, there will be some questions for which you will not have a clue (i.e., impossible questions). Do not be disturbed by these questions. Guess and move on. As a medical student, you are used to scoring well on standardized examinations (otherwise you would not be in medical school), so the USMLE Step 1 may be your first experience with facing lots of questions to which you do not know the answer. Prepare yourself for this. After narrowing down the answers as best you can, have a plan for guessing so that you do not waste time. Remember that you are not expected to know all the answers.

Another reason for not dwelling too long on any question is that certain questions may be **experimental** or may be **printed incorrectly.** Not all questions are scored. Some questions serve as "embedded pretest items" that do not count toward your overall score.[26] Students have also noted several printing errors in past USMLE Step 1 examinations. The lesson here is that you should not waste too much time with ambiguous or "flawed" questions. The reason you are having difficulty with the question may lie in the question itself, not with you!

Batch Fill-in

Most students mark their answer sheets after answering each question. However, constantly shifting back and forth between the test booklet and the answer sheet can break concentration and impart a small but significant time penalty. Batch fill-in separates the tasks of answering the questions and transcribing the answers. First, mark the answers clearly in the margin of the test booklet as you do each question, and then carefully transcribe two pages' worth of answers onto the answer sheet before turning the page. Batch fill-in may improve your concentration by keeping your eyes focused on the booklet and help you develop a good question–answer rhythm. (You may want to revert to transcribing answers question by question toward the end of each test session.) In addition, some students recommend using a dull pencil to fill in the answer sheet because it may be faster. Batch fill-in does not work for everyone; do not use batch fill-in unless you have practiced it extensively.

Margin Marking

Feel free to write in the test booklet and circle or underline key phrases. Draw diagrams or make notes concerning specific facts when encountering case histories or descriptive vignettes. Focus on specific "buzzwords" within the clinical histories. If you find it helpful, circle important directions and repeated words in the answers. Many students mark the possible answers as "T," "F," or "?" to work out difficult questions.

Guessing

There is **no penalty** for wrong answers. Thus, no answer sheet should be turned in with unanswered questions. A hunch is probably better than a random guess. If you have to guess, we suggest guessing an answer you recognize over one that is totally unfamiliar. Go where the money is. If you have studied the subject and do not recognize a particular answer, then it is more likely a distractor than a correct answer. Remember, however, that distractors are carefully written and edited to appear reasonable to all but the most competent examinees. Also be aware that students often disregard instructions, allowing for an answer choice to be selected more than once in matching sets.

Changing Your Answer

The conventional wisdom regarding "reconsidering" answers is not to change answers that you have already marked unless there is a convincing and logical reason to do so—in other words, go with your first hunch. You can test this strategy for yourself by keeping a running total of the questions on which you seriously considered changing your answer when taking practice exams. Experience eventually tells you how strongly to trust your first hunches.

Fourth-Quarter Effect (Avoiding Burnout)

Pacing and endurance are important. Practice helps develop both. Fewer and fewer examinees are leaving the examination session early. Use any extra time at the end to return to unresolved questions or carefully recheck your answers. Do not be too casual in your review or you may overlook serious mistakes. A few students report that near the end of a booklet they suddenly remember facts that help answer questions they had guessed on earlier.

Do not leave the test too early. Carefully review your answers if possible.

Remember your goals, and keep in mind the effort you have devoted to studying compared with the small additional effort required to maintain focus and concentration throughout the examination.

Never give up. If you feel yourself getting frustrated, try taking a 30-second breather. Look away from the exam booklet, breathe deeply, and slowly count to ten. Hopefully, you can return to the exam refreshed and clear. Every point you earn is to your advantage. The difference between passing and an average score is far fewer questions than you might think—about 25% of students who failed were within 15 questions of passing.

The "Glossy" Booklets

The "glossy" booklets contain approximately 20–30 questions with accompanying gross and microscopic photographs. Two such booklets appeared in the June 1997 exam. Student experience shows that 30–50% of these questions can be answered correctly independent of the photograph. Some students report trying to answer the question without the photograph and then looking at the photo to confirm their answer.

Do not panic if you are unfamiliar with a particular photograph.

Types of photographs include gross pathology (e.g., hydatidiform mole, cardiac valve vegetations), histopathology (e.g., liver cirrhosis, myocardial infarction, glomerulonephritis), blood smears (e.g., target cells, basophilic stippling), dermatopathology (e.g., lupus, Lyme disease, basal cell carcinoma), and extensive imaging (e.g., CT and MR anatomy, cerebral angiogram, plain film fractures). There are several websites that contain photographic material that may be helpful for Step 1 studying. A fast Internet connection is a must when browsing images. One site is http://www.kumc.edu/AMA-MSS/study/path_review/index.htm. Additional links to study material can be found at http://www.s2smed.com.

CLINICAL VIGNETTE STRATEGIES

In recent years, the USMLE Step 1 has become increasingly clinically oriented. Students polled from the June 1997 exam report that nearly two-thirds of the questions were presented as clinical vignettes. This change mirrors a trend in medical education in which an increasing number of medical schools expose students to clinical problem solving during the basic science years. The increasing clinical emphasis of the Step 1 may be challenging to those students who attend schools with a more traditional curriculum.

The first step toward approaching the clinical vignette is not to panic. The same basic science concepts are often being tested in the guise of a clinical vignette.

What Is a Clinical Vignette?

Be prepared to read fast and think on your feet!

A clinical vignette is a short (usually paragraph-long) description of a patient, including demographics, presenting symptoms, signs, and other information concerning the patient. Sometimes this paragraph is followed by a brief listing of the important physical findings and/or laboratory results. The task of assimilating all this information and answering the associated question in the span of one minute can be intimidating. Be prepared to read fast and think on your feet. Remember that the question is often indirectly asking something you already know.

Here are two examples of vignettes that appear complex but actually ask a relatively straightforward question.

Vignette #1

A 38-year-old African-American woman visits her physician. She explains that she has been experiencing palpitations, shortness of breath, and syncopal episodes for several months. In addition to a constant feeling of impending doom, she also has episodes of dizziness without nausea or vomiting. Her sleep pattern is normal. The physician's first course of action should be to:

    A) provide psychotherapy
    B) treat the patient with benzodiazepines
    C) perform a physical examination
    D) refer the patient to a psychiatrist
    E) teach the patient self-hypnosis

Answer: C. Regardless of whether a psychiatric or organic disorder is present, a history and physical examination should always be performed during the first visit. As the history is summarized in the vignette, the physical exam would be the first course of action before considering any of the other answer choices.

Vignette #2

J.B. is a seven-year-old Caucasian male who complains of a chronic, persistent cough. The cough is often elicited by physical activity or cold exposure. His mother says that she had an uncomplicated, full-term pregnancy and that the child has been healthy except for one episode of pneumonia when he was five years old. She also notes that his appetite is variable and that he frequently has light-colored and foul-smelling stool. On physical exam, his weight was 20.5 kg (25th percentile) and his height was 119.5 cm (25th percentile). His physician orders a sweat chloride test (Cook-Gibson method) and receives the following results:

    Right arm   103 mEq/L
    Left arm   108 mEq/L
    Normal   <70 mEq/L

What is the mode of inheritance of this disorder?

    A) autosomal dominant
    B) autosomal recessive
    C) mitochondrial
    D) X-linked recessive
    E) none of the above

Answer: B.

Strategy

Step 1 vignettes usually describe diseases or disorders in their most classic presentation.

Remember that the Step 1 vignettes usually describe diseases or disorders in their most classic presentation. Look for buzzwords or cardinal signs (e.g., malar rash for SLE or nuchal rigidity for meningitis) in the narrative history. Sometimes the data from labs and the physical exam will help you confirm or reject possible diagnoses, thereby helping you rule answer choices in or out. In some cases, they will be a dead giveaway for the diagnosis.

Sometimes making a diagnosis is not necessary at all.

Making a diagnosis from the history and data is often not the final answer. Not infrequently, the diagnosis is divulged at the end of the vignette, after you have just struggled through the narrative in order to come up with a diagnosis of your own. The question instead asks about a related aspect of the diagnosed disease.

One strategy that many students suggest is to *skim* the questions and answer choices before reading a vignette, especially if the vignette is lengthy. This will focus your attention on the relevant information and reduce the time spent on that vignette. Sometimes you may not need much of the information in the vignette to answer the question.

For vignette #2, consider the following approach.

1. Take a look at the question and answer choices first. We see that a diagnosis of some inherited disease will likely have to be made in order to answer this question.
2. As in many vignettes, the first sentence presents the patient's age, sex, and race. This information can help direct your diagnosis. For the case above, you are looking for a genetic disease in a Caucasian boy, which may already tip you off to cystic fibrosis. If you are looking for an inherited anemia, sickle-cell disease would be more likely for an African-American patient. If, by contrast, the patient were Asian or Mediterranean, then thalassemia might be more likely.
3. Next, look for the chief complaint, in this case "chronic persistent cough."
4. Even if the diagnosis of cystic fibrosis is not apparent at this point, fear not! The vignette further describes other classic symptoms of the disease (e.g., fat malabsorption due to pancreatic insufficiency, growth retardation, elevated sweat chloride levels).
5. Instead of asking for the diagnosis, the question asks its mode of inheritance. Questions like this one require the test taker to go beyond the first stage in the reasoning process. **These "two-step questions" are appearing with increasing frequency on the Step 1 exam.**

"Two-step questions" are appearing with increasing frequency on the Step 1 exam.

IRREGULAR BEHAVIOR

During 1995, more than 75 individuals were reported by proctors to be suspicious of "irregular behavior," including continuing to work after being asked to stop, taking notes, talking with other examinees, looking at other examinees, falsifying score reports, and memorizing, reproducing, and disseminating test items. If a determination of irregular behavior is made, a permanent annotation is made on the individual's USMLE record.[27] Following the June 1997 administration of the USMLE Step 1, score results were delayed several weeks due to suspected cheating.

TESTING AGENCIES

National Board of Medical Examiners (NBME)
Department of Licensing Examination Services
3750 Market Street
Philadelphia, PA 19104-3190
(215) 590-9700
http://www.nbme.org

Educational Commission for Foreign Medical Graduates (ECFMG)
3624 Market Street, Fourth Floor
Philadelphia, PA 19104-2685
(215) 386-5900 or (202) 293-9320
Fax: (215) 386-9196
http://www.ecfmg.org

Federation of State Medical Boards (FSMB)
400 Fuller Wiser Road, Suite 300
Euless, TX 76039-3855
(817) 571-2949
Fax: (817) 868-4099
http://www.fsmb.org

USMLE Secretariat
3750 Market Street
Philadelphia, PA 19104-3190
(215) 590-9600
http://www.usmle.org

REFERENCES

1. Bidese, Catherine M., *U.S. Medical Licensure Statistics and Current Licensure Requirements 1995,* American Medical Association, 1995 (ISBN 0899707270).

2. National Board of Medical Examiners, *Part I Examination Guidelines and Sample Items, 1991,* Philadelphia, 1990.

3. National Board of Medical Examiners, *Bulletin of Information and Description of National Board Examinations, 1991,* Philadelphia, 1990.

4. Federation of State Medical Boards and National Board of Medical Examiners, *United States Medical Licensing Examination: 1996 Step 1 General Instructions, Content Outline, and Sample Items,* Philadelphia, 1995.

5. Federation of State Medical Boards and National Board of Medical Examiners, *United States Medical Licensing Examination: 1995 Bulletin of Information,* Philadelphia, 1994.

6. "Report on 1996 Examinations," *The National Board Examiner,* Winter 1997, Vol. 44, No. 1, pp. 1–4.

7. FSMB and NBME, *1998 Step 1 General Instructions, Content Description, and Sample Items* (http://www.usmle.org/stp1norm.htm).

8. "Highlights of the 1991 Annual Meeting: Standard Setting System, Score Reporting and Examinee Feedback Plan, USMLE Implementation Plans," *The National Board Examiner,* Spring 1991, Vol. 38, No. 2, pp. 1–6.

9. Swanson, David B., Case, Susan M., Melnick, Donald E., et al., "Impact of the USMLE Step 1 on Teaching and Learning of the Basic Biomedical Sciences," *Academic Medicine,* September Supplement 1992, Vol. 67, No. 9, pp. 553–556.

10. "Report on 1996 Examinations," *op. cit.,* Vol. 44, No. 1, pp. 1–4.

11. National Board of Medical Examiners, *Summary of Examinee Performance,* Philadelphia, 1996.

12. FSMB and NBME, *USMLE: 1993 Step 1 General Instructions, Content Outline, and Sample Items, op. cit.*

13. http://www.nbme.org/usmleex.htm

14. Swanson et al., *op. cit.*

15. Iserson, K., *Getting into Residency,* Tucson, AZ, Galen Press, 1996 (ISBN 1883620104).

16. Case, Susan M., and Swanson, David B., "Validity of NBME Part I and Part II Scores for Selection of Residents in Orthopaedic Surgery, Dermatology, and Preventive Medicine," *Academic Medicine,* February Supplement 1993, Vol. 68, No. 2, pp. S51–S56.

17. FSMB and NBME, *USMLE: 1993 Step 1 General Instructions, Content Outline, and Sample Items, op. cit.*

18. Swanson et al., *op. cit.*

19. "Report on 1995 Examinations," *op. cit.*

20. National Board of Medical Examiners, *United States Medical Licensing Examination: 1993 Application Instructions for Step 1 and Step 2,* Philadelphia, 1992.

21. "Report on 1996 Examinations," *op. cit.*

22. Swanson et al., *op. cit.*

23. O'Donnell, M.J., Obenshain, S. Scott, and Erdmann, James B., "I: Background Essential to the Proper Use of Results of Step 1 and Step 2 of the USMLE," *Academic Medicine,* October 1993, Vol. 68, No. 10, pp. 734–739.

24. Robinson, Adam, *What Smart Students Know,* New York, Crown Publishers, 1993 (ISBN 0517880857).

25. National Board Examinations, "Preliminary Report on June 1988 Part I Performance," *The National Board Examiner,* Fall 1988, Vol. 35, No. 4, p. 3.

26. O'Donnell et al., *op. cit.*

27. http://www.usmle.org/97/irreg.htm

Special Situations

International Medical Graduate (IMG) is the term now used to describe any student or graduate of a non-US or non-Canadian medical school, regardless of whether he or she is a US citizen. The old term "Foreign Medical Graduate" (FMG) was replaced because it was misleading when applied to US citizens attending medical schools outside the United States.

The IMG's Steps to Licensure in the United States

In order to become licensed to practice in the United States, an IMG must go through the following steps (not necessarily in this order). These steps must be completed by all IMGs even if you are already a practicing physician and have completed a residency program in your own country:

■ Complete the basic sciences program of your medical school (equivalent to the first two years of US medical school).

■ Take the USMLE Step 1. You can do this while still in school or after graduating, but your medical school must certify that you have completed the basic science part of your school's curriculum in order to be eligible.

■ Complete the clinical clerkship program of your medical school (equivalent to the third and fourth years of US medical school).

■ Take the USMLE Step 2. If you are still in medical school, you must be certified by your school that you are within one year of graduating to be allowed to take Step 2.

■ Take the Educational Commission for Foreign Medical Graduates (ECFMG) English test (or an equivalent to the Test of English as a Foreign Language recognized by the ECFMG).

■ Graduate with your medical degree.

■ Once you have passed Step 1, Step 2, and the English test, you must obtain an ECFMG certificate; you can get this from ECFMG (see following) after you have sent them a copy of your degree, which they will verify with your medical school. This can take eight weeks or more. The ECFMG certificate is required for you to obtain a position in an accredited residency program; some programs do not allow you to apply unless you already have this certificate.

■ The ECFMG has announced that applicants who have not met all of the requirements for ECFMG certification on or before June 30, 1998 will be required to pass the Clinical Skills Assessment (CSA) exam (see following) in order to obtain an ECFMG certificate.

■ Apply for residency positions in your field of interest, either directly or through the National Residency Matching Program ("the Match"). You do not need to have an ECFMG certificate, to have graduated, or to have passed any USMLE Step or the English test in order to apply for residencies, either directly or through the Match, but you do need to have passed all the examinations necessary for ECFMG certification (i.e., Step 1, Step 2, English test) by a certain deadline (in 1998, this is February 19) in order to be entered into the Match itself. If you have not passed all these exams, you will be automatically withdrawn from the Match.

■ Obtain a visa to allow you to enter and work in the United States if you are not already a US citizen or green card holder (permanent resident).

■ Some states require IMGs to obtain an educational/training/limited medical license that allows them to practice as a resident in the state in which their residency program is located. The residency program may assist you with this application. Note that medical licensing is the prerogative of each individual state, not of the federal government, and that states vary in the exact laws about licensing (although all 50 states recognize the USMLE).

■ Take USMLE Step 3 during your residency, and then obtain a full medical license. Note that as an IMG you will not be able to take Step 3 and obtain an independent license until you have completed one, two, or three years of residency, depending on which state you live in. However, even if you live in a state that requires two or three years of residency in order to take Step 3, you can still take Step 3 and then obtain a license in another state. Once you have a license in any one state you are permitted to practice in federal facilities such as VA hospitals and in Indian Health Service facilities in any state. This can open the door to "moonlighting" opportunities. For details on individual state rules, write to the licensing board in the state in question or contact the FSMB (see following).

■ Complete your residency and then take the appropriate specialty board exams in order to become board certified (e.g., internal medicine, surgery). If you already have a specialty certification in your home country (e.g., in surgery, cardiology), some specialty boards may grant you six months' or one year's credit toward your total residency time.

USMLE Step 1 and the IMG

The USMLE Step 1 is administered by the ECFMG at approximately 78 examination centers in North America and around the world in June and October of each year. USMLE Step 1 is often the first, and for most IMGs the most challenging, hurdle to overcome. The USMLE is a standardized licensing system that gives IMGs a level playing field (it is the same exam series taken by US graduates, even though it is administered by the ECFMG rather than by the NBME). This means that pass marks for IMGs, for both Step 1 and Step 2, are determined by a statistical process that is based on the scores of US medical students in 1991. In general, to pass Step 1, you will probably have to score higher than the bottom 8–10% of US and Canadian graduates in Step 1. However, in 1996, only 55% of ECFMG candidates passed Step 1 on their first attempt, compared with 93% of US and Canadian medical students and graduates.

Developing good test-taking strategy is especially critical for the IMG.

41

Of note, 1994–1995 data showed that USFMGs (US citizens attending non-US medical schools) performed 0.4 SDs lower than FMGs (non-US citizens attending non-US medical schools). Although their overall scores were lower than those of FMGs, USFMGs performed relatively better on behavioral sciences.

A good Step 1 score is key to a strong IMG application.

As an IMG, you must do as well as you can on Step 1 in particular. Probably no one ever feels totally ready to take Step 1, but nearly all IMGs require a period of serious study and preparation to reach their potential. A poor score on Step 1 is a distinct disadvantage when applying for most residencies. Remember that if you pass Step 1, you cannot retake it to try to improve your score. Your goals should be to beat the mean, because you can then confidently assert that you have done better than average for US students. Good Step 1 scores lend credibility to your residency application.

Of interest is the fact that students from non-US medical schools perform worst in behavioral science and biochemistry (1.9 and 1.5 SDs below US students) and comparatively better in gross anatomy and pathology (0.7 and 0.9 SDs below US students). Although they are derived from 1994–1995, these data may be helpful in focusing your studying.

Do commercial review courses help improve your scores? Reports vary, and these courses can be expensive. Many IMGs decide to try the USMLE on their own first and then consider a review course only if they fail. But many states require that you pass within three attempts, so you do not have many chances. (For more information on review courses, see p. 359.)

The Other Exams and the IMG

- **USMLE Step 2.** In the past, this examination had a reputation for being much easier than Step 1, but this no longer seems to be the case for both IMGs and US medical students. In August 1996, 54% of ECFMG candidates passed on their first attempt, compared with 95% of US and Canadian candidates. Because this is a clinical sciences exam, cultural and geographic considerations play a greater role than they do in Step 1. For example, if your medical education gave you a lot of exposure to malaria, brucellosis, and malnutrition, but little to alcohol withdrawal, child abuse, and cholesterol screening, you must do some work to familiarize yourself with topics that are more heavily emphasized in US medicine. Also, you must have a basic understanding of the legal and social aspects of US medicine, because you will be asked questions about communicating with and advising patients.

Native English–speaking IMGs are also required to take the language test.

- **The English language test.** All IMGs must take an English test, irrespective of citizenship (including US-born US citizens) and native language. Although this exam can appear absurd to the native English speaker, it is generally considered to be a fair and appropriate test. It does not involve any use of medical knowledge or medical terminology; in the first part, candidates listen to tape recordings of typical English conversations and are asked simple questions to assess their comprehension. In the second part, written sentences are presented in which candidates are asked to choose an appropriate replacement for a missing word that is both grammatically correct and meaningful. This test is strictly pass–fail; there is no numerical grade. The test is generally not difficult for those who feel comfortable having ordinary and natural conversations with Americans. Having lived in or visited the US is almost always an advantage for the foreign-born IMG seeking US licensure. Tentative test dates are March 4 and August 26, 1998, and March 3 and August 25, 1999.

- **Clinical Skills Assessment (CSA).** Applicants for ECFMG certification will be required to pass the ECFMG **Clinical Skills Assessment,** which incorporates a Test of Spoken English. In addition, applicants must pass the basic medical and clinical science examinations and the ECFMG English test. This additional assessment will require that the examinee demonstrate proficiency on components of clinical skills such as history taking, physical examination, organization and interpretation of clinical data, as well as interpersonal skills and oral English. Applicants will be required to pass the CSA if they have not met all of the requirements for ECFMG certification on or before June 30, 1998, as set forth in the applicable edition of the ECFMG *Information Booklet.*

There is a big difference between textbook learning of a language and actually being immersed in the culture that goes with it.

To be eligible to take the CSA, applicants must be either a **student** officially enrolled in a medical school listed in the current edition of the *World Directory of Medical Schools* published by the World Health Organization and within 12 months of completion of the full didactic curriculum **or** must be a **graduate** of a medical school which was listed in the *World Directory* at the time of graduation. In addition, all applicants for the CSA must have passed the required basic medical and clinical science examinations and the ECFMG English test or Test of English as a Foreign Language (TOEFL) under the current ECFMG policies. Graduates of foreign medical schools who currently hold a Standard ECFMG Certificate or who will meet all of the current requirements for certification by June 30, 1998, will *not* be required to take the CSA but will be eligible to do so. However, such applicants will not be issued a new Standard ECFMG Certificate.

The CSA will be administered throughout the year on a daily basis in a single ECFMG test center in Philadelphia, Pennsylvania. In it, candidates are required to demonstrate their skills in the course of ten half-hour interactions with each of ten standardized "patients," all of whom are specially trained actors. The exam lasts five hours and is conducted over an entire morning or an entire afternoon session. Each "patient" grades each student. The interaction is not watched by any observers, but it will be video-

and audio-taped in case any problems or disputes arise later. You must pass the CSA to enter the residency Match.

The ECFMG CSA will include a number of clinical problems that physicians in programs of graduate medical education in the United States will likely encounter. Specifically, it will consist of clinical encounters with standardized patients during which the examinee will be asked to obtain a focused history, perform a relevant physical examination and communicate initial diagnoses and a management plan to the standardized patients. Following the clinical encounter with each patient, a written exercise will be administered to the examinee in the form of a patient progress note. The standardized patients are individuals who are trained to portray clinical problems that may include positive findings. They are trained to document and evaluate the clinical skills performance of the examinee and other related behaviors such as interpersonal skills.

The ECFMG Clinical Skills Assessment will be implemented beginning July 1, 1998. Additional information will be made available later in 1997.

Passing this exam demonstrates your ability to use English in the practice of clinical medicine with patients. This exam requires that you demonstrate proficiency in English conversation in the context of doctor–patient encounters. Fluency, intelligible pronunciation, and organized history and physical exam skills are likely to be keys to success.

Residencies and the IMG

It is undoubtedly becoming harder for IMGs to obtain residencies in the United States. After about a decade of decreasing discrimination against IMGs on the part of the AMA and residency directors, the tide has turned owing to an increasing concern about an oversupply of physicians in the US. Official bodies such as COGME (the Council on Graduate Medical Education) have thus recommended that the total number of residency slots be reduced from the current 144% of the number of US graduates to 110%. Furthermore, changes introduced in the 1996 immigration law are likely to make it much harder for noncitizens or legal residents of the US to remain in the country after completing a residency.

In the 1997 residency Match, US-citizen IMG applications rose from 735 in 1995 to 1467 in 1997, but the percentage of such IMGs accepted dropped from 49.8% to 43.5%; for non-US-citizen IMGs, applications rose from 5675 in 1995 to 8090 in 1997, while the percentage accepted fell dramatically from 50.5% to 34.5%. These percentages are likely to drop further in the future, especially as some large hospitals which traditionally hire many IMGs (such as those in New York) cut back sharply on their residency slots.

Resources for the IMG

- ECFMG
  3624 Market Street, Fourth Floor
  Philadelphia, PA 19104-2685
  (215) 386-5900 or (202) 293-9320
  Fax: (215) 386-9196

  This number is answered only between 9:00 AM and 12:30 PM, and between 1:30 PM and 5:00 PM Monday through Friday EST. The ECFMG often takes a long time to answer the phone and is often busy at peak times of the year, and there is then a long voice-mail message to listen to, so it is better to write or fax early rather than rely on a last-minute phone call. Do not contact the National Board of Medical Examiners. All IMG exam affairs are conducted by the ECFMG. The ECFMG publishes the *Handbook for Foreign Medical Graduates* and *Information Booklet* on ECFMG certification and the USMLE program; the latter gives details of dates and locations of forthcoming USMLE, CSA, and English tests for IMGs, together with application forms. It is free of charge and is also available from the public affairs offices of US embassies and consulates worldwide, as well as from Overseas Educational Advisory Centers. Single copies of the handbook may also be ordered by calling (215) 386-5900, preferably on weekends or between 6 PM and 6 AM Philadelphia time, or by fax to (215) 387-9963. Requests for multiple copies must be made by fax or mail on organizational letterhead. The full text of the booklet is also available on the ECFMG's website at http://www.ecfmg.org/content.htm#Top.

- Federation of State Medical Boards
  400 Fuller Wiser Road, Suite 300
  Euless, TX 76039-3855
  (817) 868-4000
  Fax: (817) 868-4099

  FSMB publishes Exchange, Section I, which gives detailed information on examination and licensing requirements in all US jurisdictions. The 1996–1997 edition costs $25. (Texas residents must add 7.75% state sales tax.) To obtain publications, write to Federation Publications at the above address. All orders must be prepaid by a personal check drawn on a US bank, a cashier's check, or a money order payable to the Federation. Foreign orders must be accompanied by an international money order or the equivalent, payable in US dollars through a US bank or a US affiliate of a foreign bank. For Step 3 inquiries, the telephone number is (817) 868-4000, and the fax number is (817) 868-4099.

- Some of the Step 1 commercial review courses listed in Section III are conducted outside the United States. Write or call the course providers for details.

- The ECFMG has a home page on http://www.ecfmg.org with the complete ECFMG Information Booklet available online. Late announcements (e.g., dates of mailing out score reports) are also made on this site.

- The FSMB has a home page at http://www.fsmb.org

- The Internet news groups misc.education.medical and bit.listsery.medforum can be valuable forums to exchange information on licensing exams, residency applications, and so on.

- Some immigration information for IMGs is available from the various sites of Siskind, Susser, Haas & Chang, a firm of attorneys specializing in immigration law, on the following websites, which include a searchable index and a free e-mail subscription to immigration law bulletins:
    http://www.telalink.net/~gsiskind/bulletin.html
    http://www.visalaw.com/~gsiskind/95feb/2feb95.html
    http://www.telalink.net/~gsiskind/95feb/2feb95.html
    http://www.americanlaw.com/q&a28.html

- Another source of immigration information can be found on the website of the law offices of Carl Shusterman, a Los Angeles lawyer specializing in medical immigration law:
    http://websites/earthlink.net/~visalaw

- International Medical Placement Ltd., a US company specializing in recruiting foreign physicians to work in the United States, has a site at http://www.cyberdeas.com/imp. This site includes ordering information for several publications by FMSG, Inc., including USMLE Study Guides and residency matching information, and details of USMLE lecture courses offered by the author of these publications, Dr. Stanley Zaslau. It also has information on seminars held by the company in foreign countries for physicians thinking of moving to the United States.

- *The USMLE for International Medical Graduates* by Thornborough (McGraw-Hill, ISBN 0070645639, $22.00) is expected in 1998.

- *The International Medical Graduates' Guide to U.S. Medicine: Negotiating the Maze* by Louise B. Ball (199 pages; ISBN 1-883620-16-3).

Galen Press
PO Box 64400
Tucson, AZ 85728-4400
(800) 442-5369 (United States and Canada)
(520) 577-8363
Fax: (520) 520-6459

Price: $28.95 plus $3.00 shipping and handling, add $2.95 for priority mail (US dollars); Arizona residents add 7% sales tax.

This book has a lot of detailed information, and is particularly strong on the intricacies of immigration law as it applies to foreign citizen IMGs who wish to practice in the United States—although this is a rapidly changing field, and some of this information is probably out of date already. However, much of the book's contents may be irrelevant for any one person, as many chapters are geared toward specific situations (e.g., how to sponsor a relative, how a small American town may try to sponsor a foreign physician, how a US faculty member can sponsor a foreign clinical research fellow), and there is considerable duplication across chapters.

Bottom line: Great for foreign citizens who need help in understanding how to "negotiate the maze" of medical immigration regulations, but not necessarily high yield for many other IMGs.

What Is the COMLEX Level 1?

For years, the National Board of Osteopathic Medicine Examination (NBOME) served as the osteopathic version of the USMLE, with osteopathic students usually taking Parts I and II during medical school training. Then, in 1995, the NBOME introduced a new assessment tool called the Comprehensive Osteopathic Medical Licensing Examination, or COMLEX. Like the NBOME, the COMLEX is administered over three levels. In 1995, only Level 3 was administered, but by 1998 all three levels will be implemented. The COMLEX is now the only exam offered to osteopathic students. One of the goals of this changeover is to get all states to recognize this examination as equivalent to the USMLE, thereby allowing DO students to use it for licensing. Another stated goal of the COMLEX Level 1 is to create a more primary-care-oriented exam that integrates osteopathic principles into clinical situations. In order to take the COMLEX Level 1, you must have satisfactorily completed at least half of your sophomore year in an AOA-approved medical school and have the approval of your dean.

For all three levels of the COMLEX, raw scores are converted to a score ranging from 5 to 995. For Levels 1 and 2, a score of 400 is required to pass; for Level 3, a score of 350 is required. The COMLEX uses the same conversion scales as the USMLE, and scores are usually mailed several weeks after the test date. In 1996, 92% of all first-time test takers passed the June administration of the NBOME Part I. The mean score on the June 1996 exam was 559.

If you pass a COMLEX examination, you are not allowed to retake it to improve your grade. If you fail, there is no specific limit to the number of times you can retake the exam in an effort to pass. However, all examinations must be completed in sequential order within seven years of the successful completion of Level 1. Figure 14 shows the upcoming examination dates for all levels of the COMLEX in 1998.

FIGURE 14. Test Dates for COMLEX in 1998

Level 1	June 2–3
	October 20–21
Level 2	March 24–25
	October 20–21
Level 3	February 17–18
	June 9–10

What Is the Structure of the COMLEX Level 1?

Like the USMLE Step 1, the COMLEX Level 1 is a multiple-choice examination that is given over two days and consists of four booklets, each containing approximately 220 questions. You are given four hours to complete each booklet. In the 1997 exam there were 890 questions in total. Since the number of questions may change, the best way to determine the number of questions you will encounter is to consult the most recent *Examination Guidelines and Sample Exam* (which you should receive when you register for the test).

The COMLEX Level 1 exam consists of one-best-answer questions, clinical vignettes, and matching sets. In the 1997 exam, approximately 75% of the questions were one-best-answer, 20% were clinical vignettes, and 5% were matching sets; there were no negatively phrased best-answer questions, answers such as "all the above" or "none of the above," or K-type questions. Each booklet had a similar breakdown; that is to say, at the end of each test booklet were approximately 9 to 10 clinical vignettes followed by approximately 10 matching questions.

Each clinical vignette in the NBOME Part I had three to six questions related to the clinical case described within the vignette. Generally, the first question asked for a diagnosis of the problem, with the remaining questions emphasizing history and physical presentation, patient management, and basic science principles in a clinical setting. It should be noted that if you misdiagnose the problem in the first question, you may miss many of the questions that follow.

In 1997, color photos were introduced into the examination for the first time. Accompanying each photo was a brief clinical description and then a question asking for the diagnosis of the problem. Although there were only three photos (and three questions) in the 1997 exam, many students believe that there will likely be an increase in clinical photographic material in future exams (this might include x-rays, diagrams, and histopathology). Moreover, given that the COMLEX is intended to become more primary care/clinically oriented, more clinical vignettes may well appear in future exams.

What Is the Difference Between the USMLE and the COMLEX?

Although the NBOME and USMLE exams are similar in scope, content, and emphasis, there are some differences between the two that are worth noting. For example, the COMLEX Level 1 tests osteopathic principles but does not emphasize lab techniques. Both exams often require that you apply and integrate knowledge over several areas of basic science in order to answer a question. However, many students who took both tests in 1997 report that the style of the questions differed somewhat. It was reported, for example, that USMLE questions generally required that the student reason and draw from the information given (often a two-step process), whereas those on the NBOME exam tended to be more straightforward. Furthermore, the questions in the USMLE were on average found to be considerably longer than those of the NBOME; therefore, many students felt they had plenty of time for the NBOME but felt time pressure during the USMLE.

Students also said that the NBOME made greater use of "buzzwords" (e.g., "rose spots" in typhoid fever), whereas the USMLE avoided buzzwords in favor of straight descriptions of clinical findings or symptoms (e.g., rose-colored papules on the abdomen instead of "rose spots"). Finally, the USMLE had many more photographs than did the NBOME, but this difference may narrow in 1998. The overall impression was that the USMLE was a more "thought-provoking" exam, while the COMLEX is expected to be a more "knowledge-based" one.

Who Should Take Both the USMLE and the COMLEX?

Aside from facing the COMLEX Level 1, you must decide if you will also take the USMLE Step 1. We recommend that you consider taking the USMLE in addition to the COMLEX under the following circumstances:

- **If you are applying to allopathic residencies.** Although there is growing acceptance of COMLEX certification on the part of allopathic residencies, some allopathic programs prefer or even require passage of the USMLE Step 1. These include many academic programs, programs in competitive specialties (e.g., osteopathics, ophthalmology, or ER) or programs in competitive geographic areas (such as California). Fourth-year DO students who have already matched can readily tell you which programs and specialties are looking for USMLE scores.

- **If you plan to practice in Louisiana.** The state of Louisiana requires that osteopathic physicians pass the USMLE system to obtain a license for practice. However, this state may have reciprocating agreements with other states that accept the COMLEX. Therefore, it may be possible to be licensed in another state and then petition to have your license transferred.

- **If you are unsure about your postgraduate training plans.** Successful passage of both the COMLEX Level 1 and the USMLE Step 1 is certain to provide you with the greatest range of options when applying for internship and residency training.

Unfortunately, taking both exams can be a trying experience. Students planning to take both exams in June 1998 have to deal with the USMLE Step 1 one week after having taken the COMLEX Level 1. In October, Step 1 and Level 1 examination dates are currently the same. Another option would be to take Level 1 or Step 1 in June and then wait until October to sit for the other exam. The clinical coursework that most DO students receive during the summer of their

third year (as opposed to starting clerkships) is considered helpful in integrating basic science knowledge for the COMLEX or the USMLE.

How Do I Prepare for the COMLEX Level 1?

Students' experience suggests that you should start studying for the COMLEX four to six months before the test date; an early start will allow you to devote up to a month to each subject. The recommendations made in Section I regarding study and testing methods, strategies, and resources, as well as the books suggested in Section III for the USMLE Step 1, hold true for the COMLEX as well.

Many students believe that doing old test questions is a very good way to prepare for the test. SOMA, KCOM (Kansas), and PCOM (Pittsburgh) have each put together a group of old test questions that provide an excellent way to gauge your studying. Many students reported that some questions from past exams appeared on the 1997 NBOME Part I. However, sometimes these old test review books have errors. It is therefore important to look up the information you missed.

Another important source of information can be found in the *Examination Guidelines and Sample Exam.* This booklet discusses the breakdown of each subject while also providing sample questions. However, many students felt that this breakdown provided only a general guideline. For example, a number of students felt that more than 15% of the questions on anatomy (the stated percentage in the booklet) covered neuroanatomy. Also, the sample questions did not provide examples of the clinical vignettes, which made up approximately 25% of the exam. You will receive this publication when you register for the COMLEX Level 1 exam, but you can also receive a copy and additional information by writing:

NBOME
2700 River Road, Suite 607
Des Plaines, IL 60018
(847) 635-9955
website: http://www.nbome.org

In 1997, many students reported an emphasis in certain areas. For example:

- There was an overall emphasis on microbiology and pharmacology.
- High-yield osteopathic manipulative technique (OMT) topics on the 1997 NBOME exam included sacral testing/diagnosis, sympathetic innervation of viscera, spinal motion and diagnosis, and cranial and joint/ligament testing (e.g., McMurray's test).
- Specific topics were repeatedly tested on the exam. These included measles, rubella, neurology, diabetes, acid-base physiology, and testicular cancer.

Since these topics appeared in all four booklets, it was useful for students to review these topics in between the two test days. It is important to understand that the topics emphasized on the 1997 exam may not be stressed on the 1998 exam. However, since certain topics seem to be emphasized each year, it may be to your advantage to review these topics between test days.

The National Board of Podiatric Medical Examiners (NBPME) tests (see Fig. 15 for examination dates) are designed to assess whether a candidate possesses the knowledge required to practice as a minimally competent entry-level podiatrist. In all states that recognize them, the NBPME examinations are used as part of the licensing process governing the practice of podiatric medicine. Individual states use the examination scores differently; therefore, DPM candidates should refer to the information in the *NBPME Bulletin of 1998 Examinations.*

Candidates performing at extreme levels are passed or failed at 90 minutes.

The NBPME Part I is generally taken after the completion of the second year of podiatric medical education. Unlike the USMLE Step 1, there is no behavioral science section. The exam does sample the seven basic science disciplines: general anatomy; lower extremity anatomy; biochemistry; physiology; medical microbiology and immunology; pathology; and pharmacology. Questions covering these content areas are interspersed throughout the test.

Your NBPME Appointment

In early spring, your college registrar will have you fill out an application for the NBPME Part I. After receipt of your application and registration fees, you will be mailed the *NBPME Bulletin of 1998 Examinations.* It gives you a list of Sylvan Learning Centers across the country that are participating in the computer-based testing format. You must find the location nearest you and set up an appointment to take the examination. We suggest that you do this as soon as you receive your *NBPME Bulletin* because the reservation slots fill up quickly, especially in the home cities of the seven podiatric medical schools.

On the day of the exam, arrive at the testing center at least 30 minutes before your scheduled appointment. At that time, you will be registered, escorted to a computer terminal, and given a tutorial to acquaint you with the exam format. At the end of the examination, you will be asked to complete a survey regarding your computer-based testing experience.

Computer-Based Testing

The NBPME Part I is delivered as a Computerized Mastery Test (CMT). The format is multiple choice. Each candidate is administered a base test of 90 ques-

FIGURE 15. 1998 NBPME Examination Dates

Part 1	July 9–10 (Registration Deadline—May 1)
Part 1 (retake)	September 10–11 (Registration Deadline—August 8)

tions. The maximum time permitted for this base test is 90 minutes. Following the base test, candidates performing at extreme levels (high or low) are passed or failed immediately. Candidates with an intermediate level of performance are administered additional testlets (consisting of 15 questions each) permitting them additional opportunity to demonstrate minimal competence. The maximum time allowed for each additional testlet is 15 minutes. You should try your best on each question, marking any questions that you would like to review should time permit. There is no penalty for guessing. No more than 180 questions are administered to a candidate.

Interpreting Your Score

On completion of the NBPME Part I, a pass/fail decision is reported on the computer. You need a scaled score of at least 75 to pass. Eighty-five percent of first-time test takers pass the NBPME Part I. In computing the scaled score, the number of questions vary from candidate to candidate; however, this is taken into consideration along with the number of questions answered correctly. Approximately two weeks after the examination, you will receive your official score report by mail. Passing candidates receive a message of congratulations, but no numerical score is reported. Failing candidates receive a report with one score between 55 and 74 in addition to diagnostic messages intended to help identify strengths or weaknesses in particular content areas. If you fail the NBPME Part I, you must retake the entire examination at a later date. There is no limit to the number of times you can retake the exam.

Preparation for the NBPME Part I

Students suggest that you begin studying for the NBPME Part I at least three months prior to the test date. Each of the colleges of podiatric medicine conducts a series of board reviews. Ask a third-year student which review sessions are most informative. As with the USMLE Step 1, the suggestions made in Section 1 regarding study and testing methods can be applied to the NBPME as well. This book should be used as a supplement and not as the sole source of information.

Know everything about lower extremity anatomy.

Approximately 24% of the NBPME Part I focus is lower extremity anatomy. Students should rely on the notes and material that they received from their class. Remember, lower extremity anatomy is the podiatrist's specialty—everything is important. Do not forget to study osteology. Keep your old tests and look through old lower extremity class exams because each of the podiatric colleges submits questions from its own exams. This gives you a better understanding of the types of questions that may be asked.

As with the USMLE, the NBPME requires that you apply and integrate knowledge over several areas of basic science in order to answer a question. Students report that many questions emphasize clinical presentations; however, the facts in this book are very helpful in recalling the different diseases and organisms. DPM candidates should expand on the high-yield pharmacology section and study antifungal drugs and treatment protocols for *Pseudomonas,* candidiasis, erythrasma, and so on. The high-yield section focusing on pathology is very useful; however, additional emphasis on diabetes mellitus and all its secondary manifestations should not be overlooked. Students should also focus on classic podiatric dermatopathologies, gout, and arthritis.

A sample set of questions is found in the *NBPME Bulletin of 1997 Examinations.* If you do not receive a *NBPME Bulletin* or if you have any questions regarding registration, fees, test centers, authorization forms, and score reports, please contact your college registrar or:

National Board of Podiatric Medical Examiners (NBPME)
PO Box 6516
Princeton, NJ 08541-6516
(609) 951-6335

Best of luck!

The following material is excerpted from the NBME World Wide Web site (http://www.nbme.org/testacco.htm) and is © 1996 by The Federation of State Medical Boards of the United States, Inc., and the National Board of Medical Examiners.®

Requesting Test Accommodations in USMLE for a Disability
How do I request test accommodations for Steps 1 and 2 of USMLE?

It is helpful to obtain a "Guidelines and Questionnaire" booklet. The booklet provides the procedures for requesting accommodations and for documenting your disability and your need for accommodations.

If you are a student or graduate of an LCME- or AOA-accredited medical school in the United States or Canada, you must write to or telephone the National Board of Medical Examiners:

NBME
Office of Test Accommodations
3750 Market Street
Philadelphia, PA 19104-3190
Telephone: (215) 590-9509

If you are a student or graduate of a foreign medical school, you must contact the Educational Commission for Foreign Medical Graduates to obtain this information:

ECFMG
3624 Market Street, 4th Floor
Philadelphia, PA 19104-2685
Telephone: (215) 386-5900

Be specific about your disability and your individual needs.

How can I receive extra time to take the Steps?

Extra time is one of many accommodations that might be necessary for an examinee with a disability. The Americans with Disabilities Act (ADA) requires that individuals with a disability be provided with "equal access" to the testing program. Therefore, the purpose of accommodations is to "cancel" the effect of the disability, not to provide some extra help in passing an examination.

Because the same types of impairments often vary in severity and often restrict different people to different degrees or in different ways, each request is considered individually to determine the effect of the impairment on the life of the individual and whether a particular accommodation is even appropriate for that person.

Where do I send my request for test accommodations if I am taking Step 1 or Step 2 through the NBME?

Be sure to send your request—and all other documentation, questions, or other information concerning test accommodations—only to the following address:

NBME
Office of Test Accommodations
3750 Market Street
Philadelphia, PA 19104-3190

Do **not** enclose your request or other test accommodation material with your NBME Step 1 and 2 application for registration. If you do not receive a confirmation of your request within two weeks, please call the NBME Office of Test Accommodations at (215) 590-9509 to verify that it was received.

If I am requesting an accommodation from the NBME on Step 1 or Step 2, when should I send in my request and documentation?

In order to allow the necessary time to review your request, please submit your request with all testing results and documentation as soon as you know you will be requesting accommodations for an examination. Your request and accompanying documentation must be postmarked no later than the *final application deadline* for the examination. The final application deadline is listed with the NBME registration materials for each examination administration. Requests for test accommodations cannot be processed by the NBME if postmarked after the deadline.

Can my evaluator or my medical school send in my request for test accommodations?

No. A request for accommodations, by law, must be initiated by the individual with a disability. Also, in order to protect your confidentiality, the NBME does not provide information concerning your request to third parties.

How does the NBME determine what is an appropriate accommodation for USMLE?

As part of the documentation, the examinee's evaluator should recommend appropriate accommodations to ease the impact of the impairment on the testing activity. Professional consultants in learning disabilities, attention deficit disorder, and various other psychiatric and physical conditions review the documentation and recommendations of evaluators to help match the type of assistance with the demonstrated need. The NBME consults with the examinee to determine what accommodations have been effectively used in the past.

If I apply for test accommodations on USMLE, does my disability evaluation have to be up to date?

For someone with a continuing history of accommodation, which would likely include high school and college, as well as medical school, current testing is usually not necessary if objective documentation of the past accommodations is provided. However, the impact of the disability may change over time and new testing may be necessary to demonstrate the current level of impairment and resulting need for accommodation. You will be advised if updated testing is needed.

Approximately 75% of the total number of requests for all Steps are approved.

What are some reasons my request for accommodations might not be approved?

■ Insufficient documentation of a need for accommodation. Conditions such as learning disabilities and ADHD are permanent and lifelong. A diagnosis requires an objective history of chronic symptoms from childhood to adulthood as well as evidence of significant impairment currently.

■ Lack of presence of a moderate to severe level of impairment attributable to the disorder.

■ The identified difficulty is not considered to be a disability under the law, i.e., slow reading without evidence of an underlying language processing disorder; language difficulties as a result of English as a second language.

Once my request for accommodations has been approved, do I need to arrange for accommodations the next time I register for a Step?

An examinee with a disability must provide notification of a request each time accommodations are required. For NBME examinees, a letter requesting accommodations must be sent to the Office of Test Accommodations and must be postmarked no later than the *final published deadline* for the test administration. The letter must also state whether there is any change in the accommodations required and, if so, documentation of the needed change must be provided.

Accommodations are **not** automatic, even if they have been approved for previous Step administrations.

The NBME tentatively plans to administer its first computerized exam for the USMLE Step 1 in June 1999. You should therefore be aware that if you are planning on taking the test in 1998 but ultimately delay it or fail, you may end up facing the computerized test unexpectedly. Many of the details have yet to be fully worked out or confirmed. Although the NBME does not anticipate major changes in the content of the exam, the mechanics of taking the USMLE Step 1 will change significantly.

- The exam may possibly be administered over a period of approximately one month at Sylvan Prometric Learning Centers and/or at various medical schools. The computerized exam will most likely be a pass/fail exam for which percentile scores will not be included in the official exam report.

- The exam may include "computer-adaptive sequential testing," a method in which preconstructed test modules are adaptively administered (i.e., with increasing or decreasing difficulty) in a predefined manner.

- The logistics of taking a computerized exam will necessarily require changes in test-taking strategies, since the option of flipping through a test booklet and skimming and returning to difficult questions will not be as practical.

Student Experience from the 1997 Computer-Based Step 1 Field Trial

In 1997, trial testing of the computerized exam was conducted at Sylvan Prometric Learning Centers throughout the country. The following information is based on student experiences with this computerized field test. The extent to which this will reflect the final implementation of the exam is not certain. We expect the NBME to provide additional details in 1998.

- Each cubicle was equipped with a PC terminal and a 14-inch VGA screen with a gray background. Two laminated $8\frac{1}{2}$-by-11-inch dry-erase boards were provided along with dry-erase fine-tip markers and tissues to erase the boards. Several ceiling-mounted cameras monitored each testing room.

- Each three-hour section was divided into three one-hour segments of time. With 60 minutes for 60 questions, an examinee had approximately one minute per question. There was a chance to take a short break between sections.

- A clock in the upper right-hand corner of the screen did not give any warnings during its countdown, so it was the examinee's responsibility to pay attention to the clock near the end of a one-hour section.

- A 30-minute practice tutorial was available before the actual examination for those who wished to familiarize themselves with the program's logistics and format. The tutorial demonstrated how to select answers using the mouse or keyboard. Additionally, it explained how particular questions could be marked and returned to later as well as how a pop-up window containing the table of normal values could be accessed.

- Many students felt that a working knowledge of Microsoft Windows was useful in efficiently navigating the testing interface. Of note here is the fact that an NBME study documented that US medical students have considerably more computer experience than do IMGs.

- When time expired for a given section, a window appeared to notify the examinee that the time was up. If the test taker chose to click "OK" at this point, the program immediately proceeded to the next section. If the test taker paused and waited to click "OK," then he or she could take a short break to stretch and relax. Once time on a 60-minute section had expired, the questions in that section ceased to be available for review.

- Students reported that the window containing normal values was quite cumbersome to use. The default size of the window required too much scrolling and sometimes covered the test question.

- If any question was longer than the field, a scroll bar appeared at the right. Usually, only the questions with images or figures required scrolling. For the most part, the slides and images were easy to visualize and were of reasonable quality.

- In order to advance to the next question, the test taker had to click the "Next>>" button on the toolbar at the bottom of the screen. Although it was possible to skip a question without answering it, the students polled felt that this was not advisable. It is probably better to take your best guess and click "Mark" so that the question can be optionally reviewed later.

- Any question could be viewed at any time by clicking the "Review Answers" icon on the toolbar at the bottom of the screen. From the "Review Answers" screen, it was possible to review skipped items only, marked items only, or both. In each case, the program presented the questions in numerical order, from the first unmarked or unanswered item on. Additionally, it was possible to review any particular question by typing in or clicking on its number.

Summary

- The field-test version of the Step 1 exam was reasonably well suited to linear test takers (i.e., those who answer every question in sequence).

- The field-test version of the Step 1 exam felt awkward and difficult to students who prefer a more flexible style of skimming the exam and skipping and then returning to many questions.

- Familiarity with the Microsoft Windows interface is an asset.

- Familiarity with important normal values is an asset.

Stay tuned for more detailed information from the NBME if you are planning to take Step 1 in 1999.

Database of High-Yield Facts

Anatomy
Behavioral Science
Biochemistry
Microbiology
Pathology
Pharmacology
Physiology

The 1998 edition of *First Aid for the USMLE Step 1* contains a revised and expanded database of basic science material that student authors and faculty have identified as high-yield for boards review. The facts are loosely organized according to the seven traditional basic medical science disciplines (anatomy, behavioral science, biochemistry, microbiology, pathology, pharmacology, and physiology). Each discipline is then divided into smaller subsections of loosely related facts. Individual facts are generally presented in a three-column format, with the **Title** of the fact in the first column, the **Description** of the fact in the second column, and the **Mnemonic** or **Special Note** in the third column.

Some facts do not have a mnemonic and are presented in a two-column format. Others are presented in list or tabular form in order to emphasize key associations. The database structure is useful for reviewing material already learned. This section is not ideal for learning complex or highly conceptual material for the first time. At the end of each basic science section we list supplementary high-yield topics that have appeared on recent exams in order to help focus your additional review.

The Database of High-Yield Facts is not comprehensive. Use it to complement your core study material and not as your primary study source. The facts and notes have been condensed and edited to emphasize the essential material, and as a result each entry is "incomplete." Work with the material, add your own notes and mnemonics, and realize that not all memory techniques work for all students.

We update Section II annually to keep current with new trends in boards content as well as to expand our database of high-yield information. However, we must note that inevitably many other very-high-yield entries and topics are not yet included in our database.

We actively encourage medical students and faculty to submit entries and mnemonics so that we may enhance the database for future students. We also solicit recommendations of alternate tools for study that may be useful in preparing for the examination, such as diagrams, charts, and computer-based tutorials (*see* How to Contribute, page xv).

Disclaimer
The entries in this section reflect student opinions of what is high-yield. Owing to the diverse sources of material, no attempt has been made to trace or reference the origins of entries individually. We have regarded mnemonics as essentially in the public domain. All errors and omissions will be gladly corrected if brought to the attention of the authors, either through the publisher or directly by e-mail.

Anatomy

Several topics fall under this heading, including embryology, gross anatomy, histology, and neuroanatomy. Studying all anatomy topics in great detail is generally a low-yield approach. However, do not ignore anatomy altogether. Review what you have already learned and what you wish you had learned. Do not memorize all the small details. Many questions require two steps. The first step is to identify a structure on anatomic cross-section, electron micrograph, or photomicrograph. The second step may require an understanding of the clinical significance of the structure.

When studying, try to stress clinically important material. For example, be familiar with gross anatomy that is related to specific diseases (e.g., Pancoast's tumor, Horner's syndrome), traumatic injuries (e.g., fractures, sensory and motor nerve deficits), procedures (e.g., lumbar puncture), and common surgeries (e.g., cholecystectomy). There are also many questions on the exam involving x-rays, CT scans, and neuro MRI scans. Many students suggest browsing through a well-illustrated general radiology atlas, pathology atlas, and histology atlas by just reading the captions and looking at the pictures. Focus on learning basic anatomy at key levels in the body (e.g., sagittal brain MRI; axial CT midthorax, abdomen, and pelvis). Basic neuroanatomy (especially pathways, blood supply, and functional anatomy) has good yield. Use this as an opportunity to learn associated neuropathology and neurophysiology. Basic embryology (especially congenital malformations) has good yield and is worth reviewing.

Cell Type
Embryology
Gross Anatomy
Histology
Neuroanatomy
High-Yield Clinical Vignettes
High-Yield Glossy Material
High-Yield Topics

Erythrocyte

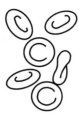

Anucleate, biconcave → large surface area: volume ratio → easy gas exchange (O_2 and CO_2). Source of energy = glucose (90% anaerobically degraded to lactate, 10% by HMP shunt). Survival time = 120 days. Membrane contains the chloride-bicarbonate antiport important in the "physiologic chloride shift," which allows the RBC to transport CO_2 from the periphery to the lungs for elimination.

Eryth = red; *cyte* = cell.
Erythrocytosis = polycythemia = increased number of red cells
Anisocytosis = varying sizes
Poikilocytosis = varying shapes
Reticulocyte = baby erythrocyte

Leukocyte

Types: granulocytes (basophils, eosinophils, neutrophils) and mononuclear cells (lymphocytes, monocytes). Responsible for defense against infections. Normally 4,000–10,000 per microliter.

Leuk = white; *cyte* = cell.

Basophil

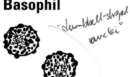

dumbbell-shaped nuclei

Mediates allergic reaction. <1% of all leukocytes. Bilobate nucleus. Densely basophilic granules containing heparin (anticoagulant), histamine (vasodilator) and other vasoactive amines, and SRS-A (slow-reacting substance of anaphylaxis).

Basophilic = staining readily with *basic* stains.

Mast cell

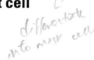

differentiate into mast cell.

Mediates allergic reaction. Degranulation = release of histamine, heparin, and eosinophil chemotactic factors. Can bind IgE to membrane. Mast cells resemble basophils structurally and functionally but are not the same cell type.

Masten = fatten.
Involved in Type I hypersensitivity reactions. Cromolyn sodium prevents mast cell degranulation.

Eosinophil

May be multilobed

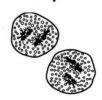

1%–6% of all leukocytes. Bilobate nucleus. Packed with large eosinophilic granules of uniform size. Defends against helminthic and protozoan infections. Highly phagocytic for antigen–antibody complexes.

Eosin = a dye; *philic* = loving.
NAACP:
   N = **N**eoplastic
   A = **A**sthma
   A = **A**llergic processes
   C = **C**ollagen vascular diseases
   P = **P**arasites

Neutrophil

Acute inflammatory response cell. 40%–75% WBCs. Phagocytic. Multilobed nucleus. Large, spherical, azurophilic 1° granules (called lysosomes) contain hydrolytic enzymes, lysozyme, myeloperoxidase.

Hypersegmented polys are seen in vit. B_{12}/folate deficiency.

Monocyte	2%–10% of leukocytes. Large. Kidney-shaped nucleus. Extensive "frosted glass" cytoplasm. Differentiates into macrophages in tissues.	*Mono* = one; single; *cyte* = cell
Lymphocyte	Small. Round, densely staining nucleus. Small amount of pale cytoplasm. B lymphocytes produce antibodies. T lymphocytes manifest the cellular immune response as well as regulate B lymphocytes and macrophages.	
B lymphocyte	Part of humoral immune response. Arises from stem cells in bone marrow. Matures in marrow. Migrates to peripheral lymphoid tissue (follicles of lymph nodes, white pulp of spleen, unencapsulated lymphoid tissue). When antigen is encountered, B cells differentiate into plasma cells and produce antibodies. Has memory. Can function as antigen-presenting cell (APC).	**B** = **B**one marrow or **B**ursa of Fabricius (in birds).
Plasma cells	Off-center nucleus, clock-face chromatin distribution, abundant RER and well-developed Golgi apparatus. B cells differentiate into plasma cells, which can produce large amounts of antibody specific to a particular antigen.	Multiple myeloma is a plasma cell neoplasm.
T lymphocyte	Mediates cellular immune response. Originates from stem cells in the bone marrow, but matures in the thymus. T cells differentiate into cytotoxic T cells (MHC I, CD8), helper T cells (MHC II, CD4), suppressor T cells, delayed hypersensitivity T cells.	**T** is for **T**hymus. **CD** is for **C**luster of **D**ifferentiation. **MHC** × **CD** = **8** (e.g., 2 × 4 = 8).
Macrophage	Phagocytizes bacteria, cell debris, and senescent red cells and scavenges damaged cells and tissues. Long life in tissues. Macrophages differentiate from circulating blood monocytes. Activated by γ-IFN. Can function as APC.	*Macro* = large; *phage* = eater.
Airway cells	Ciliated cells extend to the respiratory bronchioles; goblet cells extend only to the terminal bronchioles. Type I cells (97% of alveolar surfaces) line the alveoli. Type II cells (3%) secrete pulmonary surfactant (dipalmitoylphosphatidylcholine), which lowers the alveolar surface tension.	All the mucus secreted can be swept orally (ciliated cells run deeper). A lecithin:sphingomyelin ratio of > 1.5 in amniotic fluid is indicative of fetal lung maturity.

Juxtaglomerular apparatus (JGA)

JGA = JG cells (modified smooth muscle of afferent arteriole) and macula densa (Na^+ sensor, part of the distal convoluted tubule). JG cells secrete renin (leading to ↑ angiotensin II and aldosterone levels) in response to ↓ renal blood pressure, ↓ Na^+ delivery to distal tubule, and ↑ sympathetic tone. JG cells also secrete erythropoietin.

JGA defends glomerular filtration rate via the renin-angiotensin system.

Juxta = close by.

Microglia

migrate to brain from reticular monocyte system

CNS phagocytes. Mesodermal origin. Not readily discernible in Nissl stains. Have small irregular nuclei and relatively little cytoplasm. In response to tissue damage, transform into large ameboid phagocytic cells.

HIV-infected microglia fuse to form multinucleated giant cells in the CNS.

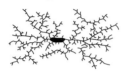

Oligodendroglia

Function to myelinate multiple CNS axons. In Nissl stains, they appear as small nuclei with dark chromatin and little cytoplasm. Predominant type of glial cell in white matter.

These cells are destroyed in multiple sclerosis.

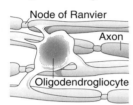

Node of Ranvier

Axon

Oligodendrogliocyte

Schwann cells

Function to myelinate PNS axons. Unlike oligodendroglia, many Schwann cells myelinate a single PNS axon. Schwann cells promote axonal regeneration.

single internodal segment

Acoustic neuroma is an example of a schwannoma.

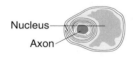

Nucleus

Axon

Cones

For bright, acute vision (color, concentrated in fovea). Comprise inner and outer segments connected by 9 + 0 modified cilium; outer segment disks continuous with plasma membrane. Contain iodopsin pigment, red-green-blue specific.

Cones are for **C**olor, and their outer segments are **C**ontinuous (with the plasma membrane, unlike rods).
Cones have a sharp tip (acuity).

Outer segment (photosensitive region, generation of receptor potential) — Sacs

Cilium

Inner segment (metabolic region) — Mitochondria

Plasma membrane

Synaptic terminal (synapses with bipolar cells)

Incident light from lens

Rods

For night vision (no color; many more than cones; none in the fovea). Comprise inner and outer segments connected by 9 + 0 modified cilium; outer segment disks not continuous with plasma membrane. Rods contain rhodopsin pigment.

Rods have **Rhod**opsin.
Rods have high sensitivity due to multiple rods synapsing on one bipolar cell (convergence).

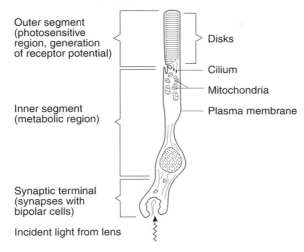

Outer segment (photosensitive region, generation of receptor potential) — Disks
— Cilium
— Mitochondria
Inner segment (metabolic region) — Plasma membrane
Synaptic terminal (synapses with bipolar cells)
Incident light from lens

ANATOMY—EMBRYOLOGY

Umbilical cord
Wharton's Jelly

Contains 2 umbilical arteries, which return deoxygenated blood from the fetus, and 1 umbilical vein, which supplies oxygenated blood from the placenta to the fetus.

Divascular
Single umbilical artery is associated with congenital and chromosomal anomalies.

Embryologic derivatives

Ectoderm	Epidermis (including hair, nails), nervous system (CNS and neural crest derivatives), pituitary.
Mesoderm	Connective tissue, muscle, bone, cardiovascular structures, lymphatics, blood, urogenital structures, and serous linings of body cavities (e.g., peritoneal), spleen, adrenal cortex.
Endoderm	Gut tube epithelium and derivatives (e.g., lungs, liver, pancreas, thymus, thyroid, parathyroid).
Notochord	Induces ectoderm to form neuroectoderm (neural plate). Its postnatal derivative is the nucleus pulposus of the intervertebral disc.

Rathke's pouch is ectoderm

Neural crest derivatives

ANS, dorsal root ganglia, melanocytes, chromaffin cells of adrenal medulla, enterochromaffin cells, pia, celiac ganglion, Schwann cells, odontoblasts, parafollicular cells (of thyroid).

Dura is of mesodermal origin.

Early development
Rule of 2s for 2nd week

2 germ layers (bilaminar disc): epiblast, hypoblast.
2 cavities: amniotic cavity, yolk sac.
2 components to placenta: cytotrophoblast, syncytiotrophoblast.

Rule of 3s for 3rd week

3 germ layers (gastrula): ectoderm, mesoderm, endoderm.

The epiblast (precursor to ectoderm) invaginates to form primitive streak. Cells from the primitive streak give rise to both intraembryonic mesoderm and endoderm.

Aortic arch derivatives

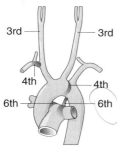

3rd — 3rd

4th — 4th

6th — 6th

1st = part of **max**illary artery.

2nd = stapedial artery and hyoid artery.

3rd = common **C**arotid artery and proximal part of internal carotid artery.

4th = on left, aortic arch; on right, proximal part of right subclavian artery.

6th = proximal part of pulmonary arteries and (on left only) ductus arteriosus.

shows right on diagram

1st arch is **max**imal.

C is 3rd letter of alphabet.

4th arch (4 limbs) = systemic.

6th arch = pulmonary and the pulmonary to systemic shunt (ductus arteriosus).

Fetal erythropoiesis

Fetal erythropoiesis occurs in:
1. **Y**olk sac (3–8 wk)
2. **L**iver (6–30 wk)
3. **S**pleen (9–28 wk)
4. **B**one marrow (28 wk onward)

Young **L**iver **S**ynthesizes **B**lood.

Fetal-postnatal derivatives

1. Umbilical vein—ligamentum teres hepatis
2. Umbilical arteries—medial umbilical ligaments
3. Ductus arteriosus—ligamentum arteriosum
4. Ductus venosus—ligamentum venosum
5. Foramen ovale—fossa ovalis
6. Allantois—urachus—median umbilical ligament
7. Notochord—nucleus pulposus

Urachal cyst or sinus is a remnant of the allantois (urine drainage from bladder).

Branchial apparatus

Branchial clefts are derived from ectoderm.

Branchial arches are derived from mesoderm and neural crests.

Branchial pouches are derived from endoderm.

CAP covers outside from inside (**C**lefts = ectoderm, **A**rches = mesoderm, **P**ouches = endoderm)

Branchial arch 1 derivatives

Meckel's cartilage: mandible, malleus, incus, sphenomandibular ligament.

Muscles: muscles of mastication (temporalis, masseter, lateral and medial pterygoids), mylohyoid, anterior belly of digastric, tensor tympani, tensor veli palatini.

Nerve: CN V$_3$

tensors are CN V.

Branchial arch 2 derivatives

Reichert's cartilage: stapes, styloid process, lesser horn of hyoid, stylohyoid ligament.

Muscles: muscles of facial expression: stapedius, stylohyoid, posterior belly of digastric.

Nerve: CN VII

Branchial arch 3 derivatives

Cartilage: greater horn of hyoid.

Muscles: stylopharyngeus.

Nerve: CN IX

Think of pharynx: stylo**pharyngeus** innervated by glosso**pharyngeal** nerve.

Branchial arches 4 to 6 derivatives	Cartilages: thyroid, cricoid, arytenoids, corniculate, cuneiform. Muscles (4th arch): most pharyngeal constrictors, cricothyroid, levator veli palatini. Muscles (6th arch): intrinsic muscles of larynx. Nerve: 4th arch—X 6th arch—X (recurrent laryngeal branch)	Arch 5 makes no major developmental contributions.
Branchial arch innervation	Arch 1 derivatives supplied by CN V_2 and V_3. Arch 2 derivatives supplied by CN VII. Arch 3 derivatives supplied by CN IX. Arch 4 derivatives supplied by CN X.	
Branchial cleft derivatives	1st cleft develops into external auditory meatus. 2nd through 4th clefts form temporary cervical sinuses, which are obliterated by proliferation of 2nd arch mesenchyme.	Persistent cervical sinus can lead to a branchial cyst in the neck. *laterally located*

Ear development	**Bones**	**Muscles**	**Miscellaneous**
	Incus/malleus—1st arch	Tensor tympani (V_3)—1st arch	External auditory meatus—1st cleft
	Stapes—2nd arch	Stapedius (VII)—2nd arch	Eardrum, eustachian tube—1st pouch

Pharyngeal pouch derivatives	1st pouch develops into middle ear cavity, eustachian tube, mastoid air cells. 2nd pouch develops into epithelial lining of palatine tonsil. 3rd pouch (dorsal wings) develops into inferior parathyroids. 3rd pouch (ventral wings) develops into thymus. 4th pouch develops into superior parathyroids. 5th pouch houses the ultimobranchial bodies, which become the C cells of the thyroid. *NC cells.* *parafollicular*	1st pouch contributes to endoderm-lined structures of ear. 3rd pouch contributes to 3 structures (thymus, L and R inferior parathyroids). Ultimobranchial bodies arise from neural crest cells but migrate into 5th pouch.
Thymus	Site of T-cell maturation. Encapsulated. From epithelium of 3rd branchial pouches. Lymphocytes of mesenchymal origin. Cortex is dense with immature T cells; medulla is pale with mature T cells and epithelial reticular cells. Positive and negative selection occurs at the corticomedullary junction.	Think of the **T**hymus as "finishing school" for **T** cells. They arrive immature and "dense" in the cortex; they are mature in the medulla.
Thyroid development	Thyroid diverticulum arises from floor of primitive pharynx, descends into neck. Connected to tongue by thyroglossal duct, which normally disappears but may persist as pyramidal lobe of thyroid. Foramen cecum is normal remnant of thyroglossal duct.	

Tongue development

1st branchial arch forms anterior ⅔ (thus pain via CN V₃, taste via CN VII). *chorda tympani*

3rd and 4th arches form posterior ⅓ (thus pain and taste mainly via CN IX, extreme posterior via CN X).

Motor innervation is via CN XII.

Taste is CN VII, IX, X; pain is CN V₃, IX, X.

Motor is CN XII.

Cleft lip and cleft palate

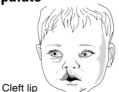

Cleft lip—failure of fusion of the maxillary and medial nasal processes.

Cleft palate—failure of fusion of the lateral palatine processes with each other, the nasal septum, and/or the median palatine process.

Cleft lip

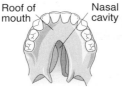

Roof of mouth   Nasal cavity

Cleft palate (partial)

Diaphragm embryology

Diaphragm is derived from:
1. **S**eptum transversum   *central tendon*
2. **P**leuroperitoneal folds
3. **B**ody wall   *foramen of Bochdalek*
4. **D**orsal mesentery of esophagus   *periphial?*

Several **P**arts **B**uild **D**iaphragm.

Abdominal contents may herniate into the thorax due to incomplete development.

Heart embryology

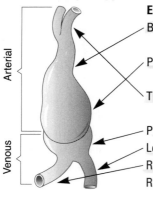

Arterial

Venous

Embryonic structure	Gives rise to
Bulbus cordis	Right ventricle and aortic outflow tract
Primitive ventricle	Left ventricle, except for the aortic outflow tract
Truncus arteriosus *great arteries*	Ascending aorta and pulmonary trunk
Primitive atria	Auricular appendages
Left horn of sinus venosus	Coronary sinus
Right horn of sinus venosus	Smooth part of the right atrium
Right common cardinal vein and right anterior cardinal vein *C.V. → VC*	Superior vena cava

Cyst/sinus/fistula/atresia

Cyst is a spherical epithelium-lined cavity.

Pseudocyst is a spherical cavity without epithelial lining.

Sinus is a blind-ending duct or space opening externally or internally.

Fistula is a patent (abnormal) canal with openings at both ends.

Atresia is a closure of a normal body opening or tubular organ.

Meckel's diverticulum

Meckel's diverticulum

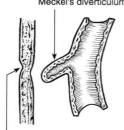

Umbilicus

Persistence of the vitelline duct or yolk stalk. May contain ectopic acid–secreting gastric mucosa and/or pancreatic tissue. Most common congenital anomaly of the GI tract. Can cause bleeding or obstruction near the terminal ileum. Contrast with omphalomesenteric cyst = cystic dilatation of vitelline duct.

The five **2**s:
- **2** inches long.
- **2** feet from the ileocecal valve.
- **2**% of population.
- Commonly presents in first **2** years of life.
- May have **2** types of epithelia.

Pancreas embryology	Pancreas is derived from the foregut. Ventral pancreatic bud becomes pancreatic head, uncinate process (lower half of head), and main pancreatic duct. Dorsal pancreatic bud becomes body, tail, isthmus, and accessory pancreatic duct.	Associate "**vent**-ral" with main duct (a **vent** is a type of duct). Everything else comes from dorsal bud. Annular pancreas, a rare malformation, can cause duodenal obstruction.

put head + un... (handwritten margin note)

Genital ducts

Mesonephric (wolffian) duct	Develops into **S**eminal vesicles, **E**pididymis, **E**jaculatory duct, and **D**uctus deferens.	**SEED**
Paramesonephric (müllerian) duct	Develops into fallopian tube, uterus, and part of vagina. Bicornuate uterus results from incomplete fusion of the paramesonephric ducts. Müllerian inhibiting substance secreted by testes suppresses development of paramesonephric ducts in males.	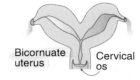 Bicornuate uterus Cervical os

Male/female genital homologues

Corpus spongiosum ≈ vestibular bulbs.
Bulbourethral glands (of Cowper) ≈ greater vestibular glands (of Bartholin).
Prostate gland ≈ urethral and paraurethral glands (of Skene).
Glans penis ≈ glans clitoris.
Ventral shaft of the penis ≈ labia minora.
Scrotum ≈ labia majora.

Congenital penile abnormalities

Hypospadias	Abnormal opening of penile urethra on inferior (ventral) side of penis due to failure of urethral folds to close.	Exstrophy of the bladder is associated with epispadias.
Epispadias	Abnormal opening of penile urethra on superior (dorsal) side of penis due to faulty positioning of genital tubercle.	

Sperm development

Spermatogenesis: spermatogonia → 1° spermatocyte → 2° spermatocyte → spermatid → (spermiogenesis) → spermatozoa. Full development takes 2 months. Spermatogenesis in seminiferous tubules.

Derivation of sperm parts

Acrosome is derived from the Golgi apparatus and flagellum (tail) from one of the centrioles. Middle piece (neck) has mitochondria.

Meiosis and ovulation

1° oocytes begin meiosis I during fetal life and complete meiosis I just prior to ovulation. Meiosis I is arrested in prophase for years until ovulation. Meiosis II is arrested in metaphase until fertilization.

Amniotic fluid abnormalities

Polyhydramnios	> 1.5–2 L of amniotic fluid; associated with esophageal/duodenal atresia, anencephaly.
Oligohydramnios	< 0.5 L of amniotic fluid; associated with bilateral renal agenesis or posterior urethral valves (in males).

~1 L of amniotic fluid is nl. (handwritten note)

Potter's syndrome Bilateral renal agenesis → oligohydramnios → limb deformities, facial deformities, pulmonary hypoplasia.

ANATOMY—GROSS ANATOMY

Erb-Duchenne palsy Traction or tear of the superior trunk of the brachial plexus (C5 and C6 roots); follows fall to shoulder or trauma during delivery.
Findings: Limb hangs by side (paralysis of abductors), medially rotated (paralysis of lateral rotators), forearm is pronated (loss of biceps).

"Waiter's tip" owing to appearance of arm.

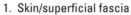

Lumbar puncture

Cauda equina   Spinous process
L3
L4
L4/5 disk
L5
Needle in subarachnoid space

CSF obtained from lumbar subarachnoid space between L4 and L5 (at the level of iliac crests). Structures pierced as follows:
1. Skin/superficial fascia
2. Ligaments (supraspinous, interspinous, ligamentum flavum)
3. Epidural space
4. Dura mater
5. Subdural space
6. Arachnoid
7. Subarachnoid space—CSF

Pia is not pierced.

Nerve injury

	Deficit in motion	Deficit in sensation
Radial	Loss of triceps brachii (triceps reflex), brachioradialis (brachioradialis reflex), and extensor carpi radialis longus (→ wrist drop); often 2° to humerus fracture	Posterior brachial cutaneous Posterior antebrachial cutaneous
Median	No loss of power in any of the arm muscles; loss of forearm pronation, wrist flexion, finger flexion, and several thumb movements; eventually, thenar atrophy	Loss of sensation over the lateral palm and thumb and the radial 2½ fingers
Ulnar	Impaired wrist flexion and adduction, and impaired adduction of thumb and the ulnar 2 fingers	Loss of sensation over the medial palm and ulnar 1½ fingers
Axillary	Loss of deltoid action (shoulder dislocation)	
Musculocutaneous	Loss of function of coracobrachialis, biceps, and brachialis muscles (biceps reflex)	
Common peroneal	Loss of dorsiflexion (→ foot drop)	**PED** = **P**eroneal **E**verts and **D**orsiflexes
Tibial	Loss of plantar flexion	**TIP** = **T**ibial **I**nverts and **P**lantarflexes; if injured, can't stand on **TIP**toes
Femoral	Loss of knee jerk	
Obturator	Loss of hip adduction	

Recurrent laryngeal nerve	Supplies all intrinsic muscles of the larynx except the cricothyroid muscle. Left recurrent laryngeal nerve wraps around the arch of the aorta and the ligamentum arteriosum. Right recurrent laryngeal nerve wraps around right subclavian artery. Damage results in hoarseness. Complication of thyroid surgery.	
Scalp and meninges: layers 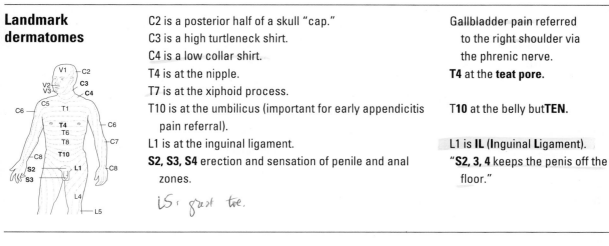	**S**kin, **C**onnective tissue, **A**poneurosis, **L**oose connective tissue, **P**ericranium; skull. **D**ura mater, subdural (SD) space, **A**rachnoid, subarachnoid (SA) space, **P**ia mater, brain.	**SCALP**–skull–**D**s**A**s**P** (PAD spelled backwards). Also, *mater* = mother (protector) of the brain, *pia* = tender, *dura* = strong (durable). Loose connective tissue is vascular.
Spinal cord lower extent	In adults, spinal cord extends to lower border of L1–L2; subarachnoid space extends to lower border of S2. Lumbar puncture is usually performed in L3–L4 or L4–L5 interspaces, at level of cauda equina.	To keep the cord alive, keep the spinal needle between L3 and L5.
Spinal nerves	There are 31 spinal nerves altogether: 8 cervical, 12 thoracic, 5 lumbar, 5 sacral, 1 coccygeal.	31, just like 31 flavors!
Trigeminal ganglion	Also called semilunar ganglion or gasserian ganglion. Located in the trigeminal cave (of Meckel). Trigeminal neuralgia = tic douloureux.	Trigeminal neuralgia can be treated with carbamazepine or surgical decompression.
Landmark dermatomes	C2 is a posterior half of a skull "cap." C3 is a high turtleneck shirt. C4 is a low collar shirt. T4 is at the nipple. T7 is at the xiphoid process. T10 is at the umbilicus (important for early appendicitis pain referral). L1 is at the inguinal ligament. **S2, S3, S4** erection and sensation of penile and anal zones.	Gallbladder pain referred to the right shoulder via the phrenic nerve. **T4** at the **teat pore.** **T10** at the belly but**TEN.** **L1 is IL (Inguinal Ligament).** "**S2, 3, 4** keeps the penis off the floor."

L5 great toe.

Eight layers of abdominal wall/ spermatic cord	1. Skin 2. Fascia: Camper's (fatty) → dartos muscle Scarpa's: → dartos fascia 3. External oblique → external spermatic fascia and superficial inguinal ring 4. Internal oblique → cremaster muscle and conjoint tendon 5. Transversus abdominis → no contribution except to conjoint tendon 6. Transversalis fascia → internal spermatic fascia and deep inguinal ring 7. Extraperitoneal fat 8. Peritoneum → tunica vaginalis testis and processus vaginalis	Scarpa's fascia is continuous with Colles' fascia of perineum. *allows extravasated urine into abd. wall*

Inguinal hernias

Direct hernia	Protrudes through the inguinal (Hesselbach's) triangle (bounded by inguinal ligament, inferior epigastric artery, and lateral border of rectus abdominis). Direct hernia bulges directly through abdominal wall medial to inferior epigastric artery. Goes through the superficial inguinal ring only. Usually in older men.
Indirect hernia	Indirect hernia goes through deep inguinal ring and superficial inguinal ring and into scrotum. Due to failure of closure of processus vaginalis. Indirect hernia enters deep inguinal ring lateral to inferior epigastric artery. Usually in young boys.

Mastication muscles	Three muscles close jaw: masseter, temporalis, medial pterygoid. One opens: lateral pterygoid. All are innervated by the trigeminal nerve (V_3).	**L**ateral **L**owers (when speaking of pterygoids with respect to jaw motion).
Muscles with *glossus*	All muscles with root *glossus* in their names (except palatoglossus, innervated by vagus nerve) are innervated by hypo*glossal* nerve.	Palat: vagus nerve. *Glossus*: hypo*glossal* nerve.
Muscles with *palat* *Tensor: CN V* *tensor veli palatini* *knot tympani*	All muscles with root *palat* in their names (except tensor veli palatini, innervated by mandibular branch of CN V) are innervated by vagus nerve.	Palat: vagus nerve (except tensor, who was too tense).
Rotator cuff muscles	Shoulder muscles that form the rotator cuff: **S**upraspinatus, **I**nfraspinatus, **t**eres minor, **S**ubscapularis	**S I t S** (small t is for teres minor).

Acromion **S**upraspinatus
Coracoid
Infra-spinatus
Biceps tendon
Teres minor
Sub-scapularis

Posterior   **Anterior**

Thenar-hypothenar muscles	Thenar: **O**pponens pollicis, **A**bductor pollicis brevis, **F**lexor pollicis brevis. Hypothenar: **O**pponens digiti minimi, **A**bductor digiti minimi, **F**lexor digiti minimi.	Both groups perform the same functions: **O**ppose, **A**bduct, and **F**lex **(OAF)**.

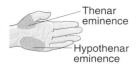

Thenar eminence

Hypothenar eminence

Unhappy triad/knee injury	This common football injury (caused by clipping from the lateral side) consists of damage to medial collateral ligament (MCL), medial meniscus, and anterior cruciate ligament (ACL). PCL = posterior cruciate ligament. LCL = lateral collateral ligament.	Positive anterior drawer sign indicates tearing of the anterior cruciate ligament.

Lateral condyle
Medial condyle
ACL
PCL
LCL
MCL
Lateral meniscus
Medial meniscus

Ligaments of the uterus	Pubocervical ligament, transverse cervical (cardinal) ligament, sacrocervical ligament, round ligament of uterus, round ligament of ovary. Round ligament of uterus is homologous (but not analogous) to gubernaculum testis: runs from labia majora to uterus. Round ligament of ovary runs from uterus to ovary. Broad ligament contains the round ligaments of the uterus, the uterine tubes, the round ligament of the ovary, the epoöphoron, and multiple lymphatic vessels and nerve fibers.	

Round ligament of uterus
Suspensory ligament of ovary
Uterine tube
Ovary
Fimbria
Posterior surface of uterus
Broad ligament
Uterosacral ligament

Carotid sheath	Three structures inside: 1. Internal jugular **V**ein (lateral) 2. Common carotid **A**rtery (medial) 3. Vagus **N**erve (posterior) CN XI *temporarily*	**VAN**

Femoral sheath	Femoral sheath contains femoral artery, femoral vein, and femoral canal (containing deep inguinal lymph nodes). Femoral nerve lies outside femoral sheath.	Lateral to medial: **N-(AVEL) = Nerve–(A**rtery–**V**ein–**E**mpty space–**L**ymphatics).

Diaphragm structures	Structures perforating diaphragm: At T**8**: IVC At T**10**: esophagus, vagus (two trunks) At T**12**: aorta (red), thoracic duct (white), azygous vein (blue) Diaphragm is innervated by **C3, 4,** and **5**. Pain from the diaphragm can be referred to the shoulder. *same dermatome.*	1-2-3 (number of major items): **8** (IVC), **10** (esophagus, vagus), **12** (red-white-blue). "**C3, 4, 5** keeps the diaphragm alive."

Coronary artery anatomy

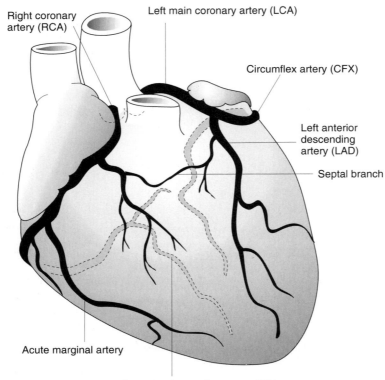

Right coronary artery (RCA)

Left main coronary artery (LCA)

Circumflex artery (CFX)

Left anterior descending artery (LAD)

Septal branch

Acute marginal artery

Posterior descending artery (PD)

In the majority of cases, the SA and AV nodes are supplied by the RCA. Eighty percent of the time, the RCA supplies the inferior portion of the left ventricle via the PD artery (= Ⓡ dominant).

Portal-systemic anastomoses

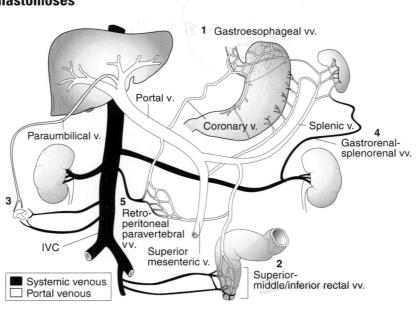

1 Gastroesophageal vv.

Portal v.

Paraumbilical v.

Coronary v.

Splenic v.

4 Gastrorenal-splenorenal vv.

3

5 Retro-peritoneal paravertebral vv.

IVC

Superior mesenteric v.

2 Superior-middle/inferior rectal vv.

■ Systemic venous
□ Portal venous

1. Left gastric-azygous → *esophageal* varices.
2. Superior-middle/inferior rectal → *hemorrhoids.*
3. Paraumbilical-inferior epigastric → *caput* medusae (navel).
4. Retroperitoneal → renal.
5. Retroperitoneal → paravertebral.

Gut, butt, and caput, the anastomoses 3. Commonly seen in alcoholic cirrhosis.

Bronchopulmonary segments	Each bronchopulmonary segment has a 3° (segmental) bronchus and two arteries (bronchial and pulmonary) in the center; veins and lymphatics drain along the borders.	**A**rteries run with **A**irways.
Lung relations	Right lung has three lobes, left has two lobes and lingula (homologue of right middle lobe). Right lung more common site for inhaled foreign body owing to less acute angle of right main stem bronchus.	Left lung is missing a lobe owing to space occupied by heart. The relation of the pulmonary artery to the bronchus at each lung hilus is described by **RALS**—**R**ight **A**nterior; **L**eft **S**uperior *epibronchial artery*

Retroperitoneal structures

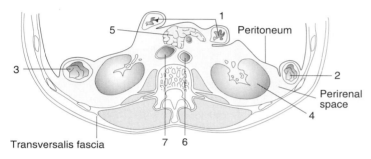

Peritoneum

Perirenal space

Transversalis fascia

1—Duodenum (2nd, 3rd, 4th parts)
2—Ascending colon
3—Descending colon
4—Kidney and ureters
5—Pancreas
6—Aorta
7—Inferior vena cava
8—Adrenal glands
9—Rectum

Digestive tract anatomy

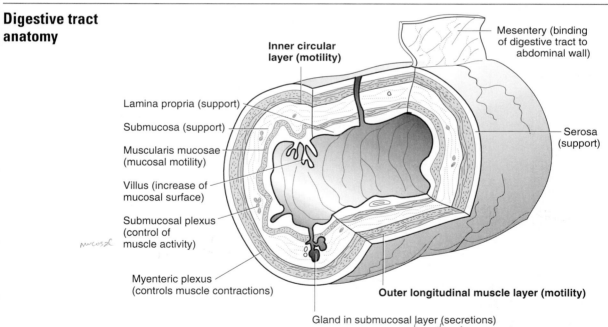

Inner circular layer (motility)

Mesentery (binding of digestive tract to abdominal wall)

Lamina propria (support)

Submucosa (support)

Muscularis mucosae (mucosal motility)

Villus (increase of mucosal surface)

Submucosal plexus (control of muscle activity)

mucosal

Myenteric plexus (controls muscle contractions)

Serosa (support)

Outer longitudinal muscle layer (motility)

Gland in submucosal layer (secretions)
duodenum only

Pectinate line

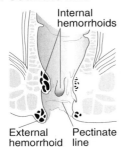

Internal hemorrhoids

External hemorrhoid   Pectinate line

Above pectinate line: Internal hemorrhoids (not painful), adenocarcinoma, visceral innervation, blood supply, and lymphatic drainage.

Below pectinate line: External hemorrhoids (painful), squamous cell carcinoma, somatic innervation, blood supply, and lymphatic drainage.

Internal hemorrhoids receive visceral innervation. External hemorrhoids receive somatic innervation and are therefore painful.

Autonomic innervation of the male sexual response

Erection is mediated by the **P**arasympathetic nervous system.

Emission is mediated by the **S**ympathetic nervous system.

Ejaculation is mediated by visceral and somatic nerves.

Point and **S**hoot.

Kidney anatomy and glomerular structure

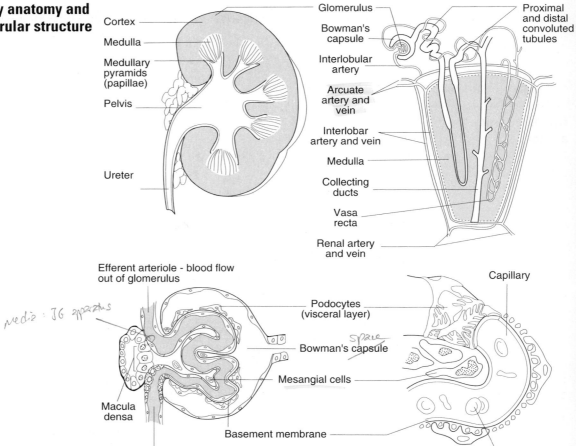

Cortex

Medulla

Medullary pyramids (papillae)

Pelvis

Ureter

Glomerulus

Bowman's capsule

Interlobular artery

Arcuate artery and vein

Interlobar artery and vein

Medulla

Collecting ducts

Vasa recta

Renal artery and vein

Proximal and distal convoluted tubules

Efferent arteriole - blood flow out of glomerulus

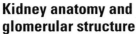

medis : JG apparatus

Macula densa

Afferent arteriole - blood flow to the glomerulus

Podocytes (visceral layer)

space

Bowman's capsule

Mesangial cells

Basement membrane

Capillary

Red blood cells

Ureters: course

Ureters pass **under** uterine artery and **under** ductus deferens (retroperitoneal).

Water (ureters) **under** the bridge (artery, ductus deferens).

Clinically important landmarks

Pudendal nerve block—ischial spine.
Appendix—⅔ of the way from the umbilicus to the anterior superior iliac spine (McBurney's point).
Lumbar puncture—iliac crest.

Triangles

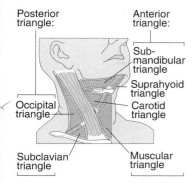

Posterior triangle:
Anterior triangle:
Sub-mandibular triangle
Suprahyoid triangle
Occipital triangle
Carotid triangle
Subclavian triangle
Muscular triangle

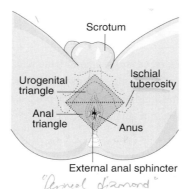

Scrotum
Urogenital triangle
Ischial tuberosity
Anal triangle
Anus
External anal sphincter
"Perineal diamond"

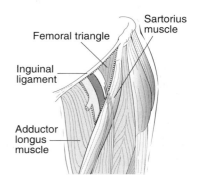

Sartorius muscle
Femoral triangle
Inguinal ligament
Adductor longus muscle

ANATOMY—HISTOLOGY

Special stains

Eosin	Acidic, anionic dye, binds acidophilic tissue with positive charge. Stains smooth ER.
Hematoxylin, methylene blue, toluidine blue	Basic, cationic dyes, bind basophilic nucleic acids with negative charge. Stains DNA, RNA, ribosomes, heparin-containing granules.
PAS	Stains glycogen and basement membranes.
Mallory's trichrome	Stains collagen.
Nissl	Stains cell bodies and dendrites of neurons.
Wright	Stain for peripheral blood smear.
Silver	Stains neuronal processes (Alzheimer's plaques, tangles) and reticular fibers. Also *Pneumocystis carinii* sporozoites and legionellae. *Other parasites/protozoans*
Giemsa	Stains blood, spleen, bone marrow, and some parasites.
Congo red	Amyloid (apple-green birefringence under polarized light).
Prussian blue	Iron.
India ink	Cryptococcus (meningitis in HIV patients).
Ziehl-Neelsen	Acid-fast stain for tubercle bacilli. *& Nocardia.*

Prussian blue — Think of Russia and the Iron Curtain.

Peripheral nerve layers

Endoneurium invests single nerve fiber.
Perineurium (permeability barrier) surrounds a fascicle of nerve fibers.
Epineurium (dense connective tissue) surrounds entire nerve (fascicles and blood vessels).

Perineurium = permeability barrier; must be rejoined in microsurgery for limb reattachment.
Endo = inner.
Peri = around.
Epi = outer.

Meissner's corpuscles

footballs

Small, encapsulated sensory receptors found in dermis of palm, soles, and digits of skin. Involved in light discriminatory touch of glabrous (hairless) skin.

Pacinian corpuscles

onions

Large, encapsulated sensory receptors found in deeper layers of skin at ligaments, joint capsules, serous membranes, mesenteries. Involved in pressure, coarse touch, vibration, and tension.

Inner ear

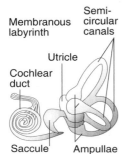

Membranous labyrinth

Semi-circular canals

Utricle

Cochlear duct

Saccule

Ampullae

The bony labyrinth is filled with perilymph (Na^+ rich: similar to ECF) and includes the cochlea (hearing), the vestibule (linear acceleration), and the semicircular canals (angular acceleration).

The membranous labyrinth is filled with endolymph (K^+ rich: similar to ICF) and contains the cochlear duct, utricle, saccule, and semicircular canals. Hair cells are the sensory elements in both the cochlear and vestibular apparatus.

Peri—think outside of cell (Na^+).
Endo—think inside of cell (K^+).
Endolymph is made by the stria vascularis.
Utricle and saccule contain maculae: for linear acceleration.
Semicircular canals contain **a**mpullae: **a**ngular acceleration.

Enteric plexuses

Red Aorbach - muscular (°)

Myenteric — Also known as Auerbach's plexus. Contains cell bodies of some parasympathetic terminal effector neurons. Located between inner and outer layers of smooth muscle in GI tract wall. Coordinates muscle activity along entire gut wall.

Think of Auerbach, the quarterback (Staubach), a (muscular) football player.

Submucosal — Also known as Meissner's plexus. Contains cell bodies of some parasympathetic terminal effector neurons. Located between mucosa and inner layer of smooth muscle in GI tract wall. Regulates local secretions, blood flow, and absorption.

Collagen types

Type I: bone, tendon, skin, dentin, fascia, late wound repair.

Type II: cartilage (including hyaline), vitreous body, nucleus pulposus.

Type III (reticulin): skin, blood vessels, uterus, fetal tissue, granulation tissue.

Type IV: basement membrane or basal lamina.

Type X: epiphyseal plate. *previous exams*

Type I: B**ONE**

Type II: car**TWO**lage

Epidermis layers	From base to surface: stratum **G**erminativum, stratum **S**pinosum, stratum **G**ranulosum, stratum **L**ucidum, stratum **C**orneum. *C nuclei clear at*	**G**entle **S**kin **G**ets **L**avish **C**are.
Glomerular basement membrane	Formed from fused endothelial and podocyte basement membranes and coated with negatively charged heparan sulfate. Responsible for actual filtration of plasma according to net charge and size.	In **ne**phrotic syndrome, **ne**gative charge is lost (and plasma protein is lost in urine as a consequence).
Cilia structure	9 + 2 arrangement of microtubules. Peripheral 9 are unconventional. Central 2 are conventional. Dynein is an ATPase that links peripheral 9 doublets and causes bending of cilium by differential sliding of doublets.	**9 + 2 arrangement.** Kartagener's syndrome is due to a dynein arm defect, resulting in immotile cilia.
Intermediate filament	Permanent structure. Long fibrous molecules with 10-nm diameter. Linked to plasma membrane at desmosomes by desmoplakin. Very insoluble. No cytoplasmic pool of monomeric subunits. Intermediate filaments are tissue specific. Rich in cysteine.	
Epithelial cells	Contain cytokeratin. — *Mallory hyaline bodies*	
Connective tissue	Contains vimentin.	
Muscle cells	Contain desmin.	
Neuroglia	Contain glial fibrillary acidic proteins (GFAP).	
Neurons	Contain neurofilaments.	
Nucleus	Contains nuclear lamin.	
Nissl bodies	Nissl bodies (in neurons) = rough ER; not found in axon or axon hillock. Synthesize enzymes (e.g., ChAT) and peptide neurotransmitters.	
Functions of Golgi apparatus	1. Distribution center of proteins and lipids from ER to the plasma membrane, lysosomes, and secretory vesicles 2. Modifies N-oligosaccharides on asparagine. 3. Adds O-oligosaccharides to serine and threonine residues 4. Proteoglycan assembly from proteoglycan core proteins 5. Sulfation of sugars in proteoglycans and of selected tyrosine on proteins 6. Addition of mannose-6-phosphate on specific lysosomal proteins, which targets the protein to the lysosome	I-cell disease is caused by the failure of addition of mannose-6-phosphate to lysosome proteins, causing these enzymes to be secreted outside the cell instead of being targeted to the lysosome.
Rough endoplasmic reticulum (RER)	Rough ER is the site of synthesis of secretory (exported) proteins and of N-linked oligosaccharide addition to many proteins.	Mucus-secreting goblet cells of the small intestine are rich in RER.

Smooth endoplasmic reticulum (SER)	SER is the site of steroid synthesis and detoxification of drugs and poisons.	Liver hepatocytes and steroid-hormone–producing cells of the adrenal cortex are rich in SER.
Sinusoids of liver	Irregular "capillaries" with round pores 100–200 nm in diameter without diaphragm. No basement membrane. Not a barrier to macromolecules of plasma (full access to surface of liver cells through space of Disse).	
Sinusoids of spleen	Long, vascular channels in red pulp. With fenestrated "barrel hoop" basement membrane. Macrophages found nearby. *PALS : T cells*	T cells are found in the PALS and the red pulp of the spleen. B cells are found in follicles within the white pulp of the spleen.
Pancreas endocrine cell types	Islets of Langerhans are collections of endocrine cells (most numerous in tail of pancreas). α = glucagon; β = insulin; δ = somatostatin. Islets arise from pancreatic buds.	

Adrenal cortex and medulla

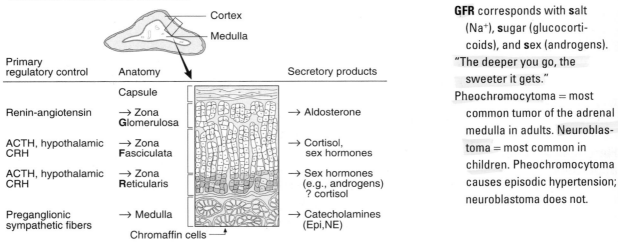

Primary regulatory control	Anatomy	Secretory products
	Capsule	
Renin-angiotensin	→ Zona **G**lomerulosa	→ Aldosterone
ACTH, hypothalamic CRH	→ Zona **F**asciculata	→ Cortisol, sex hormones
ACTH, hypothalamic CRH	→ Zona **R**eticularis	→ Sex hormones (e.g., androgens) ? cortisol
Preganglionic sympathetic fibers	→ Medulla	→ Catecholamines (Epi,NE)

Chromaffin cells ⟶

GFR corresponds with **s**alt (Na⁺), **s**ugar (glucocorticoids), and **s**ex (androgens).
"The deeper you go, the sweeter it gets."
Pheochromocytoma = most common tumor of the adrenal medulla in adults. Neuroblastoma = most common in children. Pheochromocytoma causes episodic hypertension; neuroblastoma does not.

Types of secretion	Merocrine (eccrine) = by exocytosis (i.e., proteins). Apocrine = secretion with loss of cytoplasm from apical side (i.e., sweat). Holocrine = secretion with destruction of the cell (i.e., products of sebaceous glands).	**Apo**crine = **Api**cal cytoplasm. **Holo**crine = **Whole** cytoplasm.
Brunner's glands	Secrete alkaline mucus. Located in submucosa of duodenum (the only GI submucosal glands). Duodenal ulcers cause hypertrophy of Brunner's glands.	**BAGS: B**runner's **A**lkaline **G**lands, **S**ubmucosal.

Lymph node   A secondary lymphoid organ that has many afferents, one or more efferents. Encapsulated. With trabeculae. Functions are nonspecific filtration by macrophages, storage/proliferation of B and T cells, Ab production.

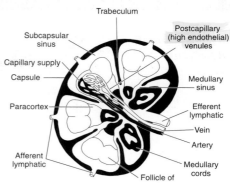

Follicle   Site of B-cell localization and proliferation. In outer cortex. 1° follicles are dense and dormant. 2° follicles have pale central germinal centers and are active.

Medulla   Consists of medullary cords (closely packed lymphocytes and plasma cells) and medullary sinuses. Medullary sinuses communicate with efferent lymphatics and contain reticular cells and macrophages.

Paracortex   Houses T cells. Region of cortex between follicles and medulla. Contains high endothelial venules through which T and B cells enter from blood. In an extreme cellular immune response, paracortex becomes greatly enlarged. Not well developed in patients with DiGeorge's syndrome.

Peyer's patch   Unencapsulated lymphoid tissue found in lamina propria and submucosa of intestine. Covered by single layer of cuboidal enterocytes (no goblet cells) with specialized M cells interspersed. M cells take up antigen. Stimulated B cells leave Peyer's patch and travel through lymph and blood to lamina propria of intestine, where they differentiate to IgA-secreting plasma cells. IgA receives protective secretory piece, then is transported across epithelium to gut to deal with intraluminal Ag.

Think of **IgA**, the **I**ntra-**g**ut–**A**ntibody. And always say, "secretory IgA."

Hypothalamus: functions	**T**hirst and water balance (supraoptic nucleus). **A**denohypophysis control via releasing factors. **N**eurohypophysis releases hormones synthesized in hypothalamic nuclei.	The hypothalamus wears **TAN HATS.**
	Hunger (lateral nucleus) and satiety (ventromedial nucleus). **A**utonomic regulation (anterior hypothalamus regulates parasympathetic activity), circadian rhythms (suprachiasmatic nucleus).	If you zap your **ventromedial** nucleus, you grow **ven**trally and **medial**ly (hyperphagia and obesity). **L**ittle (**L**ateral) food makes you hungry.
	Temperature regulation: Posterior hypothalamus—heat conservation and production when cold. **A**nterior hypothalamus—coordinates **C**ooling when hot. **S**exual urges and emotions (**s**eptate nucleus).	If you zap your **P**osterior hypothalamus, you become a **P**oikilotherm (cold-blooded snake). **A/C** = anterior coolin
Posterior pituitary (neurohypophysis)	Receives hypothalamic axonal projections from supraoptic (ADH) and paraventricular (oxytocin) nuclei.	Oxytocin: *oxys* = quick; *tocos* = birth.
Functions of thalamic nuclei	Lateral geniculate nucleus = visual. Medial geniculate nucleus = auditory. Ventral posterior nucleus, lateral part = proprioception, pressure, pain, touch vibration of body. Ventral posterior nucleus, medial part = facial sensation, including pain. Ventral anterior/lateral nuclei = motor.	**L**ateral to **L**ook. **M**edial for **M**usic.

Limbic system: functions	Responsible for **F**eeding, **F**ighting, **F**eeling, **F**light, and sex.	The famous **5 F's**.
CNS/PNS supportive cells	**A**strocytes—physical support, repair, K⁺ metabolism. **M**icroglia—phagocytosis. **O**ligodendroglia—central myelin production. **S**chwann cells—peripheral myelin production. **E**pendymal cells—inner lining of ventricles.	"**A MOSE** (like 'most') wonderful array of neural supportive cells."
Blood–brain barrier	Formed by three structures: 1. Arachnoid 2. Choroid plexus epithelium 3. Intracerebral capillary endothelium Glucose and amino acids cross by carrier-mediated transport mechanism. Nonpolar/lipid–soluble substances cross more readily than polar/water–soluble ones.	Other barriers include: 1. Blood–bile barrier 2. Blood–testis barrier 3. Blood–PNS barrier Example: L-dopa, rather than dopamine, is used to treat parkinsonism because dopamine does not cross blood-brain barrier.
Chorea	Sudden, jerky, purposeless movements. Characteristic of basal ganglia lesion (e.g., Huntington's disease).	*Chorea* = dancing (Greek). Think choral dancing or choreography.
Athetosis	Slow, writhing movements, especially of fingers. Characteristic of basal ganglia lesion.	*Athetos* = not fixed (Greek). Think snakelike.
Hemiballismus	Sudden, wild flailing of one arm. Characteristic of subthalamic nucleus lesion.	Half ballistic (as in throwing a baseball).
Tremors: cerebellar versus basal	Cerebellar tremor = intention tremor. Basal ganglion tremor = resting tremor.	Basal = at rest (**Park**inson's disease) when **Park**ed.

Cerebral cortex functions

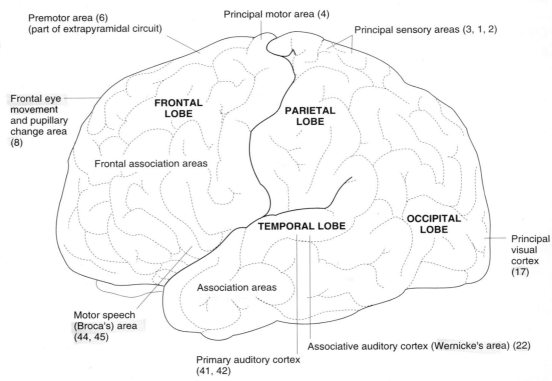

Premotor area (6)
(part of extrapyramidal circuit)

Principal motor area (4)

Principal sensory areas (3, 1, 2)

Frontal eye movement and pupillary change area (8)

FRONTAL LOBE

PARIETAL LOBE

Frontal association areas

TEMPORAL LOBE

OCCIPITAL LOBE

Association areas

Principal visual cortex (17)

Motor speech (Broca's) area (44, 45)

Primary auditory cortex (41, 42)

Associative auditory cortex (Wernicke's area) (22)

Brain lesions

Area of lesion	Consequence
Broca's area	Motor (expressive) aphasia
Wernicke's area	Sensory (fluent) aphasia
Amygdala (bilateral)	Klüver-Bucy syndrome (hyperorality, hypersexuality, disinhibited behavior)
Frontal lobe	Frontal release signs (e.g., personality changes and deficits in concentration, orientation, judgment)
Right parietal lobe	Spacial neglect syndrome (agnosia of the contralateral side of the world) *left-sided neglect.*
Reticular activating system	Coma
Mamillary bodies (bilateral)	Wernicke–Korsakoff's encephalopathy (confabulations, anterograde amnesia).

BROca's is **BRO**ken speech.
Wernicke's is **W**ordy but makes no sense. *"word salad".*

Cavernous sinus

CN III, IV, V$_1$, V$_2$, VI all pass through the cavernous sinus. Only CN VI is "free-floating." Also contains cavernous portion of internal carotid artery.

The nerves that control extraocular muscles (plus V$_1$ and V$_2$) pass through the cavernous sinus.

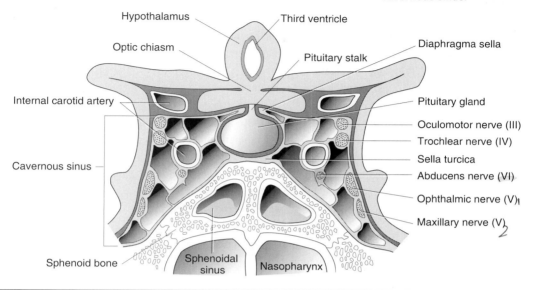

- Hypothalamus
- Third ventricle
- Optic chiasm
- Pituitary stalk
- Diaphragma sella
- Internal carotid artery
- Pituitary gland
- Oculomotor nerve (III)
- Trochlear nerve (IV)
- Sella turcica
- Cavernous sinus
- Abducens nerve (VI)
- Ophthalmic nerve (V)$_1$
- Maxillary nerve (V)$_2$
- Sphenoid bone
- Sphenoidal sinus
- Nasopharynx

Foramina: middle cranial fossa

1. Optic canal (CN II, ophthalmic artery, central retinal vein)
2. **S**uperior orbital fissure (CN III, IV, V$_1$, VI, ophthalmic vein)
3. Foramen **R**otundum (CN V$_2$)
4. Foramen **O**vale (CN V$_3$)
5. Foramen spinosum (middle meningeal artery)

All structures pass through sphenoid bone. Divisions of CN V exit owing to **S**tanding **R**oom **O**nly (**S**uperior orbital fissure, foramen **R**otundum, foramen **O**vale).

Foramina: posterior cranial fossa

1. Internal auditory meatus (CN VII, VIII)
2. Jugular foramen (CN IX, X, XI, jugular vein)
3. Hypoglossal canal (CN XII)
4. Foramen magnum (spinal roots of CN XI, brain stem, vertebral arteries)

All structures pass through temporal or occipital bones.

Extraocular muscles and nerves

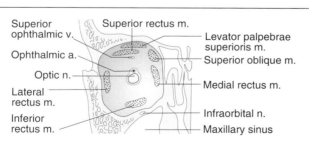

- Superior ophthalmic v.
- Superior rectus m.
- Levator palpebrae superioris m.
- Ophthalmic a.
- Superior oblique m.
- Optic n.
- Medial rectus m.
- Lateral rectus m.
- Inferior rectus m.
- Infraorbital n.
- Maxillary sinus

Lateral **R**ectus is CN VI, **S**uperior **O**blique is CN IV, **R**est are CN III. The "chemical formula" **LR$_6$SO$_4$R$_3$**; the rest is CN III.

Internuclear ophthalmoplegia

Lesion in the medial longitudinal fasciculus (MLF). Results in medial rectus palsy on attempted lateral gaze. Nystagmus in abducting eye. Convergence is normal. MLF syndrome is seen in many patients with multiple sclerosis.

Cranial nerves

		Function	Type		
Olfactory	I	Smell	**S**ensory	**S**ome
Optic	II	Sight	**S**ensory	**S**ay
Oculomotor	III	Eye movement, pupil constriction, accommodation, eyelid opening	**M**otor	**M**arry
Trochlear	IV	Eye movement	**M**otor	**M**oney
Trigeminal	V	Mastication, facial sensation	**B**oth	**B**ut
Abducens	VI	Eye movement	**M**otor	**M**y
Facial	VII	Facial movement, anterior 2/3 taste, lacrimation, salivation (submaxillary and submandibular salivary glands)	**B**oth	**B**rother
Vestibulocochlear	VIII	Hearing, balance	**S**ensory	**S**ays
Glossopharyngeal	IX	Posterior 1/3 taste, swallowing, salivation (parotid gland), monitoring carotid body and sinus	**B**oth	**B**ig
Vagus	X	Taste, swallowing, palate elevation, talking, thoracoabdominal viscera *aortic arch BP, chemoreceptors*	**B**oth	**B**rains
Accessory	XI	Head turning, shoulder shrugging, talking *— enters part of CN X*	**M**otor	**M**atter
Hypoglossal	XII	Tongue movements	**M**otor	**M**ost

Cranial nerves and passageways

Cribriform plate	I
Optic canal	II
Superior orbital fissure	III, IV, V$_1$, VI
Foramen rotundum	V$_2$
Foramen ovale	V$_3$
Internal auditory meatus	VII, VIII
Jugular foramen	IX, X, XI
Hypoglossal canal	XII

Brainstem anatomy

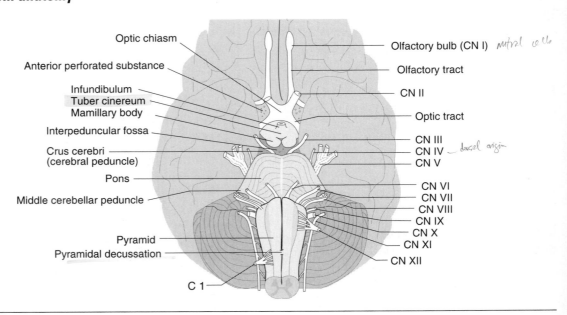

Optic chiasm
Anterior perforated substance
Infundibulum
Tuber cinereum
Mamillary body
Interpeduncular fossa
Crus cerebri (cerebral peduncle)
Pons
Middle cerebellar peduncle
Pyramid
Pyramidal decussation
C 1

Olfactory bulb (CN I) *mitral cells*
Olfactory tract
CN II
Optic tract
CN III
CN IV *— dorsal origin*
CN V
CN VI
CN VII
CN VIII
CN IX
CN X
CN XI
CN XII

Visual field defects

1. Right anopsia
2. Bitemporal hemianopsia
3. Left homonymous hemianopsia
4. Left upper quadrantic anopsia (right temporal lesion)
5. Left lower quadrantic anopsia (right parietal lesion)

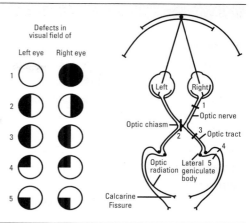

Defects in visual field of

Left eye   Right eye

KLM sounds: kuh, la, mi

Kuh-kuh-kuh tests palate elevation (CN X—vagus).
La-la-la tests tongue (CN XII—hypoglossal).
Mi-mi-mi tests lips (CN VII—facial).

Say it aloud.

Vagal nuclei

Nucleus **S**olitarius	Visceral **S**ensory information (e.g., taste, gut distention, etc.).
Nucleus a**M**biguus	**M**otor innervation of pharynx, larynx, and upper esophagus.
Dorsal motor nucleus	Sends autonomic (parasympathetic) fibers to heart, lungs, and upper GI.

Lesions and deviations

CN XII lesion (LMN): tongue deviates **toward** side of lesion.
CN V motor lesion: jaw deviates **toward** side of lesion.
Unilateral lesion of cerebellum: patient tends to fall **toward** side of lesion.
CN X lesion: uvula deviates **away** from side of lesion.

Spinal cord and associated tracts

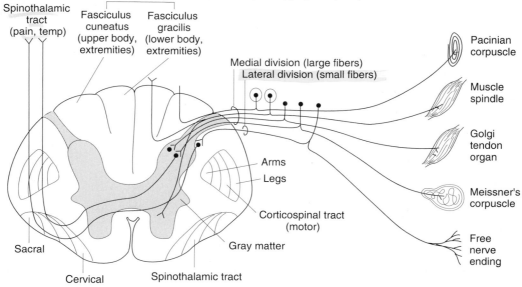

89

| **Dorsal column organization** | In dorsal columns, lower limbs are inside to avoid crossing the upper limbs on the outside. Fasciculus gracilis = legs. Fasciculus cuneatus = arms. | Dorsal column is organized like you are, with hands at sides—arms outside and legs inside. *Gracilis* (Latin) = graceful, slender, like ballerina's legs. |

| **Brown-Séquard syndrome** 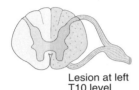 Lesion at left T10 level | Hemisection of spinal cord. Findings below the lesion: 1. Ipsilateral motor paralysis and spasticity (pyramidal tract)-not shown *already crossed* 2. Ipsilateral loss of tactile, vibration, proprioception sense (dorsal column) 3. Contralateral pain and temperature loss (spinothalamic tract) 4. Ipsilateral loss of all sensation at level of lesion | 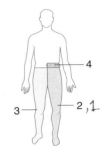 |

| **Lower motor neuron (LMN) signs** | LMN injury signs: atrophy, flaccid paralysis, absent deep tendon reflexes. Fasciculations may be present. | **Lower** MN ≈ everything **lower**ed (less muscle mass, **decreased** muscle tone, **decreased** reflexes, **down**going toes). |

| **Upper motor neuron (UMN) signs** | UMN injury signs: little atrophy, spastic paralysis (clonus), hyperactive deep tendon reflexes, possible positive Babinski. *atrophy of disuse.* | **Upper** MN ≈ everything **up** (tone, DTRs, toes). |

Spindle muscle control

| Reflex arc | Muscle spindle stretch stimulates Ia afferents. Ia stimulates alpha motor neurons of agonist muscle to contract extrafusal muscle fibers. | Tendon Muscle fiber (extrafusal) Ia afferent γ motor neuron α motor neuron Muscle spindle (intrafusal) |
| Gamma loop | Gamma motor neurons from CNS contract intrafusal muscle fibers → stretch spindle → reflex arc → stimulate alpha motor neuron. Responsible for maintaining tone. | |

Brachial plexus

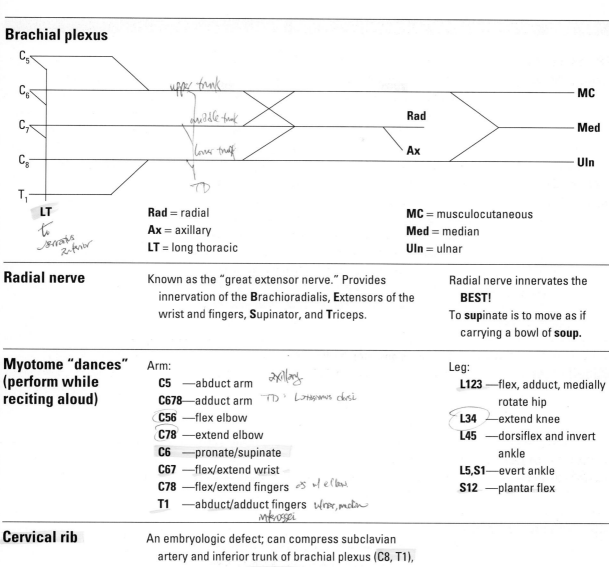

C5
C6
C7
C8
T1

upper trunk
middle trunk
lower trunk
TD
LT
to serratus anterior

Rad
Ax

MC
Med
Uln

Rad = radial
Ax = axillary
LT = long thoracic

MC = musculocutaneous
Med = median
Uln = ulnar

Radial nerve

Known as the "great extensor nerve." Provides innervation of the **B**rachioradialis, **E**xtensors of the wrist and fingers, **S**upinator, and **T**riceps.

Radial nerve innervates the **BEST!**

To **sup**inate is to move as if carrying a bowl of **soup.**

Myotome "dances" (perform while reciting aloud)

Arm:

C5	—abduct arm axillary
C678	—adduct arm TD > Latissimus dorsi
C56	—flex elbow
C78	—extend elbow
C6	—pronate/supinate
C67	—flex/extend wrist
C78	—flex/extend fingers as of elbow.
T1	—abduct/adduct fingers Ulnar, median interossei

Leg:

L123	—flex, adduct, medially rotate hip
L34	—extend knee
L45	—dorsiflex and invert ankle
L5,S1	—evert ankle
S12	—plantar flex

Cervical rib

An embryologic defect; can compress subclavian artery and inferior trunk of brachial plexus (C8, T1), resulting in thoracic outlet syndrome:

1. Atrophy of the thenar and hypothenar eminences
2. Atrophy of the interosseous muscles
3. Sensory deficits on the medial side of the forearm and hand
4. Disappearance of the radial pulse upon moving the head toward the opposite side

Facial lesion

Central facial

Paralysis of the contralateral facial muscles except the frontalis and orbicularis oculi muscles. Because the motor neurons supplying the frontalis and orbicularis oculi muscles receive bilateral cortical innervation, the muscles are not paralyzed by lesions involving one motor cortex or its corticobulbar pathways.

Bell's palsy

Peripheral facial paralysis.

Can occur idiopathically.

Seen as a complication in diabetes, tumors, sarcoidosis, AIDS, and Lyme disease.

Bell's phenomenon—when an attempt is made to close the eyelid, the eyeball on the affected side may turn upward.

AD: 2 only affects lower facial nn.

pmy effect dr. (LMN) —— Complete destruction of the facial nucleus itself or its branchial efferent fibers (facial nerve proper) paralyzes all ipsilateral facial muscles.

submandibular branch

Face area of motor cortex

Cortico-bulbar tract (UMN lesion= **central facial**)

Facial nucleus

Upper division

Lower division

Muscles of facial expression:

Frontalis
Orbicularis oculi
Buccinator
Orbicularis oris
Platysma

CN VII (LMN lesion= **Bell's palsy**)

Clinical reflexes

Biceps = C5 nerve root. *C5, C6*

Triceps = C7 nerve root. *C7, C8*

Patella = L4 nerve root. *L3, L4*

Achilles = S1 nerve root. *S1, S2*

Babinski = dorsiflexion of the big toe and fanning of other toes; sign of upper motor neuron lesion.

These abstracted case vignettes are designed to demonstrate the thought processes necessary to answer multistep clinical reasoning questions.

- Baby vomits milk when fed and has a gastric air bubble → what kind of tracheoesophageal fistula is present? → blind esophagus with lower segment of esophagus attached to trachea.
- Patient cannot flex or abduct arm and has a cupped hand → where is the lesion? → upper trunk of brachial plexus. *Erb Duchenne palsy*
- Patient describes a cold, tingling hand with muscle weakness → brachial plexopathy or subclavian steal?
- 18-year-old presents with stab wound to the hand; can still use a pen → which tendon or muscle is most likely to have been damaged?
- Rock star loses hearing → where is the damage? → cochlea.
- 40-year-old dancer reports decreased plantar flexion and decreased sensation over the back of her thigh, calf, and lateral half of her foot → what spinal nerve is involved? *S1*
- Patient presents with decreased pain and temperature sensation over the lateral aspects of both arms → where is the lesion? → cervical spinal cord. *? syringomyelia*
- Penlight in patient's right eye produces bilateral pupillary constriction. When moved to the left eye, there is paradoxical bilateral pupillary dilatation → what is the defect? → atrophy of the left optic nerve.
- Patient describes decreased prick sensation on the lateral aspect of her leg and foot → a deficit in what muscular action can also be expected? → dorsiflexion of foot. *—L5, S1 also plantar flexion (S1, S2)*
- Elderly lady presents with arthritis and tingling over lateral digits of her right hand → what is the diagnosis? → carpal tunnel syndrome.
- Woman involved in motor vehicle accident cannot control left sternocleidomastoid or trapezius muscles → what structure is damaged? → jugular foramen. *(CN XI would be a less presumptuous answer.*
- Tongue of man with right-sided Horner's syndrome points to the right → where is the lesion? → medulla. *location of hypoglossal nucleus (dorsal). hypothalamospinal tract lesion.*
- Man presents with one wild, flailing arm → where is the lesion? → subthalamic nucleus. *hemiballismus*
- Pregnant woman in third trimester has normal blood pressure when standing and sitting. When supine, blood pressure drops to 90/50 → what is the diagnosis? → compression of the inferior vena cava.
- Soccer player who was kicked in the leg suffered a damaged medial meniscus → what else is likely to have been damaged? → anterior cruciate ligament. *2/3 of unhappy triad*
- Gymnast dislocates her shoulder anteriorly → what nerve is most likely to have been damaged? → axillary nerve.
- Patient with cortical lesion does not know that he has a disease → where is the lesion? → right parietal lobe. *left-sided neglect.*

- Carotid angiography → identify the anterior cerebral artery → occlusion of this artery will produce a deficit where? → contralateral leg, middle cerebral artery, etc.
- H&E of normal liver → identify the central vein, portal triad, bile canaliculi, etc.
- X-ray of fractured humerus → what nerve is most likely damaged? → radial nerve. *radial tract° in humerus*
- X-ray of hip joint → what part undergoes avascular necrosis with fracture at the neck of the femur? → femoral head.
- Abdominal CT cross section → obstruction of what structure results in enlarged kidneys? → inferior vena cava.
- Intravenous pyelogram with right ureter dilated → where is the obstruction? → ureterovesicular junction → stone.
- Illustration of fetal head → medial maxillary eminence gives rise to what? *intermaxillary segment, incisors, 1° p*
- Abdominal MRI cross section → locate the splenic artery, portal vein, etc.
- EM of cell → lysosomes (digestion of macromolecules), RER (protein synthesis), SER (steroid synthesis).
- Coronal MRI section of the head at the level of the eye → where is medial rectus muscle? → what is its function?
- Optic nerve path → defect where would cause diminished pupillary reflex in right eye? Defect where would cause right homonymous hemianopsia?
- Aortogram → identify adrenal artery, renal arteries, SMA, etc.
- Chest x-ray → pleural effusion with layering → where is the fluid located? → costodiaphragmatic recess.
- MRI abdominal cross section → what structure is derivative of the common cardinal veins? → inferior vena cava.
- Sagittal MRI of brain of patient with hyperphagia, increased CSF pressure, and visual problems → where is the lesion?

VM hypothalamus   blockade of 3rd ventricle (?)   optic chiasm compression/ CN II compression

pituitary or hypothal. tumor

Embryology

1. Development of the heart, lung, liver, kidney (i.e., what are the embryologic structures that give rise to these organs?).
2. Etiology and clinical presentation of important congenital malformations (e.g., neural tube defects, cleft palate, tetralogy of Fallot, tracheoesophageal fistula, horseshoe kidney).
3. Development of the central nervous system (e.g., telencephalon, diencephalon, mesencephalon).
4. Derivatives of the foregut, midgut, and hindgut as well as their vascular supply.
5. Derivatives of the somites, and malformations associated with defects in somite migration.
6. Fetal circulation (path of oxygenated and deoxygenated blood, fetal circulatory structures and their adult derivatives).
7. Changes in the circulatory/respiratory system on the first breath of a newborn.
8. Development of the embryonic plate in weeks two and three.

Gross Anatomy

1. Anatomic landmarks in relation to medical procedures (e.g., direct and indirect hernia repair, lumbar puncture, pericardiocentesis).
2. Anatomic landmarks in relation to major organs (e.g., lungs, heart, kidneys).
3. Common injuries of the knee (including clinical examination), hip, shoulder, and clavicle; paying attention to the clinical deficits caused by these injuries (e.g., shoulder separation, hip fracture).
4. Clinical features and anatomic correlations of specific brachial plexus lesions (e.g., waiter's tip, wrist drop, claw hand, scapular winging).
5. Clinical features of common peripheral nerve injuries (e.g., common vs. deep peroneal nerve palsy, radial nerve palsy).
6. Etiology and clinical features of common diseases affecting the hands (e.g., carpal tunnel syndrome, cubital tunnel syndrome, Dupuytren's contracture).
7. Anatomic basis for the blood–testis barrier.
8. Major blood vessels and collateral circulatory pathways of the gastrointestinal tract (e.g., collaterals between the superior and inferior mesenteric arteries).
9. Bone structures (metaphysis, epiphysis, diaphysis), including histologic features; linear (epiphysis) and annular (diaphysis) bone growth.

Histology

1. Histology of the respiratory tract (i.e., differentiate between the bronchi, terminal bronchioles, respiratory bronchioles, and alveoli). Also differentiate between cell types in the alveolus.
2. Structure, function, and electron microscopic (EM) appearance of major cellular organelles and structures (e.g., lysosomes, peroxisomes, glycogen, mitochondria, ER, Golgi apparatus, nucleus, nucleolus).
3. Structure, function, and EM appearance of cell–cell junctional structures (e.g., tight junctions, gap junctions, desmosomes).
4. Histology of lymphoid organs (e.g., lymph nodes, tonsils, thymus, spleen).
5. Resident phagocytic cells of different organisms (e.g., Langerhan's cells, Kupffer cells, alveolar macrophages, microglia).

Histology *(continued)*

6. Histology of muscle fibers and changes seen with muscle contraction (sarcomere structure, different bands, rigor mortis).
7. Bone ossification (intramembranous vs. endochondral).

Neuroanatomy

1. Etiology and clinical features of important brain, cranial nerve, and spinal cord lesions (e.g., brain stem lesions and "crossed signs," dorsal root lesions, effects of schwannoma, Weber and Parinaud syndromes).
2. Production, circulation, and composition of cerebrospinal fluid.
3. Neuroanatomy of hearing (central and peripheral hearing loss).
4. Extraocular muscles (which muscle abducts, adducts, etc.) and their innervation.
5. Structure and function of a chemical synapse (e.g., neuromuscular junction).
6. Major neurotransmitters, receptors, second messengers, and effects.
7. Blood supply of the brain (anterior, middle, posterior cerebral arterial areas, "watershed" areas) and neurologic deficits corresponding to various vascular occlusions).
8. Functional anatomy of the basal ganglia (e.g., globus pallidus, caudate, putamen).
9. Anatomic landmarks near the pituitary gland.
10. Brain MRI/CT, including morphologic changes in disease states (e.g., Huntington's chorea, MS, aging).
11. Clinical exam of pupillary light reflex: pathway tested, important anatomic lesions, swinging light test.

Radiology

1. X-rays; plain films.
    a. fractures (skull, humerus, etc.) and associated clinical findings.
    b. PA and lateral chest films, including important landmarks (costodiaphragmatic recess, major blood vessels, cardiac chambers, and abnormalities seen with different diseases (consolidation, pneumothorax, mitral stenosis, cardiomyopathy).
    c. abdominal films, including vasculature (locate important vessels in contrast films) and other important structures.
    d. joint films (e.g., shoulder, wrist, knee, hip, spine); including important injuries/diseases (e.g., osteoarthritis, herniated disc).
2. CT/MRI studies.
    a. brain cross-sections (e.g., hematomas, brain lesions, extra-ocular muscles).
    b. chest cross-section (e.g., superior vena cava, aortic arch, heart).
    c. abdominal cross-section (e.g., liver, kidney, pancreas, aorta, inferior vena cava, rectus abdominis muscle, splenic artery).

Behavioral Science

A heterogeneous mix of epidemiology/biostatistics, psychiatry, psychology, sociology, psychopharmacology, and more falls under this heading. Many medical students do not study this discipline diligently because the material is felt to be "easy" or "common sense." In our opinion, this is a missed opportunity. Each question gained in behavioral science is equal to a question in any other section in determining the overall score. At many medical schools, this material is not covered in a single course. Many students feel that some behavioral science questions are less concrete and require awareness of social aspects of medicine. For example: If a patient does or says something, what should you do or say back? Medical ethics and medical law are also appearing with increasing frequency. In addition, the key aspects of the doctor–patient relationship (e.g., communication skills, open-ended questions, facilitation, silence) are high yield. Basic biostatistics and epidemiology are very learnable and high yield. Be able to apply biostatistical concepts such as specificity and predictive values in a problem-solving format. Also review the clinical presentation of personality disorders.

Epidemiology
Ethics
Life Cycle
Physiology
Psychiatry
Psychology
High-Yield Clinical Vignettes
High-Yield Topics

Prevalence versus incidence	Prevalence is total number of cases in a population at a given time.	
	Incidence is number of new cases in a population per unit time.	**Incidence** is new **incidents.**

Sensitivity	Number of true positives divided by number of all people with the disease.	**PID** = **P**ositive **I**n **D**isease (note that PID is a **sensitive** topic).
	False negative ratio is equal to 1 − sensitivity.	
	High sensitivity is desirable for a screening test.	

Specificity	Number of true negatives divided by number of all people without the disease.	**NIH** = **N**egative **I**n **H**ealth.
	False positive ratio is equal to 1 − specificity.	
	High specificity is desirable for a confirmatory test.	

Predictive value

Positive predictive value

Number of true positives divided by number of people who tested positive for the disease.

The probability of having a condition, given a positive test.

Negative predictive value

Number of true negatives divided by number of people who tested negative for the disease.

The probability of not having the condition, given a negative test.

Unlike sensitivity and specificity, predictive values are dependent on the prevalence of the disease.

The higher the prevalence of a disease, the higher the positive predictive value of the test.

Disease

Test	⊕	⊖
⊕	a	b
⊖	c	d

$$\text{Sensitivity} = \frac{a}{a+c}$$

$$\text{Specificity} = \frac{d}{b+d}$$

$$\text{PPV} = \frac{a}{a+b}$$

$$\text{NPV} = \frac{d}{c+d}$$

Odds ratio and relative risk

Odds ratio

Approximates the relative risk if the prevalence of the disease is not too high. Used for retrospective studies (e.g., case-control studies).

OR = ad / bc

Relative risk

Disease risk in exposed group/disease risk in unexposed group. Used for cohort studies.

Disease

Exposure	⊕	⊖
⊕	a	b
⊖	c	d

$$RR = \frac{\left[\dfrac{a}{a+b}\right]}{\left[\dfrac{c}{c+d}\right]} \qquad \text{Attributable Risk} = \left[\frac{a}{a+b}\right] - \left[\frac{c}{c+d}\right]$$

Standard deviation versus error	n = sample size, σ = standard deviation, SEM = standard error of the mean, $SEM = \sigma/\sqrt{n}$ Therefore, SEM < σ and SEM ↓ as n ↑.	Normal (Gaussian) distribution:
Distribution: skew, bimodal	Terms that describe statistical distributions: Normal ≈ Gaussian ≈ bell-shaped. (Mean = median = mode.) Bimodal is simply two humps. Positive skew is asymmetry with tail on the right. Negative skew has tail on the left.	Positive skew = tail on more positive side (mean > median > mode). Negative skew = tail on more negative side (mean < median < mode).
Precision vs. accuracy	Precision is: 1. The consistency and reproducibility of a test (reliability) 2. The absence of random variation in a test Accuracy is the trueness of test measurements.	Random error = reduced precision in a test. Systematic error = reduced accuracy in a test.
Reliability and validity	Reliability = reproducibility (dependability) of a test. Validity = whether the test truly measures what it purports to measure. Appropriateness of a test.	Test is reliable if repeat measurements are the same. Test is valid if it measures what it is supposed to measure.
Correlation coefficient (r)	r is always between −1 and 1. Absolute value indicates strength of correlation. Pearson coefficient is used when values are evaluated directly. Spear**man (rank)** coefficient is used when values are placed in rank order and ranks are analyzed. Coefficient of determination = r^2.	Spear**men** stand in **ranks.**
_t_-test versus ANOVA versus χ^2	_t_-test checks difference between two **mean**s. ANOVA analyzes variance of three or more variables. χ^2 checks difference between two or more percentages or proportions of categorical outcomes (not mean values).	Mr. **T** is **mean**. **ANOVA = AN**alysis **O**f **VA**riance of three or more variables. χ^2 = compare percentages (%) or proportions.
Meta-analysis	Pooling data from several studies (often via a literature search) to achieve greater statistical power.	Cannot overcome limitations of individual studies or bias in study selection.

Case-control study	Observational study. Sample chosen based on presence (cases) or absence (controls) of disease. Information collected about risk factors.	Often retrospective.
Cohort study	Observational study. Sample chosen based on presence or absence of risk factors. Subjects followed over time for development of disease.	The Framingham heart study was a large prospective cohort study.
Clinical trial	Experimental study. Compares therapeutic benefit of 2 or more treatments.	Highest quality study.

Statistical hypotheses

Null (H_0)	Hypothesis of no difference (e.g., there is no association between the disease and the risk factor in the population).	Reality
Alternative (H_1)	Hypothesis that there is some difference (e.g., there is some association between the disease and the risk factor in the population).	

Study results / Reality:

	H_1	H_0
H_1	Power $(1 - \beta)$	α
H_0	β	

Type I error (α)	Stating that there **is** an effect or difference when there really is not (to mistakenly accept the experimental hypothesis and reject the null hypothesis). α is the probability of making a type I error and is equal to p (usually $< .05$). p = probability of making a type I error.	If $p < .05$, then there is less than a 5% chance that the data will show something that is not really there. α = you "saw" a difference that did not exist—for example, convicting an innocent man.
Type II error (β)	Stating that there **is not** an effect or difference when there really is (to fail to reject the null hypothesis when in fact H_0 is false). β is the probability of making a type II error.	β = you did not "see" a difference that does exist—for example, setting a guilty man free. $1 - \beta$ is "power" of study, or probability that study will see a difference if it is there.
Power	Probability of rejecting null hypothesis when it is in fact false. It depends on: 1. Total number of end points experienced by population 2. Difference in compliance between treatment groups (differences in the mean values between groups)	If you increase sample size, you increase power. There is power in numbers. Power = $1 - \beta$.

Low birth weight	Defined as under 2500 g. Associated with greater incidence of physical and emotional problems. Caused by prematurity or intrauterine growth retardation. Complications include infections, respiratory distress syndrome, necrotizing enterocolitis, and persistent fetal circulation.	

embryonic pd.

Fetal alcohol syndrome	Newborns of mothers who consumed significant amounts of alcohol (teratogen) during pregnancy (highest risk at 3–8 weeks) have a higher incidence of congenital abnormalities, including pre- and postnatal developmental retardation, microcephaly, facial abnormalities, limb dislocation, and heart and lung fistulas. Mechanism may include inhibition of cell migration. The number one cause of congenital malformations in the United States.	

Apgar score (at birth)	Score 0–2 at 1 and 5 min in each of five categories: 1. Heart rate (0, <100, 100+) 2. Respiratory effort (0, irregular, regular) 3. Muscle tone (limp, some, active) 4. Reflex irritability (0, grimace, grimace + cough) 5. Color (blue/pale, trunk pink, all pink) 10 is perfect score.	After Virginia **Apgar,** a famous neonatologist. **A** = **A**ppearance (color) **P** = **P**ulse **G** = **G**rimace **A** = **A**ctivity **R** = **R**espiration

Heroin addiction	Approximately 500,000 US addicts. Heroin is schedule I (not prescribable). Evidence of addiction is narcotic abstinence syndrome (dilated pupils, lacrimation, rhinorrhea, sweating, yawning, irritability, and muscle aches). Also look for track marks (needle sticks in veins). Related diagnoses are hepatitis, abscesses, overdose, hemorrhoids, AIDS, and right-sided endocarditis.	Naloxone (Narcan) and naltrexone competitively inhibit opioids. Methadone (long-acting oral opiate) for heroin detoxification or long-term maintenance.

Reportable diseases	Only some infectious diseases are reported, including AIDS (but not HIV positivity), chickenpox, gonorrhea, hepatitis A and B, measles, mumps, rubella, salmonella, shigella, syphilis, tuberculosis.	

Leading causes of death in the US by age

Infants	Congenital anomalies, sudden infant death syndrome, short gestation/low birth weight, respiratory distress syndrome, maternal complications of pregnancy.	AIDS is leading cause of death between the ages of 25 and 44.
Age 1–14	Injuries, cancer, congenital anomalies, homicide, heart disease.	
Age 15–24	Injuries, homicide, suicide, cancer, heart disease.	
Age 25–64	Cancer, heart disease, injuries, stroke, suicide.	
Age 65+	Heart disease, cancer, stroke, COPD, pneumonia.	

Disease prevention

1°—Prevent disease occurrence (e.g., vaccination).

2°—Early detection of disease (e.g., Pap smear).

3°—Reduce disability from disease (e.g., exogenous insulin for diabetes).

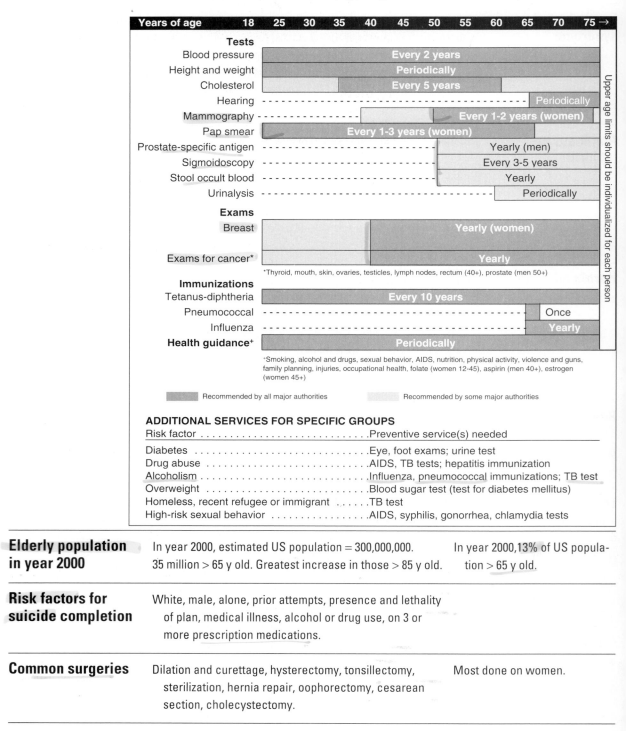

Years of age	18 25 30 35 40 45 50 55 60 65 70 75 →

Tests
- Blood pressure — Every 2 years
- Height and weight — Periodically
- Cholesterol — Every 5 years
- Hearing — Periodically
- Mammography — Every 1-2 years (women)
- Pap smear — Every 1-3 years (women)
- Prostate-specific antigen — Yearly (men)
- Sigmoidoscopy — Every 3-5 years
- Stool occult blood — Yearly
- Urinalysis — Periodically

Exams
- Breast — Yearly (women)
- Exams for cancer* — Yearly

*Thyroid, mouth, skin, ovaries, testicles, lymph nodes, rectum (40+), prostate (men 50+)

Immunizations
- Tetanus-diphtheria — Every 10 years
- Pneumococcal — Once
- Influenza — Yearly

Health guidance⁺ — Periodically

⁺Smoking, alcohol and drugs, sexual behavior, AIDS, nutrition, physical activity, violence and guns, family planning, injuries, occupational health, folate (women 12-45), aspirin (men 40+), estrogen (women 45+)

Upper age limits should be individualized for each person

☐ Recommended by all major authorities   ☐ Recommended by some major authorities

ADDITIONAL SERVICES FOR SPECIFIC GROUPS

Risk factor . . . . .Preventive service(s) needed

Diabetes . . . . .Eye, foot exams; urine test
Drug abuse . . . . .AIDS, TB tests; hepatitis immunization
Alcoholism . . . . .Influenza, pneumococcal immunizations; TB test
Overweight . . . . .Blood sugar test (test for diabetes mellitus)
Homeless, recent refugee or immigrant . . . . . .TB test
High-risk sexual behavior . . . . .AIDS, syphilis, gonorrhea, chlamydia tests

---

Elderly population in year 2000

In year 2000, estimated US population = 300,000,000. 35 million > 65 y old. Greatest increase in those > 85 y old.

In year 2000, 13% of US population > 65 y old.

Risk factors for suicide completion

White, male, alone, prior attempts, presence and lethality of plan, medical illness, alcohol or drug use, on 3 or more prescription medications.

Common surgeries

Dilation and curettage, hysterectomy, tonsillectomy, sterilization, hernia repair, oophorectomy, cesarean section, cholecystectomy.

Most done on women.

Divorce statistics	US has highest rate. Teenage marriages at high risk. More common when religions are mixed. Peaks at second/third year of marriage. Higher with low SES. Unrelated to industrialization. Divorcees remarry very frequently.	
Drug agencies	FDA = Food and Drug Administration (safety and efficacy of drugs).	FDA = protection.
	DEA = Drug Enforcement Administration (security of controlled substances).	DEA = prosecution.
	NIDA = National Institute on Drug Abuse (education, prevention).	NIDA = prevention.
Medicare, Medicaid	Medicare and Medicaid are federal programs that originated from amendments to the Social Security Act. Medicare Part A = hospital; Part B = supplemental. Medicaid is federal and state assistance for those on welfare or who are indigent.	**Medicare** is **care** for the elderly. **Medicaid** is **aid** for the poor.

<h3 style="background:black;color:white;">BEHAVIORAL SCIENCE—ETHICS</h3>

Futility	If medical situation is futile, physician may refuse patient's or family's request for intervention or may spare the patient an invasive intervention. Strict futility defined: 1. Intervention does not make sense pathophysiologically 2. Maximal treatment is failing 3. The intervention has already failed the patient 4. Intervention will not achieve the goals of care	
Autonomy	Obligation to respect patients as individuals and to honor their preferences in medical care.	
Informed consent	Legally requires: 1. Discussion of pertinent information 2. Obtaining the patient's agreement to the plan of care 3. Freedom from coercion	Patients must understand the risks, benefits, and alternatives, which include no intervention.
Exceptions to informed consent	1. Patient lacks decision-making capacity (not legally competent) 2. Implied consent in an emergency 3. Therapeutic privilege—withholding information when disclosure would severely harm the patient or undermine informed decision-making capacity 4. Waiver—patient waives the right of informed consent	
Decision-making capacity	1. Patient makes and communicates a choice 2. Patient is informed 3. Decision is stable over time 4. Decisions consistent with patient's values and goals 5. Decisions not a result of delusions or hallucinations	The patient's family cannot require that a doctor withhold information from the patient.

Advance directives If medical situation is not futile but the patient is not capable of making an informed decision, is there an advance directive outlining the patient's wishes? If an advance directive does not exist, a physician may appoint and work with a surrogate decision maker.

Oral advance directive Incapacitated patient's prior oral statements commonly used as guide. Problems arise from variance in interpretation of these statements. However, if patient was informed, directive is specific, patient makes a choice, and decision is repeated over time, the oral directive is more valid.

Written advance directive
1. Living wills—Patient directs physician to withhold or withdraw life-sustaining treatment if the patient develops a terminal disease or enters a persistent vegetative state.
2. Durable power of attorney—Patient designates a surrogate to make medical decisions in the event that the patient loses decision-making capacity. Patient may also specify decisions in clinical situations. More flexible than a living will.

Nonmaleficence "Do no harm." However, if benefits of an intervention outweigh the risks, a patient may make an informed decision to proceed.

Beneficence Physicians have a special ethical responsibility to act in the patient's best interest (physician is a fiduciary). Patient autonomy may conflict with beneficence. If the patient makes an informed decision, ultimately the patient has the right to decide.

Confidentiality Confidentiality respects patient privacy and autonomy. Disclosing information to family and friends should be guided by what the patient would want. The patient may also waive the right to confidentiality (e.g., insurance companies).

Exceptions to confidentiality
1. Potential harm to third parties is serious
2. Likelihood of harm is high
3. No alternative means exist to warn or to protect those at risk
4. Third party can take steps to prevent harm
Examples include:
1. Infectious diseases—physicians may have a duty to warn public officials and identifiable people at risk
2. The Tarasoff decision—law requiring physician to protect potential victim from harm; may involve breach of confidentiality
3. Child and/or elder abuse
4. Impaired automobile drivers
5. Suicidal/homicidal patient
6. Domestic violence

Malpractice Civil suit under negligence requires:
1. Physician breach of duty to patient
2. Patient suffers harm
3. Breach of duty causes harm

The **4 D's: D**ereliction of **D**uty **D**irectly led to **D**amage

Anaclitic depression	Anaclitic depression = depression in an infant owing to continued separation from caregiver. Can result in failure to thrive. Infant becomes withdrawn and unresponsive.	*Ana* = against; *clitic* = lean.

Regression in children	Children regress to younger behavior under stress: physical illness, punishment, birth of a new sibling, tiredness. An example is bedwetting in a child when hospitalized.	

Infant deprivation effects	Long-term deprivation of affection results in: 1. Decreased muscle tone 2. Poor language skills 3. Poor socialization skills 4. Lack of basic trust 5. Anaclitic depression Severe deprivation can result in infant death.	Studied by René Spitz. The **4 W's: W**eak, **W**ordless, **W**anting (socially), **W**ary. Deprivation for longer than 6 months can lead to irreversible changes.

Developmental stages

	Infant	Toddler	Preschool	Latency	Adolescence	Early Adult	Mid-Adult	Late Adult
Piaget	Sensorimotor		Pre-operational	Concrete operational (conscience)	Formal operational (abstract concepts)			
Erikson	Trust vs. mistrust	Autonomy vs. doubt / shame	Initiative vs. guilt	Industry vs. inferiority	Identity vs. role confusion	Intimacy vs. isolation	Generativity vs. self-absorption	Ego integrity vs. despair
Freud	Oral	Anal	Phallic	Latency	Genital			
Age:	1	3	6	11	14 17 20		30	65

Developmental milestones

	Approximate age	Milestone
Infant	3 mo	Holds head up
	4–5 mo	Rolls front to back, sits when propped
	7 mo	Sits alone, orients to voice
	7–9 mo	Stranger anxiety
	15 mo	Walking, few words
Toddler	12–24 mo	Object permanence
	18–24 mo	Rapprochement
	24–30 mo	Parallel play
	24–36 mo	Core gender identity
Preschool	30–36 mo	Toilet training
	3 y	Group play
	4 y	Cooperative play
School age	6–11 y	Development of conscience (superego), same-sex friends, identification with same-sex parent
Adolescence (puberty)	11 y (girls) 13 y (boys)	Abstract reasoning (formal operations)

Kübler-Ross dying stages

Denial, **A**nger, **B**argaining, **G**rieving, **A**cceptance.

Death **A**rrives **B**ringing **G**rave **A**djustments.

Grief

Normal bereavement characterized by shock, denial, guilt and somatic symptoms. Typically lasts 6 mo–1 yr.

Pathologic grief includes excessively intense or prolonged grief, or grief that is delayed, inhibited or denied.

BEHAVIORAL SCIENCE—PHYSIOLOGY

Endorphins and enkephalins

Both have opiate-like activities, are blocked by naloxone, lose activity over time.

Enkephalins are pentapeptides (small).

β-endorphin (31 amino acids) is derived from POMC.

Endorphin = **End**ogenous m**orphine**. Also, Morpheus was the god of sleep.

Neurotransmitter changes with disease

Depression—decreased NE and serotonin (5-HT).

Alzheimer's dementia—decreased ACh.

Huntington's disease—decreased GABA, decreased ACh.

Bipolar affective disorder—decreased serotonin (5-HT).

Schizophrenia—increased dopamine.

Parkinson's disease—decreased dopamine.

Frontal lobe functions

Concentration, **O**rientation, **L**anguage, **A**bstraction, **J**udgment, **M**otor regulation, **M**ood.

Lack of social judgment is most notable in frontal lobe lesion.

COLA-JMM

Hypothalamic nuclei

Satiety	Ventromedial nucleus controls appetite.	Ablating **ventromedial** nucleus will cause you to grow **ventral**ly and **medial**ly (you get fat).
Hunger	Lateral nucleus	

Sleep stages

	Description	Waveform
0—eyes open	Awake, alert, active mental concentration	Beta (highest frequency, lowest amplitude)
0—eyes closed	Awake	Alpha
1 (5%)	Light sleep	Theta
2 (45%)	Deeper sleep	Sleep spindles and K-complexes
3–4 (25%)	Deepest, non-REM sleep; sleepwalking; night terrors, bedwetting (slow-wave sleep)	Delta (lowest frequency, highest amplitude)
REM (25%)	Dreaming, loss of motor tone, possibly memory processing function, erections, ↑ brain O_2 use	Beta

1. Serotonergic predominance of raphe nucleus key to initiating sleep
2. Norepinephrine reduces REM sleep
3. Extraocular movements during REM due to activity of PPRF (parapontine reticular formation/conjugate gaze center)
4. REM sleep having the same EEG pattern as while awake and alert has spawned the terms "paradoxical sleep" and "desynchronized sleep"
5. Benzodiazepines shorten stage 4 sleep; thus useful for night terrors and sleepwalking
6. Imipramine is used to treat enuresis since it decreases stage 4 sleep

REM sleep	Increased and variable pulse, rapid eye movements (REM), increased and variable blood pressure, penile/clitoral tumescence. 25% of total sleep. Occurs every 90 minutes; duration increases through the night. REM sleep decreases with age. Acetylcholine is the principal neurotransmitter involved in REM sleep.	REM sleep is like sex: ↑pulse, penile/clitoral tumescence, ↓ with age.
REM rebound	Body compensates for missed REM sleep. Drugs that decrease the amount of REM sleep (e.g., barbiturates, alcohol, phenothiazines, and MAO inhibitors) cause an increased amount of REM sleep after the specific drug is discontinued.	Benzodiazepines decrease the amount of REM sleep without causing REM rebound.
Sleep apnea	Central sleep apnea: no respiratory effort. Obstructive sleep apnea: respiratory effort against airway obstruction. Person stops breathing for at least 10 sec during sleep. Associated with obesity, loud snoring, systemic/pulmonary hypertension, arrhythmias, and possibly sudden death. Individuals may become chronically tired.	

Narcolepsy	Person falls asleep suddenly. May include hypnagogic (just before sleep) or hypnopompic (with awakening) hallucinations. The person's nocturnal and narcoleptic sleep episodes start off with REM sleep. Cataplexy (sudden collapse when awake) in some patients. Strong genetic component. Treat with stimulants (e.g., amphetamines).
Sleep patterns of depressed patients	Patients with depression typically have the following changes in their sleep stages: 1. Reduced slow-wave sleep 2. Decreased REM latency 3. Early morning waking (important screening question)

Sensory deprivation effects

1. Suppression of EEG
2. Decreased galvanic skin response
3. Decreased respiration
4. Increased urinary epinephrine

Seen in the ICU setting or after excessive studying.

Stress effects	Stress induces production of free fatty acids, 17-OH corticosteroids, lipids, cholesterol, catecholamines; affects water absorption, muscular tonicity, gastrocolic reflex, and mucosal circulation.

BEHAVIORAL SCIENCE—PSYCHIATRY

Forensic psychiatry	Confidentiality: breachable in child abuse, emergencies, communicable diseases. Good samaritan law protects roadside MD from malpractice liability. Involuntary hold: danger to self, others, unable to provide food/clothing/shelter.

Cultural/ethnic psychiatry

Specific diseases:
Amok = killing rampage (seen in southeast Asia).
Latah = echolalia, coprolalia (Malaysia).
Koro = fear of penile regression, death (seen in Chinese men).

The origin of "running amok."
Echolalia = repetition of another person's words or phrases.
Coprolalia = "filthy" language.

Orientation as to person

Is the patient aware of him- or herself as a person?
Does the patient know his or her own name?
Anosognosia = unaware that one is ill.
Autopagnosia = unable to locate one's own body parts.
Depersonalization = body seems unreal or dissociated.

Generally, the last thing to go (first = time, second = place, last = person).

Orientation as to place	Deficiency in orientation as to place, including jamais vu (person is in a familiar surrounding but feels he or she has never been there before) and déjà vu (person is in an unfamiliar situation and feels he or she has been there before).

Amnesia types	*Antero*grade amnesia is being unable to remember things that occurred after a CNS insult (no new memory).	*Antero* = after
	Korsakoff's amnesia is a classic anterograde amnesia that is caused by thiamine deficiency (bilateral destruction of the mamillary bodies), is seen in alcoholics, and is associated with confabulations.	
	*Retro*grade amnesia is being unable to remember things that occurred before a CNS insult.	*Retro* = before

Substance dependence

Maladaptive pattern of substance use.
Defined as 3 or more of the following signs in 1 year:
1. Tolerance
2. Withdrawal
3. Substance taken in larger amounts than intended
4. Persistent desire or attempts to cut down
5. Lots of energy spent trying to obtain substance
6. Important social, occupational, or recreational activities given up or reduced because of substance use
7. Use continued in spite of knowing the problems that it causes

Substance abuse

Maladaptive pattern leading to clinically significant impairment or distress. Symptoms have not met criteria for substance dependence. One or more of the following in 1 year:
1. Recurrent use resulting in failure to fulfill major obligations at work, school, or home
2. Recurrent use in physically hazardous situations
3. Recurrent substance-related legal problems
4. Continued use in spite of persistent problems caused by use

Signs and symptoms of substance abuse

Drug	Intoxication	Withdrawal
Alcohol	Disinhibition, emotional lability, incoordination, slurred speech, ataxia, coma, blackouts (retrograde amnesia).	Tremor, tachycardia, hypertension, malaise, nausea, seizures, delirium tremens (DTs), tremulousness, agitation, hallucinations.
Opioids	CNS depression, nausea and vomiting, constipation, pupillary constriction, seizures (overdose is life-threatening).	Anxiety, insomnia, anorexia, sweating/piloerection ("cold turkey"), fever, rhinorrhea, nausea, stomach cramps, diarrhea ("flu-like" symptoms). *hallucinations?*
Amphetamines	Psychomotor agitation, impaired judgment, pupillary dilation, hypertension, tachycardia, euphoria, prolonged wakefulness and attention, cardiac arrhythmias, delusions, hallucinations, fever.	Post-use "crash," including anxiety, lethargy, headache, stomach cramps, hunger, severe depression, dysphoric mood, fatigue, insomnia/hypersomnia.
Cocaine	Euphoria, psychomotor agitation, impaired judgment, tachycardia, pupillary dilation, hypertension, hallucinations (including tactile), paranoid ideations, angina and sudden cardiac death.	Hypersomnolence, fatigue, depression, malaise, severe craving, suicidality.
PCP	Belligerence, impulsiveness, fever, psychomotor agitation, vertical and horizontal nystagmus, tachycardia, ataxia, homicidality, psychosis, delirium.	Recurrence of symptoms due to reabsorption in GI tract; sudden onset of severe, random, homicidal violence.
LSD	Marked anxiety or depression, delusions, visual hallucinations, flashbacks.	
Marijuana	Euphoria, anxiety, paranoid delusions, perception of slowed time, impaired judgment, social withdrawal, increased appetite, dry mouth, hallucinations.	
Barbiturates	Low safety margin, respiratory depression.	Anxiety, seizures, delirium, life-threatening cardiovascular collapse.
Benzodiazepines	Amnesia, ataxia, somnolence, minor respiratory depression. Additive effects with alcohol.	Rebound anxiety, seizures, tremor, insomnia.
Caffeine	Restlessness, insomnia, increased diuresis, muscle twitching, cardiac arrhythmias.	Headache, lethargy, depression, weight gain.
Nicotine	Restlessness, insomnia, anxiety, arrhythmias.	Irritability, headache, anxiety, weight gain, craving, tachycardia.

Delirium tremens   Severe alcohol withdrawal syndrome that peaks 2–5 d after last drink.
Confusion, delusions, hallucinations, autonomic system hyperactivity, tremors.

Delirium	Decreased attention span and level of arousal, disorganized thinking, hallucination, illusions, misperceptions, disturbance in sleep–wake cycle, cognitive dysfunction.	Deli**rium** = changes in senso**rium**
	Key to diagnosis: waxing and waning level of consciousness, develops rapidly.	Most common psychiatric illness on medical and surgical floors. Often reversible.
	Often due to substance use/abuse or medical illness.	

| **Dementia** | Development of multiple cognitive deficits: memory, aphasia, apraxia, agnosia, loss of abstract thought, behavioral/personality changes, impaired judgment. | De**mem**tia characterized by **mem**ory loss. Commonly irreversible. |
| | Key to diagnosis: rule out delirium—patient is alert, no change in level of consciousness. More often gradual onset. | |

Major depressive episode

Characterized by 5 of the following for 2 weeks, including (1) depressed mood or (2) anhedonia:

1. **S**leep disturbances   **SIG: E**nergy **CAPS**ules
2. Loss of **I**nterest
3. **G**uilt
4. Loss of **E**nergy
5. Loss of **C**oncentration
6. Change in **A**ppetite
7. **P**sychomotor retardation
8. **S**uicidal ideations
9. Depressed mood

Major depressive disorder, recurrent—requires 2 or more episodes with a symptom-free interval of 2 months.

Manic episode

Distinct period of abnormally and persistently elevated, expansive or irritable mood lasting at least 1 week. During mood disturbance, 3 or more of the following:

1. **D**istractibility   **DIG FAST**
2. **I**nsomnia: ↓ need for sleep
3. **G**randiosity: inflated self-esteem
4. **F**light of ideas
5. Increase in goal-directed **A**ctivity/psychomotor agitation
6. Pressured **S**peech
7. **T**houghtlessness: seeks pleasure without regard to consequences

Hypomanic episode

Like manic episode except mood disturbance not severe enough to cause marked impairment in social and/or occupational functioning or to necessitate hospitalization, and there are no psychotic features.

Bipolar disorder

Six separate criteria sets exist for bipolar I disorders with combinations of manic, hypomanic, and depressed episodes. Lithium is drug of choice. Different studies have linked bipolar disorder to chromosomes X, 11, 18, and 23.

Cyclothymic disorder

A period of at least 2 years with hypomanic symptoms and depressive symptoms that do not meet criteria for major depressive episode.

Malingering

Patient fakes or claims to have a disorder in order to attain a specific gain (e.g., financial).

Factitious disorder

Consciously creates symptoms in order to assume "sick role" and to get medical attention. Also known as Münchausen syndrome. Münchausen syndrome by proxy typically seen in a child; caused by the parent.

Somatoform disorders

Several types:
1. Conversion—symptoms suggest neurologic or physical disorder but tests and physical exam are negative
2. Somatoform pain disorder—conversion disorder with pain as presenting complaint
3. Hypochondriasis—misinterpretation of normal physical findings, leading to preoccupation with and fear of having a serious illness in spite of medical reassurance
4. Somatization—variety of complaints in multiple organ systems
5. Body dysmorphic disorder—patient convinced that part of own anatomy is malformed
6. Pseudocyesis—false belief of being pregnant associated with objective signs of pregnancy

Gain: 1°, 2°, 3°

1° gain = what the symptom does for the patient's internal psychic economy.
2° gain = what the symptom gets the patient (sympathy, attention).
3° gain = what the caretaker gets (like an MD on an interesting case).

Panic disorder

Discrete periods of intense fear or discomfort peaking in 10 minutes with 4 of the following:
1. Palpitations, racing heart
2. Sweating
3. Trembling
4. Shortness of breath
5. Choking feeling
6. Chest pain/discomfort
7. Nausea/abdominal distress
8. Dizziness, faintness, lightheadedness
9. Derealization
10. Fear of losing control
11. Fear of dying
12. Paresthesias
13. Chills or hot flashes

Panic disorder must be diagnosed in context of occurrence (e.g., panic disorder with agoraphobia). High prevalence during Step 1 exam.

Specific phobia

Fear that is excessive or unreasonable, cued by presence or anticipation of a specific object or entity. Exposure provokes anxiety response. Person (not necessarily children) recognizes fear is excessive. Fear interferes with normal routine. Treatment options include systematic desensitization.

Social phobia

Fear of one or more social performance situations. Person fears acting in a way that is embarrassing or humiliating.

Obsession	Recurrent, intrusive and persistent thoughts, impulses, or images that cannot be ignored or suppressed by logical effort. Associated with anxiety.					

Obsession — Recurrent, intrusive and persistent thoughts, impulses, or images that cannot be ignored or suppressed by logical effort. Associated with anxiety.

Compulsion — Repetitive behaviors or mental acts that person feels driven to perform. Committing act produces transient relief from anxiety.

Obsessive-compulsive disorder — Obsessions and compulsions. Patient may have poor insight. Treatment options include clomipramine, fluvoxamine, paroxetine, behavioral therapy, and insight-based psychotherapy.

Post-traumatic stress disorder — Person experienced or witnessed event that involved actual or threatened death or serious injury. Response involves intense fear, helplessness, or horror. Traumatic event is persistently reexperienced, and person persistently avoids stimuli associated with the trauma. Person experiences persistent symptoms of increased arousal. Disturbance lasts longer than 1 month and causes distress or social/occupational impairment.

Personality — Personality trait—an enduring pattern of perceiving, relating to, and thinking about the environment and oneself that is exhibited in a wide range of important social and personal contexts.
Personality disorder—when these patterns become inflexible and maladaptive, causing impairment in social or occupational functioning or subjective distress.

Personality types-enneagram — A dynamic personality typology (developed by Oscar Ichazo and refined by Richard Riso, Russ Hudson, and Helen Palmer) that describes nine distinct patterns of thinking and acting based on distinct motivations. Describes a continuum of healthy, average, and unhealthy function (approximate DSM-IV) within each personality type.

#	Riso label	Palmer label	Key traits (healthy and average function)	Gift	Unconscious drive	Approximate DSM-IV correlates (unhealthy)
1	Reformer	Perfectionist	Principled, orderly, perfectionistic and self-righteous	Discernment	Anger	Compulsive and depressive
2	Helper	Giver	Caring, generous, possessive and manipulative	Empathy	Pride	Histrionic
3	Motivator	Performer	Adaptable, ambitious, image-conscious and arrogant	Efficacy	Self-deceit	Narcissistic
4	Individualist	Romantic	Intuitive, expressive, self-absorbed and self-indulgent	Equanimity	Envy	Avoidant, depressive, narcissistic
5	Investigator	Observer	Perceptive, original, detached and eccentric	Detachment	Avarice	Schizoid, avoidant, schizotypal
6	Loyalist	Trooper	Engaging, committed, defensive and suspicious	Loyalty	Fear/doubt	Paranoid, dependent, passive-aggressive
7	Enthusiast	Epicure	Enthusiastic, accomplished, uninhibited and excessive	Optimism	Gluttony	Manic-depressive, histrionic
8	Leader	Boss	Self-confident, decisive, dominating and confrontational	Strength	Lust (excess)	Antisocial
9	Peacemaker	Mediator	Peaceful, reassuring, complacent and neglectful	Acceptance	Sloth	Dependent, schizoid, passive-aggressive

Personality types—Myers–Briggs	A personality typology originating from Carl Jung and further developed by Isabel Myers; based on four axis of personality traits.
	For each axis, one characteristic is dominant (thus, there are 16 possible types, such as E-N-T-J and I-N-T-P).

	Extroversion (from outside world)/**I**ntroversion (from internal world)	How a person is energized.
	Sensing (five senses)/**IN**tuition (unconscious perceiving)	What a person pays attention to.
	Thinking (logical and objective)/**F**eeling (personal value oriented)	How a person makes decisions.
	Judgement (organized life)/**P**erception (spontaneous life)	Lifestyle adopted by a person.

Cluster A *eccentric* **personality disorder**	Paranoid, schizoid, schizotypal
	Characteristics: paranoid, suspicious, social isolation, odd beliefs, shy, withdrawn, impoverished personal relationships.
	Clinical dilemma: patient is suspicious of and does not trust doctor.

Cluster B *dramatic* **personality disorder**	Borderline, histrionic, narcissistic, antisocial
	Characteristics: dramatic, self-indulgent, hostile, aggressive, exploitative relationships, attention seeking.
	Clinical dilemma: patient changes rules on doctor. Clingy and demands attention. Feels that he/she is VIP and special. Manipulates doctor. Narcissist demands "best specialist in the country."

Cluster C **personality disorder**	Obsessive-compulsive, avoidant, dependent, passive–aggressive
	Characteristics: fear of doing wrong thing, anxiety repressed, regulations, unable to express affect.
	Clinical dilemma: patient may subtly sabotage his/her own treatment. Person is very controlling.

Hallucination versus illusion versus delusion	Hallucinations are perceptions in the absence of external stimuli.
	Illusions are misinterpretations of actual external stimuli.
	Delusions are false beliefs not shared with other members of culture/subculture that are firmly maintained in spite of obvious proof to the contrary.

Delusion vs. loose association	A delusion is a disorder in the content of thought (the actual idea).
	A loose association is a disorder in the form of thought (the way ideas are tied together).

Hallucination types	Visual hallucination is common in acute organic brain syndrome.
	Auditory hallucination is common in schizophrenia.
	Olfactory hallucination often occurs as an aura of a psychomotor epilepsy.
	Gustatory hallucination is rare.
	Tactile hallucination (e.g., formication) is common in delirium tremens. Also seen in cocaine abusers ("cocaine bugs").
	Hypnagogic hallucination occurs while going to sleep.
	Hypnopompic hallucination occurs while waking from sleep.

Schizophrenia

Waxing and waning vulnerability to psychosis.

Positive symptoms: hallucinations, delusions, strange behavior, loose associations.

Negative symptoms: flat affect, social withdrawal, thought blocking, lack of motivation.

The **4 A's** described by Bleuler:
1. **A**mbivalence (uncertainty)
2. **A**utism (self-preoccupation and lack of communication)
3. **A**ffect (blunted)
4. **A**ssociations (loose)

Fifth A should be **A**uditory hallucinations.

Genetic factors outweigh environmental factors in the etiology of schizophrenia.

Lifetime prevalence = 1.5% (males = females, blacks = whites). Presents earlier in men.

Five subtypes:
1. Disorganized
2. Catatonic
3. Paranoid
4. Undifferentiated
5. Residual

Schizoaffective disorder: a combination of schizophrenia and a mood disorder.

Antipsychotic mechanism

Antipsychotics most commonly work by blocking dopamine (D_2 and probably D_4) receptors. Examples: haloperidol, chlorpromazine, thiothixene.

Phobias

More than 100, so use etymology to figure them out.
Examples include:
Gamophobia (*gam* = gamete) = fear of marriage.
Algophobia (*alg* = pain) = fear of pain.
Acrophobia (*acro* = height) = fear of heights.
Agoraphobia (*agora* = open market) = fear of open places.

Systematic desensitization is a treatment used for phobias.

Electroconvulsive therapy

ECT

Treatment option for major depressive disorder. ECT is painless and produces a seizure with transient memory loss and disorientation. Complications can result from anesthesia. The major adverse effect of ECT is retrograde amnesia.

BEHAVIORAL SCIENCE—PSYCHOLOGY

Structural theory of the mind

Freud's three structures of the mind:

Id	Primal urges, sex, and aggression. (I want it.)
Superego	Moral values, conscience. (You know you can't have it.)
Ego	Bridge and mediator between the unconscious mind and the external world. (Deals with the conflict.)

Ego defenses

All ego defenses are automatic and unconscious reactions to psychological stress.

	Description	Example
Acting out	Unacceptable feelings and thoughts are expressed through actions.	Tantrums.
Denial	Avoidance of awareness of some painful reality.	A common reaction in newly diagnosed AIDS and cancer patients.
Displacement	Process whereby avoided ideas and feelings are transferred to some neutral person or object.	Seen in dreams (e.g., murderous wishes toward mother are redirected at crossing guard in dream).
Dissociation	Temporary, drastic change in personality, memory, consciousness, or motor behavior to avoid emotional stress.	Extreme forms can result in multiple personalities (dissociative identity disorder).
Fixation	Partially remaining at a more childish level of development.	
Identification	Modeling behavior after another person.	Spouse develops symptoms that deceased patient had.
Isolation (of affect)	Separation of feelings from ideas and events.	Describing murder in graphic detail with no emotional response.
Projection	An unacceptable internal impulse is attributed to an external source.	Common in paranoid states.
Rationalization	Proclaiming logical reasons for actions actually performed for other reasons, usually to avoid self-blame.	
Reaction formation	Process whereby a warded-off idea or feeling is replaced by an (unconsciously derived) emphasis on its opposite.	A patient with libidinous thoughts enters a monastery.
Regression	Turning back the maturational clock and going back to earlier modes of dealing with the world.	Seen in children under stress (e.g., bedwetting) and in patients on peritoneal dialysis.
Repression	Involuntary withholding of an idea or feeling from conscious awareness.	
Sublimation	Process whereby one replaces an unacceptable wish with a course of action that is similar to the wish but does not conflict with one's value system.	Aggressive impulses used to succeed in business ventures.
Suppression	Voluntary (unlike other defenses) withholding of an idea or feeling from conscious awareness.	

"mature" - may deal of feelings later.

Oedipus complex	Repressed sexual feelings of a child for the opposite-sex parent, accompanied by rivalry with same-sex parent. First described by Freud.
Sick role	Exempts sick person from duties, allows person to expect care and sympathy, and obligates sick person to try to get well (i.e., working toward being healthy, cooperation with health care personnel in getting well, and compliance with the treatment regimen).
Dyad	A pair of people within an interactional situation (e.g., husband–wife, mother–child, therapist–patient). *often w/in families. (Breakdown of communication → system triangles*
Factors in hopelessness	Four dynamic factors in the development of hopelessness: **IGAD!** *w/ allianced oppositions* 1. Sense of **I**mpotence (powerlessness) 2. Sense of **G**uilt 3. Sense of **A**nger 4. Sense of loss/**D**eprivation leading to depression
Conditioners: fear	Moderate fear is better than severe or mild fear in changing behavior.	As in studying for big exams.
Classical conditioning	Learning in which a response (salivation) is elicited by a conditioned stimulus (bell) that previously was presented in conjunction with an unconditioned stimulus (food).	Programmed by habit, without any element of reward. As in Pavlov's **classical** experiments with dogs (ringing the bell provoked salivation).
Operant conditioning	Learning in which a particular action is elicited because it produces a reward.	Voluntary action and a reward.

Reinforcement schedules

Continuous	Shows the most rapid extinction when discontinued.	This explains why people can get addicted to slot machines at casinos and yet get upset when vending machines don't work.
Variable ratio	Shows the slowest extinction when discontinued.	

Gestalt therapy	Stresses treatment of the whole person, highlights sensory awareness of the here and now, uses role playing. Developed by Friedrich Perls.
Psychoanalysis	A form of insight therapy—intensive, lengthy, costly, great demands on patient, developed by Freud. May be appropriate for changing chronic character problems.
Topography (in psychoanalysis)	Conscious = what you are aware of. Preconscious = what you are able to make conscious with effort (like your phone number). Unconscious = what you are not aware of; the central goal of Freudian psychotherapy is to make the patient aware of what is hidden in his/her unconscious.

Existential psychotherapy	Emphasis on confrontation and feeling experiences; each individual is responsible for his or her own existence.

Intelligence testing

Stanford–Binet and Wechsler are the most famous tests.

Mean is defined at 100, with standard deviation of 15.

IQ lower than 70 (or 2 standard deviations below the mean) is one of the criteria for diagnosis of mental retardation.

IQ scores are correlated with genetic factors but are more highly correlated with school achievement.

Intelligence tests are objective (not projective) tests.

Projective tests

Projective tests use ambiguous stimuli.

Examples: Rorschach (ink blot), TAT, sentence completion, word association, draw-a-person.

The patient projects his or her personality into the test.

Sexual dysfunction

Differential diagnosis includes:

1. Drugs (e.g., antihypertensives, neuroleptics, ethanol)
2. Diseases (e.g., depression, diabetes)
3. Psychological (e.g., performance anxiety)

Changes in the elderly

1. Sexual changes

   Men: slower erection/ejaculation, longer refractory period

   Women: vaginal shortening, thinning, and dryness; sexual interest does not decrease
2. Sleep patterns: $\downarrow$ REM sleep, $\downarrow$ slow-wave sleep, $\uparrow$ sleep latency
3. Common medical conditions: arthritis, hypertension, heart disease
4. Suicide rate increases
5. Psychiatric problems (e.g., depression) become more prevalent

These abstracted case vignettes are designed to demonstrate the thought processes necessary to answer multistep clinical reasoning questions.

- Woman with anxiety about a gynecologic exam is told to relax and to imagine going through the steps of the exam → what process does this exemplify? → systematic desensitization.
- Diabetic who misses doses of insulin is using what defense mechanism? *denial*
- 65-year-old man is diagnosed with incurable, metastatic pancreatic adenocarcinoma → his family asks you, the doctor, not to tell the patient → what do you do? → talk to the family and then tell the patient.
- Husband claims that his wife is having an affair. His only evidence is a blank piece of paper and a prank phone call → what psychological problem is he likely to have? *delusional disorder / paranoid schizophrenia*
- Man admitted for chest pain is medicated for ventricular tachycardia. The next day he jumps out of bed and does 50 pushups to show the nurses he has not had a heart attack → what defense mechanism is he using? → denial or reaction formation.
- A large group of people is followed over 10 years. Every two years, it is determined who develops heart disease and who does not → what type of study is this? → cohort study.
- Girl can speak in complete sentences, has an imaginary friend, and considers boys "yucky" → how old is she? → 6–11 years old.
- Man has flashbacks about his girlfriend's death two months following a hit-and-run accident. He often cries and wishes for the death of the culprit → what is the diagnosis? → normal bereavement.
- During a particular stage of sleep, man has variable blood pressure, penile tumescence, and variable EEG → what stage of sleep is he in? → REM sleep.
- Fellow medical student has recently been missing morning classes, is becoming disheveled in his appearance, and gets obnoxiously drunk at parties → what should be done first? → tell student to get counseling.
- 11-year-old girl exhibits Tanner stage 4 sexual development (almost full breasts and pubic hair) → what is the diagnosis? → advanced stage, early in her development.
- Man consistently wakes up early in the morning and has had anhedonia since several relatives died over the last year. Despite his friends' suggestions that he get counseling, the man insists that he has "lost his wind" and seeks medication for GI upset → what is the reason for his actions? → fear of being labeled mentally ill.
- Person demands only the best and most famous doctor in town → what is the personality disorder? → narcissistic. *Hardly; pretty common among those of $/power.*
- 10-year-old kid "spaces out" in class (e.g., stops talking midsentence and then continues as if nothing happened). During spells, there is slight quivering of lips → what is the diagnosis? → absence seizure. *— ethosuximide*

Epidemiology/Biostatistics

1. Differences in the incidence of disease among various ethnic groups.
2. Leading causes and types of cancers in men versus women.
3. Prevalence of common psychiatric disorders (e.g., alcoholism, major depression, schizophrenia).
4. Differences in death rates among ethnic and racial groups.
5. Definitions of morbidity, mortality, and case fatality rate.
6. Epidemiology of cigarette smoking, including prevalence and success rates for quitting.
7. Modes of human immunodeficiency virus (HIV) transmission among different populations (e.g., perinatal, heterosexual, homosexual, intravenous).
8. Simple pedigree analysis (understand symbols) for inheritance of genetic diseases (e.g., counseling, risk assessment).
9. Different types of studies (e.g., randomized clinical trial, cohort, case series).
10. Definition and use of standard deviation, p value, r value, mean, mode, and median.
11. Effects of changing a test's criteria on number of false positives and number of false negatives.

Neurophysiology

1. Physiologic changes (e.g., neurotransmitter levels) in common neuropsychiatric disorders (e.g., Alzheimer's disease, Huntington's disease, schizophrenia, bipolar disorder).
2. Changes in cerebrospinal fluid composition with common psychiatric diseases (e.g., depression).
3. Physiologic, physical, and psychologic changes associated with aging (e.g., memory, lung capacity, glomerular filtration rate, muscle mass, pharmacokinetics of drugs).
4. Differences between anterior and posterior lobes of the pituitary gland (e.g., embryology, innervation, hormones).

Psychiatry/Psychology

1. Indicators of prognosis in psychiatric disorders (e.g., schizophrenia, bipolar disorder).
2. Genetic components of common psychiatric disorders (e.g., schizophrenia, bipolar disorder).
3. Diseases associated with different personality types.
4. Clinical features and treatment of phobias.
5. Clinical features of child abuse (shaken-baby syndrome).
6. Clinical features of common learning disorders (e.g., dyslexia, mental retardation).
7. Therapeutic application of learning theories (e.g., classical and operant conditioning) to psychiatric illnesses (e.g., disulfiram therapy for alcoholics).
8. Problems associated with the physician–patient relationship (e.g., reasons for patient noncompliance).
9. Management of the suicidal patient.
10. Addiction: risk factors, family history, behavior, factors contributing to relapse.
11. How physicians and medical students should help peers with substance abuse problems.

Biochemistry

This high-yield material includes molecular biology, genetics, cell biology, and principles of metabolism (especially vitamins, cofactors, minerals and single-enzyme-deficiency diseases). The topics are especially high-yield and are worth learning in detail. When studying metabolic pathways, emphasize important regulatory steps and enzyme deficiencies that result in disease. For example, understanding the defect in Lesch-Nyhan syndrome and its clinical consequences is higher yield than memorizing every intermediate in the purine salvage pathway. Do not spend time on hard-core organic chemistry, mechanisms, and physical chemistry. Detailed chemical structures are infrequently tested. Familiarity with the latest biochemical techniques that have medical relevance—such as enzyme-linked immunosorbent assay (ELISA), immunoelectrophoresis, Southern blotting, and PCR—is useful. Beware if you placed out of your medical school's biochemistry class, for the emphasis of the test differs from the emphasis of many undergraduate courses. Review the related biochemistry when studying pharmacology or genetic diseases as a way to reinforce and integrate the material.

DNA and RNA
Genetic Errors
Metabolism
Protein/Cell
Vitamins
High-Yield Topics

Chromatin structure

Condensed by (−) charged DNA looped twice around (+) charged H2A, H2B, H3, and H4 histones (nucleosome bead). **H1** ties nucleosomes together in a string (30-nm fiber). In mitosis, DNA condenses to form mitotic chromosomes.

Think of beads on a string.

Heterochromatin	Condensed, transcriptionally inactive.
Euchromatin	Less condensed, transcriptionally active.

Eu = true, "truly transcribed."

Nucleotides

Purines (**A, G**) have two rings. Pyrimidines (**C, T, U**) have one ring. Guanine has a ketone. Thymine has a methyl. Uracil found in RNA; thymine in DNA.
G-C bond (3 H-bonds) stronger than A-T bond (2 H-bonds).

CUT the **PY** (pie): **PY**rimidines.
PURe **A**s **G**old: **PUR**ines.
THYmine has a me**THY**l.
Crypts (**C**ytosine) and **T**ombs (**T**hymine) are found **U**nder (**U**racil) the **P**yramids (**P**yrimidines).

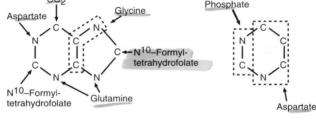

AUG codon

AUG (or rarely GUG) is the mRNA initiation codon. AUG codes for methionine, which may be removed before translation is completed. In prokaryotes the initial AUG codes for a formyl-**met**hionine (**f-met**).

AUG in**AUG**urates protein synthesis.

Genetic code: features

Unambiguous = each codon specifies only one amino acid.
Degenerate = more than one codon may code for same amino acid.
Commaless, nonoverlapping (except some viruses).
Universal (exceptions include mitochondria, archaebacteria, *Mycoplasma*, and some yeasts).

Mutations in DNA

Silent = same aa, often base change in third position of codon.
Missense = changed aa. (Conservative = new aa is similar in chemical structure.)
Nonsense = change resulting in early stop codon.
Frameshift = change resulting in misreading of all nucleotides downstream, usually resulting in a truncated protein.

Severity of damage: nonsense > missense > silent.

Transition versus transversion

Transition = substituting purine for purine or pyrimidine for pyrimidine.
Transversion = substituting purine for pyrimidine or vice versa.

Transversion = **Trans**conversion (one type to another).

DNA replication

Origin of replication: continuous DNA synthesis on leading strand and discontinuous (Okazaki fragments) on lagging strand. DNA polymerase reaches primer of preceding fragment; 5′ → 3′ exonuclease activity of DNA polymerase degrades RNA; DNA ligase seals; 3′ → 5′ exonuclease activity of DNA polymerase "proofreads" each added nucleotide.

Eukaryotic genome has multiple origins of replication. Bacteria, viruses, and plasmids have only one origin of replication.

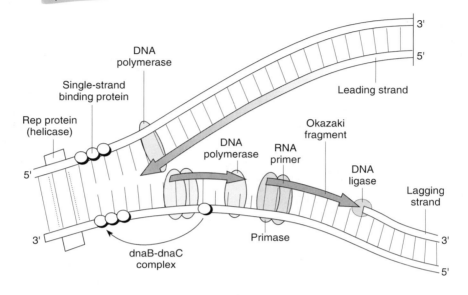

Polymerases: DNA

Functions in *E. coli:*
DNA polymerase I removes RNA primers, fills gaps, and participates in repair.
DNA polymerase II function is unknown.
DNA polymerase III (holoenzyme) elongates most efficiently, makes bulk of DNA (high fidelity).

Enzymes that proofread cannot initiate (because initiation is a sloppy process). **Primase** makes an RNA **primer** on which DNA polymerase can initiate replication.

Polymerase chain reaction (PCR)

Molecular biology laboratory procedure that is used to synthesize many copies of a desired fragment of DNA.

Steps:
1. DNA is denatured by heating to generate 2 separate strands
2. During cooling, excess of premade primers anneal to a specific sequence on each strand to be amplified
3. Heat-stable DNA polymerase replicates the DNA sequence following each primer

These steps are repeated multiple times for DNA sequence amplification.

GENETIC DISEASES DETECTABLE BY PCR

Disease	Gene
SCID	Adenosine deaminase
Lesch–Nyhan syndrome	HGPRT
Cystic fibrosis	CFTR
Familial hypercholesterolemia	LDL-R
Retinoblastoma	Rb
Sickle cell anemia and β-thalassemia	β-globin gene
Hemophilia A and B	Factor VIII (A) and IX (B)
Von Willebrand's disease	VWF
Lysosomal storage diseases	See "sphingolipidoses" on p. 130
Glycogen storage diseases	See p. 128

Molecular biology techniques

Southern blot — A **DNA** sample is electrophoresed on a gel and then transferred to a filter. The filter is then soaked in a denaturant and subsequently exposed to a labeled DNA probe that recognizes and anneals to its complementary strand. The resulting double-stranded labeled piece of DNA is visualized when the filter is exposed to film.
DNA–DNA hybridization
Southern = **S**ame

Northern blot — Similar technique, except that Northern blotting involves radioactive DNA probe binding to sample **RNA.**
DNA–RNA hybridization

Western blot — Sample protein is separated via gel electrophoresis and transferred to a filter. Labeled antibody is used to bind to relevant **protein.**
Antibody–protein hybridization

Southwestern blot — Protein sample is run on a gel, transferred to a filter, and exposed to labeled DNA. Used to detect DNA–protein interactions as with transcription factors (e.g., p53, *jun*).
DNA–protein interaction

DNA repair: single strand	Single-strand, excision-repair–specific glycosylase recognizes and removes damaged base. Endonuclease makes a break several bases to the 5′ side. Exonuclease removes short stretch of nucleotides. DNA polymerase fills gap. DNA ligase seals.	If both strands are damaged, repair may proceed via recombination with undamaged homologous chromosome.
DNA/RNA synthesis direction	DNA and RNA are both synthesized $5′ \rightarrow 3′$. Remember that the 5′ of the incoming nucleotide bears the triphosphate (energy source for bond). The 3′ hydroxyl of the nascent chain is the target.	Imagine the incoming nucleotide bringing a gift (triphosphate) to the 3′ host. **"BYOP** (phosphate) from **5** to **3.″**
Polymerases: RNA	**Eukaryotes:** RNA polymerase I makes **r**RNA. RNA polymerase II makes **m**RNA. RNA polymerase III makes **t**RNA. No proofreading function, but can initiate chains. RNA polymerase II opens DNA at promoter site (A-T-rich upstream sequence—TATA and CAAT). α-amanitin inhibits RNA polymerase II. **Prokaryotes:** RNA polymerase makes all three kinds of RNA.	I, II, and III are numbered as their products are used in protein synthesis. Or I, II, III = remote. OR **1, 2, 3 = RMT** (rhyme).

Regulation of gene expression

Promoter	Site where RNA polymerase and multiple other transcription factors bind to DNA upstream from gene locus.	Promoter mutation commonly results in dramatic decrease in amount of gene transcribed.
Enhancer	Stretch of DNA that alters gene expression by binding transcription factors. May be located close to, far from, or even within (in an intron) the gene whose expression it regulates.	

Introns versus exons	Exons contain the actual genetic information coding for protein. Introns are intervening noncoding segments of DNA.	**INT**rons **INT**errupt (or **INT**ervene). **IN**trons stay **IN** the nucleus whereas **EX**ons **EX**it and are **EX**pressed.
Types of RNA	mRNA is the **largest** type of RNA. rRNA is the most **abundant** type of RNA. tRNA is the **smallest** type of RNA.	**M**assive, **R**ampant, **T**iny.
Splicing of mRNA	Introns are precisely spliced out of primary mRNA transcripts. A lariat-shaped intermediate is formed. Small nuclear ribonucleoprotein particles (snRNP) facilitate splicing by binding to primary mRNA transcripts and forming spliceosomes.	*Lariat* = lasso.

RNA processing (eukaryotes)

Occurs in nucleus. After transcription:
1. Capping on 5′ end (7-methyl-G)
2. Polyadenylation on 3′ end (≈200 A's)
3. Splicing out of introns occurs

Initial transcript is called heterogeneous nuclear RNA (hnRNA).

Capped and tailed transcript is called mRNA. w/ exons removed

Only processed RNA is transported out of the nucleus. The cap goes on a head (the beginning of the strand) and the polyA tail goes at the end of the strand.

---

tRNA structure

75–90 nucleotides, cloverleaf form, anticodon end is opposite 3′ aminoacyl end. All tRNAs, both eukaryotic and prokaryotic, have CCA at 3′ end along with a high percentage of chemically modified bases. The amino acid is covalently bound to the 3′ end of the tRNA.

---

tRNA charging

Aminoacyl-tRNA synthetase (one per aa, uses ATP) scrutinizes aa before and after it binds to tRNA. If incorrect, bond is hydrolyzed by synthetase. The aa-tRNA bond has energy for formation of peptide bond. A mischarged tRNA reads usual codon but inserts wrong amino acid.

Aminoacyl-tRNA synthetase and binding of charged tRNA to the codon are responsible for accuracy of amino acid selection.

---

tRNA wobble

Third nucleotide of mRNA codon "wobble" pairs, allowing formation of non–Watson-Crick base pairs. A tRNA normally reads one to three specific codons— but each codon it reads designates the same one amino acid. Economizes number of tRNAs needed.

"G-U" is wobble ("gee, you wobble"), rest is standard A-U and G-C. Inosine has three-way wobble: I-U, I-C, or I-A.

Modes of inheritance

Autosomal dominant

50% of offspring inherit disease. Often due to defects in structural genes. Many generations, both male and female, affected.

Often pleiotropic and, in many cases, present clinically after puberty. Family history crucial to diagnosis.

Autosomal recessive

25% of offspring from 2 carrier parents are affected. Often due to enzyme deficiencies. Usually seen in only one generation.

Commonly more severe than dominant disorders; patients often present in childhood.

X-linked recessive

Sons of heterozygous mothers have a 50% chance of being affected. No male-to male transmission.

Commonly more severe in males. Heterozygous females may be affected.

Mitochondrial inheritance

Transmitted only through mother. All offspring of affected females may show signs of disease.

Leber's hereditary optic neuropathy, mitochondrial myopathies.

Genetic terms

Variable expression	Nature and severity of the phenotype varies from one individual to another.
Incomplete penetrance	Not all individuals with a mutant genotype show the mutant phenotype.
Pleiotropy	One gene has more than one effect on an individual's phenotype.
Imprinting	Differences in phenotype depend on whether the mutation is of maternal or paternal origin (e.g., Angelman's syndrome [maternal], Prader-Willi syndrome [paternal]).
Anticipation	Severity of disease worsens or age of onset of disease is earlier in succeeding generations (e.g., Huntington's disease).
Loss of heterozygosity	If a patient inherits or develops a mutation in a tumor suppressor gene, the complementary allele must be deleted/mutated before cancer develops. This is not true of oncogenes.

DNA repair defects

Xeroderma pigmentosum (skin sensitivity to UV light), ataxia-telangiectasia (x-rays), Bloom's syndrome (radiation), and Fanconi's anemia (cross-linking agents).

Xeroderma pigmentosum

Defective excision repair such as uvr ABC exonuclease. Results in inability to repair thymidine dimers, which form in DNA when exposed to UV light.

Associated with dry skin and with melanoma and other cancers.

Fructose intolerance

Hereditary deficiency of aldolase B. Fructose-1-phosphate accumulates, causing a decrease in available phosphate, which results in inhibition of glycogenolysis and gluconeogenesis, thus causing severe hypoglycemia.

Must decrease intake of both fructose and sucrose (glucose + fructose).

Galactosemia

Absence of galactose-1-phosphate uridyltransferase. Autosomal recessive. Damage is caused by accumulation of toxic substances (including galactitol) rather than absence of an essential compound.

Symptoms: cataracts, hepatosplenomegaly, mental retardation.

Treatment: exclude galactose and lactose (galactose + glucose) from diet.

Lactase deficiency

Age-dependent and/or hereditary lactose intolerance (blacks, Asians).

Symptoms: bloating, cramps, osmotic diarrhea.

Treatment: avoid milk or add lactase pills to diet.

Pyruvate dehydrogenase deficiency

Causes backup of substrate (pyruvate and alanine), resulting in lactic acidosis.

Findings: neurologic defects.

Treatment: increased intake of ketogenic nutrients.

Lysine and leucine—the only purely ketogenic amino acids.

Glucose-6-phosphate dehydrogenase deficiency

G6PD is rate-limiting enzyme in HMP shunt (which yields NADPH). ↓ NADPH in RBCs leads to **hemolytic anemia** due to poor RBC defense against oxidizing agents (fava beans, sulfonamides, primaquine) and antituberculosis drugs. X-linked recessive disorder. Heinz bodies: altered hemoglobin precipitates within RBCs.

G6PD deficiency more prevalent among blacks. NADPH is necessary to keep glutathione reduced, which in turn keeps the heme iron reduced so that O_2 can bind.

Glycolytic enzyme deficiency	Hexokinase, glucose-phosphate isomerase, aldolase, triose-phosphate isomerase, phosphate-glycerate kinase, enolase, and pyruvate kinase deficiencies are associated with hemolytic anemia.	RBCs depend on glycolysis (energy and reducing equivalents).
Glycogen storage diseases	12 types, all resulting in abnormal glycogen metabolism and an accumulation of glycogen within cells.	
Type I	Von Gierke's disease = glucose-6-phosphatase deficiency. Findings: severe fasting hypoglycemia, ↑↑ glycogen in liver.	Von Gierke's: liver.
Type II	Pompe's disease = lysosomal α-1,4-glucosidase deficiency. Findings: cardiomegaly and systemic findings, leading to early death.	Pompe's: liver, heart, and muscle. *Rule of 2*
Type V	McArdle's disease = skeletal muscle glycogen phosphorylase deficiency. Findings: ↑ glycogen in muscle but cannot break it down, leading to painful cramps, myoglobinuria with strenuous exercise. *or renal?*	McArdle's: muscle.
Hartnup's disease	Defect in GI uptake of neutral amino acids. Symptoms mimic pellagra (diarrhea, dementia, dermatitis) because of malabsorption of tryptophan (precursor of niacin). Carcinoid syndrome may also cause pellagra. *excess Trp → 5-HT; not enough → niacin.*	**Hard-N-Up** = **Hard N**eutral **U**ptake
Homocystinuria	Defect in cystathionine synthase. Two forms: 1. Deficiency (treatment: ↓ Met and ↑ Cys in diet) 2. Decreased affinity of synthase for pyridoxal phosphate (treatment: ↑↑ vitamin B_6 in diet)	Results in excess homocystine in the urine. Cysteine becomes essential. *from Met*
Maple syrup urine	Blocked degradation of **branched** amino acids (**I**le, **V**al, **Le**u) due to ↓ α-ketoacid dehydrogenase. Causes severe CNS defects, mental retardation, and death.	Urine smells like maple syrup. Think of cutting (blocking) **branches** of a maple tree. **I** lo**V**e **Lu**cy
Phenylketonuria	Normally, phenylalanine is converted into tyrosine (nonessential aa). In PKU, there is ↓ phenylalanine hydroxylase or ↓ tetrahydrobiopterin cofactor. Tyrosine becomes essential and phenylalanine builds up, leading to excess phenylketones. Findings: mental retardation, fair skin, eczema, musty body odor. Treatment: ↓ phenylalanine and ↑ tyrosine in diet (no Nutrasweet).	Screened for at birth. Phenylketones = phenylacetate, phenyllactate, and phenylpyruvate in urine.

Alkaptonuria	Congenital deficiency of homogentisic acid oxidase in the degradative pathway of tyrosine. Resulting alkapton bodies cause **dark urine**. Also, the connective tissue is dark. Benign disease.	*Alkapton* = alkali-hapten bodies (homogentisic acid) bind to alkali. These are in the urine.
Albinism	Congenital deficiency of tyrosinase. Results in an inability to synthesize melanin from tyrosine. Can result from a lack of migration of neural crest cells.	Lack of melanin results in an increased risk of skin cancer.
Adenosine deaminase deficiency	ADA deficiency can cause SCID. Excess ATP and dATP imbalances nucleotide pool via feedback inhibition of ribonucleotide reductase. This prevents DNA synthesis and thus lowers lymphocyte count. First disease to be treated by experimental human gene therapy.	SCID = severe combined (T and B) immunodeficiency disease. SCID happens to kids.
Lesch-Nyhan syndrome	Purine salvage problem owing to absence of HGPRTase, which converts hypoxanthine to inosine monophosphate (IMP) and guanine to guanosine monophosphate (GMP). X-linked recessive. Findings: retardation, self-mutilation, aggression, hyperuricemia, choreoathetosis.	**LNS** = **L**acks **N**ucleotide **S**alvage (purine). *hypoxanthine/guanine phosphoribotransferase lacks phosphoribosyl moiety*
Ehlers-Danlos syndrome	10 types, all resulting in faulty collagen synthesis. Skin is stretchy (hyperextensible) with poor wound healing, joints are hypermobile. Inheritance varies from autosomal dominant (type IV) to autosomal recessive (type VI) to X-linked recessive (type IX). Type I findings: Diaphragmatic hernia. Type IV findings: Ecchymoses, arterial rupture. Type VI findings: Retinal detachment, corneal rupture.	Sounds like "feller's damn loose" (loose joints).
Cystinuria	Common (1/7000) inherited defect of tubular amino acid transporter for **C**ystine, **O**rnithine, **L**ysine, and **A**rginine in kidneys. Excess cystine in urine can lead to the precipitation of cystine kidney stones.	**COLA**
Osteogenesis imperfecta	Clinically characterized by multiple fractures occurring with minimal trauma (brittle bone disease), which may occur during the birth process, as well as by blue sclerae due to the translucency of the connective tissue over the choroid. Caused by a variety of gene defects resulting in abnormal collagen synthesis.	May be confused with child abuse.

Sphingolipidoses

Each is caused by a deficiency in one of the many lysosomal enzymes.

Fabry's disease	Caused by deficiency of α-galactosidase A, resulting in accumulation of ceramide trihexoside. Finding: renal failure.	X-linked recessive.
Gaucher's disease	Caused by deficiency of β-glucocerebrosidase, leading to glucocerebroside accumulation in brain, liver, spleen, and bone marrow (Gaucher's cells with characteristic "crinkled paper" enlarged cytoplasm). Type I, the more common form, is compatible with a normal life span.	Autosomal recessive.
Niemann-Pick disease	Deficiency of sphingomyelinase causes buildup of sphingomyelin and cholesterol in reticuloendothelial and parenchymal cells and tissues. Patients die by age 3.	Autosomal recessive. No man picks (Nieman-Pick) his nose with his sphinger.
Tay-Sachs disease	Absence of hexosaminidase A results in GM$_2$ ganglioside accumulation. Death occurs by age 3. Cherry-red spot visible on macula. Carrier rate is 1 in 30 in Jews of European descent (1 in 300 for others).	Autosomal recessive. **Tay-saX** sounds like he**X**osaminidase.
Metachromatic leukodystrophy	Deficiency of arylsulfatase A results in the accumulation of sulfatide in the brain, kidney, liver, and peripheral nerves.	Autosomal recessive.
Krabbe's disease	Absence of galactosylceramide β-galactosidase leads to the accumulation of galactocerebroside in the brain. Optic atrophy, spasticity, early death.	Autosomal recessive.

BIOCHEMISTRY—METABOLISM

ATP

Base (adenine), ribose, 3 phosphoryls. 2 phosphoanhydride bonds, 7 kcal/mol each.
Aerobic metabolism produces 38 ATP via malate shuttle, 36 ATP via G3P shuttle.
Anaerobic glycolysis produces only 2 ATP per glucose molecule.
ATP hydrolysis can be coupled to energetically unfavorable reactions.

Activated carriers

Phosphoryl (ATP)
Electrons (NADH, NADPH, FADH$_2$)
Acyl (coenzyme A, lipoamide)
CO$_2$ (biotin)
One-carbon units (tetrahydrofolates)
CH$_3$ groups (SAM)   *S-adenosyl-methionine*   *"Sam The methyl donor man"*
Aldehydes (TPP)   *thiamine pyrophosphate*
Glucose (UDP-glucose)
Choline (CDP-choline)

Extracellular messengers

	Examples	Mechanism
	Nicotinic receptor, norepinephrine receptor on K^+ channel in the heart	Open or close ion channels in cell membrane
	Thyroid hormones, retinoic acid, steroid hormones, vitamin D_3	Act via cytoplasmic or nuclear receptors to increase transcription of target genes
	Angiotensin II, α_1-receptor, ADH	Activate phospholipase C with intracellular production of DAG, IP_3, protein kinase C and Ca^{++}
	β_1-receptor, β_2-receptor ($\uparrow$ cAMP), α_2-receptor ($\downarrow$ cAMP)	Activate or inhibit adenylate cyclase
	ANP, nitric oxide (EDRF)	Increase cyclic GMP in the cell
	Insulin, EGF, PDGF, M-CSF	Increased tyrosine kinase activity
	TGF-β	Increased serine kinase activity

NAD^+/NADPH	NAD^+ is generally used in **catabolic** processes to carry reducing equivalents away as NADH. **NADPH** is used in **anabolic** processes as a supply of reducing equivalents.	NADPH is a product of the HMP shunt and the malate *malic enzyme* dehydrogenase reaction.
***S*-adenosyl-methionine**	ATP + methionine $\rightarrow$ SAM. SAM transfers methyl units to a wide variety of acceptors (e.g., in synthesis of phosphocreatine, high-energy phosphate active in muscle ATP production). Regeneration of methionine (and thus SAM) is dependent on vitamin B_{12}.	SAM the methyl donor man.

Metabolism sites

Pyruvate DH

Mitochondria	Fatty acid **O**xidation (β-oxidation), **A**cetyl-CoA production, **K**rebs cycle.	**Mit**y **OAK**
Cytoplasm	Glycolysis, fatty acid synthesis, HMP shunt, protein synthesis (RER), steroid synthesis (SER).	
Both	Gluconeogenesis, urea cycle.	

Hexokinase versus glucokinase	Hexokinase is found throughout body. Glucokinase (lower affinity [$\uparrow K_m$] but higher capacity [$\uparrow V_{max}$]) is found only in the liver.	Only hexokinase is feedback inhibited by G6P.

Regulation of metabolic pathways

Pathway	Major regulatory enzyme(s)	Activator	Inhibitor	Effector hormone	Remarks
Citric acid cycle	Citrate synthase		ATP, long-chain acyl-CoA		Regulated mainly by the need for ATP and therefore by the supply of NAD^+
Glycolysis and pyruvate oxidation	Phosphofructokinase	AMP, fructose 2,6-bisphosphate in liver, fructose-1,6-bisphosphate in muscle	Citrate (fatty acids, ketone bodies), ATP, cAMP	Glucagon ↓	Induced by insulin
	Pyruvate dehydrogenase	CoA, NAD, ADP, pyruvate	Acetyl-CoA, NADH, ATP (fatty acids, ketone bodies)	Insulin ↑ (in adipose tissue)	Also important in regulating the citric acid cycle
Gluconeogenesis	Pyruvate carboxylase Phosphoenolpyruvate carboxykinase	Acetyl-CoA cAMP?	ADP	Glucagon?	Induced by glu-cocorticoids, glucagon, cAMP
	Fructose-1,6-bisphosphatase	cAMP	AMP, fructose 2,6-bisphosphate	Glucagon	Suppressed by insulin
Glycogenesis	Glycogen synthase		Phosphorylase (in liver) cAMP, Ca^{2+} (muscle)	Insulin ↑ Glucagon ↓ (liver) Epinephrine ↓	Induced by insulin
Glycogenolysis	Phosphorylase	cAMP, Ca^{2+} (muscle)		Insulin ↓ Glucagon ↑ (liver) Epinephrine ↑	
Pentose phosphate pathway	Glucose-6-phosphate dehydrogenase	$NADP^+$	NADPH		Induced by insulin
Lipogenesis	Acetyl-CoA carboxylase	Citrate	Long-chain acyl-CoA, cAMP	Insulin ↑ Glucagon ↓ (liver)	Induced by insulin
Cholesterol synthesis	HMG-CoA reductase		Cholesterol, cAMP	Insulin ↑ Glucagon ↓ (liver)	Inhibited by certain drugs, eg, lovastatin

Handwritten annotations: "PFK-1", "2 phos is no! ... by PFK", "(A → ⊕ carbohydrate", "'sugar on Camp Street'", "C Arbohydrate, not lipids"

132

Metabolism in major organs

Organ	Major function	Major pathways	Main substrates	Major products	Specialist enzymes
Liver	Service for the other organs and tissues	Most represented, including gluconeogenesis; β-oxidation; ketogenesis; lipoprotein formation; urea, uric acid & bile acid formation; cholesterol synthesis	Free fatty acids, glucose (well fed), lactate, glycerol, fructose, amino acids (Ethanol)	Glucose, VLDL (triacylglycerol), HDL, ketone bodies, urea, uric acid, bile acids, plasma proteins (Acetate)	Glucokinase, glucose-6-phosphatase, glycerol kinase, phosphoenolpyruvate carboxykinase, fructokinase, arginase, HMG-CoA synthase and lyase, 7α-hydroxylase
Brain	Coordination of the nervous system	Glycolysis, amino acid metabolism	Glucose, amino acids, ketone bodies (in starvation) Polyunsaturated fatty acids in neonate	Lactate	
Heart	Pumping of blood	Aerobic pathways, eg, β-oxidation and citric acid cycle	Free fatty acids, lactate, ketone bodies, VLDL and chylomicron triacylglycerol, some glucose		Lipoprotein lipase Respiratory chain well developed
Adipose tissue	Storage and breakdown of triacylglycerol	Esterification of fatty acids and lipolysis	Glucose, lipoprotein triacylglycerol	Free fatty acids, glycerol	Lipoprotein lipase, hormone-sensitive lipase
Muscle Fast twitch Slow twitch	Rapid movement Sustained movement	Glycolysis Aerobic pathways, eg, β-oxidation and citric acid cycle	Glucose Ketone bodies, triacylglycerol in VLDL and chylomicrons, free fatty acids	Lactate	Lipoprotein lipase Respiratory chain well developed

Glycolysis regulation, irreversible enzymes

D-glucose ⟶ Glucose-6-phosphate
    Hexokinase

Glucose-6-P $\ominus$

Fructose-6-P ⟶ Fructose-1,6-BP
    Phosphofructokinase *PFK-1*
    (rate-limiting step) $\oplus$

ATP $\ominus$, AMP $\oplus$, citrate $\ominus$,
fructose 2, 6-BP $\oplus$

Phosphoenolpyruvate ⟶ Pyruvate
    Pyruvate kinase

ATP $\ominus$, alanine $\ominus$, *Ala ↔ Pyr*
fructose-1,6-BP $\oplus$

Pyruvate ⟶ Acetyl-CoA
    Pyruvate
    dehydrogenase

ATP $\ominus$, NADH $\ominus$,
acetyl-CoA $\ominus$

Gluconeogenesis, irreversible enzymes

Pyruvate carboxylase — In mitochondria. Pyruvate → oxaloacetate.
Requires biotin, ATP. Activated by acetyl-CoA. $\oplus$

PEP carboxykinase — In cytosol. Oxaloacetate → phosphoenolpyruvate.
Requires GTP.

Fructose-1,6-bisphosphatase — In cytosol. Fructose-1,6-bisphosphate → fructose-6-P

Glucose-6-phosphatase — In cytosol. Glucose-6-P → glucose

Above enzymes found only in liver, kidney, intestinal epithelium. Muscle cannot participate in gluconeogenesis.

Hypoglycemia is caused by a deficiency of these key gluconeogenic enzymes listed above (e.g., von Gierke's disease, which is caused by a lack of glucose-6-phosphatase in the liver).

Pentose phosphate pathway

Produces ribose-5-P from G6P for nucleotide synthesis.

Produces NADPH from NADP$^+$ for fatty acid and steroid biosynthesis and for maintaining reduced glutathione inside RBCs.

Part of HMP shunt.

All reactions of this pathway occur in the cytoplasm.

Sites: lactating mammary glands, liver, adrenal cortex—all sites of fatty acid or steroid synthesis. *ALSO RBCs.*

Cori cycle

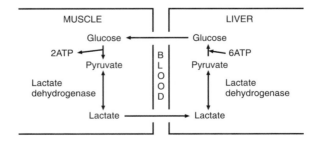

Transfers excess reducing equivalents from RBCs and muscle to liver, allowing muscle to function anaerobically (net 2 ATP).

Pyruvate dehydrogenase complex

The complex contains three enzymes that require five cofactors: pyrophosphate (from **Thiamine**), **Lipoic** acid, **Co**A (from pantothenate), **FAD** (riboflavin), **NAD** (niacin). Reaction: pyruvate + NAD^+ + CoA → acetyl-CoA + CO_2 + NADH.

The complex is similar to the α-ketoglutarate dehydrogenase complex (same cofactors, similar substrate and action).

Tender **L**oving **C**are **F**or **N**obody

TCA cycle

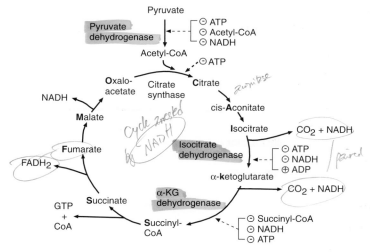

Produces 3NADH, 1FADH$_2$, 2CO$_2$, 1GTP per acetyl CoA = 12ATP/acetyl CoA (2x everything per glucose)

α-Ketoglutarate dehydrogenase complex cofactors:
1. Thiamine pyrophosphate
2. Lipoamide
3. CoA
4. FAD
5. NAD$^+$

Citric **A**cid **I**s **K**rebs' **S**tarting **S**ubstrate **F**or **M**itochondrial **O**xidation.

Electron transport chain and oxidative phosphorylation

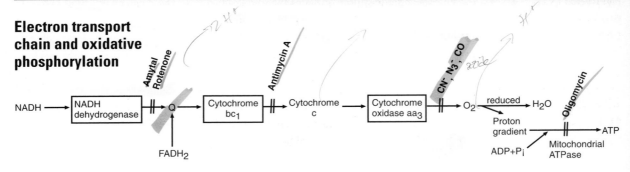

Electron transport chain

$1\ NADH \rightarrow 3ATP;\ 1\ FADH_2 \rightarrow 2ATP$

Oxidative phosphorylation poisons

1. Electron transport inhibitors (rotenone, antimycin A, CN⁻, CO) directly inhibit electron transport, causing ↓ of proton gradient and block of ATP synthesis.
2. ATPase inhibitor (oligomycin) directly inhibits mitochondrial ATPase, causing ↑ of proton gradient, but no ATP is produced because electron transport stops.
3. Uncoupling agents (2,4-DNP) increase permeability of membrane, causing ↓ of proton gradient and ↑ oxygen consumption. ATP synthesis stops. Electron transport continues.

Liver: fed state vs fasting state

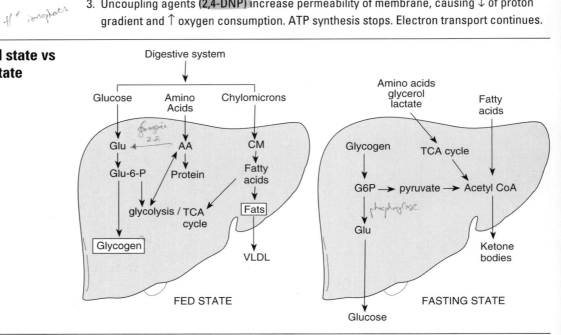

RBC energetics

RBCs have no mitochondria (no TCA) and thus depend on glycolysis (ATP) for energy and HMP shunt (NADPH) for reducing equivalents.

Brain and RBCs rely on glucose for energy. (Brain can use ketone bodies in starvation.)

Fatty acid metabolism sites

Fatty acid synthesis = cytosol.
Fatty acid degradation = mitochondria.
Fatty acid entry into mitochondrion is via carnitine shuttle (inhibited by cytoplasmic malonyl-CoA).

Fatty acid degradation occurs where its products will be consumed—in the mitochondrion.

Sphingolipid components

Sphingosine precursors are serine + palmitate.
Ceramide = sphingosine + fatty acid.
Sphingomyelin = ceramide + phosphoryl choline.
Cerebroside = ceramide + glucose/galactose.
Ganglioside = ceramide + oligosaccharide + sialic acid.

Cholesterol synthesis

Rate-limiting step is catalyzed by HMG-CoA reductase, which converts HMG-CoA to mevalonate. Two-thirds of plasma cholesterol is esterified by lecithin-cholesterol acyltransferase (LCAT), also known as phosphatidylcholine-cholesterol acyltransferase (PCAT).

Lovastatin inhibits HMG-CoA reductase.

Lipoproteins

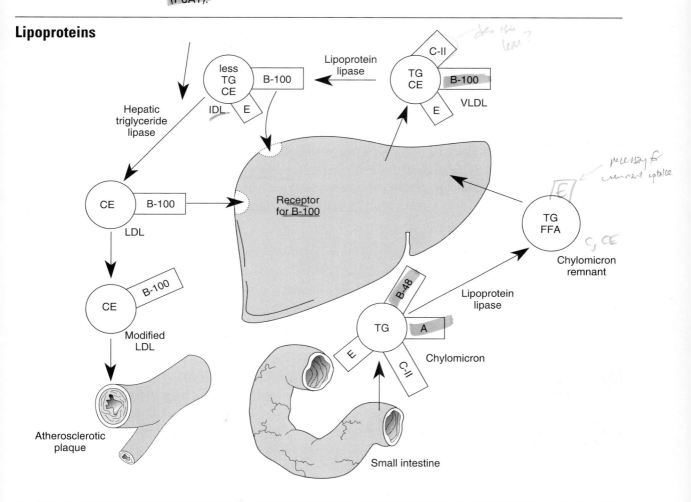

Lipoprotein functions

	Function and route	Apolipoproteins
Chylomicron	Delivers dietary triglycerides to peripheral tissues and dietary cholesterol to liver. Secreted by intestinal epithelial cells. Excess causes pancreatitis, lipemia retinalis, and eruptive xanthomas.	B-48 mediates secretion. A's are used for formation of new HDL. C-II activates lipoprotein lipase. E mediates remnant uptake by liver.
VLDL	Delivers hepatic triglycerides to peripheral tissues. Secreted by liver. Excess causes pancreatitis.	B-100 mediates secretion. C-II activates lipoprotein lipase. E mediates remnant uptake by liver.
LDL	Delivers hepatic cholesterol to peripheral tissues. Formed by lipoprotein lipase modification of VLDL in the peripheral tissue. Taken up by target cells via receptor-mediated endocytosis. Excess causes atherosclerosis, xanthomas, and arcus corneae. *arcus senilis(?)*	B-100 mediates binding to cell surface receptor for endocytosis.
HDL	Mediates centripetal transport of cholesterol (reverse cholesterol transport). Acts as a repository for apoC and apoE (which are needed for chylomicron and VLDL metabolism). Secreted from both liver and intestine.	A's help form HDL structure. A-I in particular activates LCAT (which catalyzes esterification of cholesterol). CETP mediates transfer of cholesteryl esters to other lipoprotein particles.

Major apolipoproteins

A-I: **A**ctivates LCAT.
B-100: **B**inds to LDL receptor. *+ impt. for secretion*
C-II: **C**ofactor for lipoprotein lipase.
E: Mediates **E**xtra (remnant) uptake.

Aminolevulinate (ALA) synthase

Rate-limiting step for heme synthesis. The end product (heme) feedback inhibits this enzyme. Found in the mitochondria, where it converts succinyl CoA and glycine to ALA.

Heme synthesis

Occurs in the liver and bone marrow. Committed step is glycine + succinyl CoA → δ-aminolevulinate. Catalyzed by ALA synthase. Accumulation of intermediates causes porphyrias. Lead inhibits ALA dehydratase and ferrochelatase, preventing incorporation of iron and causing anemia and porphyria.

Underproduction of heme causes microcytic hypochromic anemia.

Heme catabolism

Heme is scavenged from RBCs and Fe^{2+} is reused. Heme → biliverdin → bilirubin (sparingly water soluble, toxic to CNS, transported by albumin). Bilirubin removed from blood by liver, conjugated with glucuronate and excreted in bile. In the intestine it is processed into its excreted form. Some urobilinogen, an intestinal intermediate, is reabsorbed into blood and excreted as urobilin into urine.

Hyperbilirubinemia	From conjugated (direct) and/or unconjugated (indirect) bilirubin. Causes: massive hemolysis, block in subsequent catabolism of heme, displacement from binding sites on albumin (e.g., liver damage or bile duct obstruction). Bilirubin is yellow, causing jaundice.	**UN**conjugated is **IN**direct and **IN**soluble. Conjugated bilirubin is excreted in the urine.
Essential amino acids	Ketogenic: **L**eu, **L**ys. Glucogenic/ketogenic: **I**le, **P**he, **T**rp. Glucogenic: **M**et, **T**hr, **V**al, **A**rg, **H**is.	All essential amino acids: **PriVaTe TIM HALL.** Arg and His are required during periods of growth.
Acidic and basic amino acids	At body pH (7.4), acidic amino acids Asp and Glu are negatively charged; basic amino acids Arg and Lys are positively charged. Basic amino acid His at pH 7.4 has no net charge. Arginine is the most basic amino acid. Arg and Lys are found in high amounts in histones, which bind to negatively charged DNA.	Asp = aspartic ACID, Glu = glutamic ACID. Arg and Lys have an extra NH_3 group. The **ASP**iring **GLU**tton was **ACID**ic so others **BASIC**ally **ARG**ued with, **LY**ed to, and **HIS**sed at him.
Protein synthesis: ATP versus GTP	P site = peptidyl, A site = aminoacyl. ATP is used in tRNA charging, whereas GTP is used in binding of tRNA to ribosome and for translocation.	P = peptidyl, A = amino acid or acceptor site (on deck). Erythromycin inhibits the translocation step of protein synthesis.
Protein synthesis direction	Synthesis proceeds from N terminus to C terminus. mRNA is read $5' \rightarrow 3'$. Signal sequences are found on the N terminus of newly synthesized secretory and nuclear proteins.	The ami**N**o a**C**ids are tied together from **N** to **C**.
Urea cycle		**O**rdinarily, **C**areless **C**rappers **A**re **A**lso **F**rivolous **A**bout **U**rination.

Arachidonic acid products

Phospholipase A_2 liberates arachidonic acid from cell membrane.

Lipoxygenase pathway yields **L**eukotrienes.

L for **L**ipoxygenase and **L**eukotriene.

Cyclooxygenase pathway yields thromboxanes, prostaglandins, and prostacyclin.

Tx A_2 stimulates platelet aggregation.

PG I_2 inhibits platelet aggregation.

Platelet-**G**athering **I**nhibitor

LT B_4 is a neutrophil chemotactic agent.

LT C_4, D_4, and E_4 (SRS-A) function in bronchoconstriction, vasoconstriction, contraction of smooth muscle, and increased vascular permeability.

Insulin

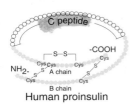

C peptide

NH_2-

Cys Cys Cys
S—S
A chain
Cys Cys
-COOH
Cys S
S
B chain
Human proinsulin

Made in β cells of pancreas. No effect on glucose uptake by brain, RBCs, and hepatocytes. Required for adipose and skeletal muscle uptake of glucose. Inhibits glucagon release by α cells of pancreas. Serum C-peptide is not present with exogenous insulin intake.

Brain, liver, and RBCs take up glucose independent of insulin. **In**sulin moves glucose **In**to cells.

Ketone bodies

In liver: fatty acid and amino acids → acetoacetate + β-hydroxybutyrate (to be used in muscle and brain). Ketone bodies found in prolonged starvation and diabetic ketoacidosis. Excreted in urine. Made from HMG-CoA. Ketone bodies are metabolized by the brain to 2 molecules of acetyl CoA.

Breath smells like acetone (fruity odor). Urine test for ketones does not detect β-hydroxybutyrate (favored by high redox state).

Ethanol hypoglycemia

Ethanol metabolism increases NADH/NAD^+ ratio in liver, causing diversion of pyruvate to lactate and OAA to malate, thereby inhibiting gluconeogenesis and leading to hypo-glycemia.

Ethanol metabolism

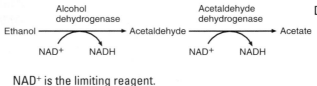

Alcohol dehydrogenase

Acetaldehyde dehydrogenase

Ethanol ——→ Acetaldehyde ——→ Acetate

NAD^+ NADH NAD^+ NADH

NAD^+ is the limiting reagent.

Alcohol dehydrogenase operates via zero order kinetics.

Disulfiram (Antabuse) inhibits acetaldehyde dehydrogenase (acetaldehyde accumulates, contributing to hangover symptoms).

Kwashiorkor versus marasmus

Kwashiorkor = protein malnutrition resulting in skin lesions, edema, liver malfunction (fatty change). Clinical picture is small child with swollen belly.

Marasmus = protein-calorie malnutrition resulting in tissue wasting.

Kwashiorkor results from a protein-deficient **MEAL:**
Malabsorption
Edema
Anemia
Liver (fatty)

Signal molecule precursors	ATP → cAMP via adenylate cyclase.
	GTP → cGMP via guanylate cyclase.
	Glutamate → GABA via glutamate decarboxylase (requires vit. B_6).
	Tyrosine → DOPA via tyrosine hydroxylase, the rate-limiting enzyme of catecholamine biosynthesis.
	Choline → ACh via choline acetyltransferase (ChAT).
	Arachidonate → prostaglandins, thromboxanes, leukotrienes via cyclooxygenase/lipoxygenase.
	Fructose-6-P → fructose-1,6-bis-P via phosphofructokinase (PFK), the rate-limiting enzyme of glycolysis.
	1,3-BPG → 2,3-BPG via bisphosphoglycerate mutase.

| **Tyrosine derivatives** | Tyrosine derivatives are thyroxine, dopamine, epinephrine, melanin. | Tire-sine ("tired without") substances that get you going: thyroxine, epinephrine, dopamine (as in Parkinson's), melanin (gets you outdoors). |

Enzyme kinetics

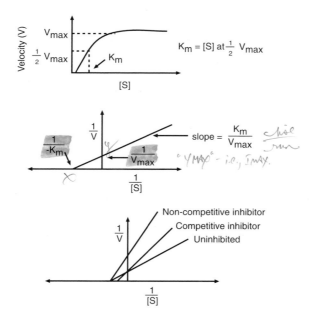

$K_m = [S]$ at $\frac{1}{2}$ V_{max}

slope = $\frac{K_m}{V_{max}}$

Competitive inhibitors:
Resemble substrates; bind reversibly to active sites of enzymes. High substrate concentration overcomes effect of inhibitor. V_{max} remains unchanged, K_m increases compared to uninhibited.

Noncompetitive inhibitors:
Do not resemble substrate; bind to enzyme but not at active site. Inhibition cannot be overcome by high substrate concentration. V_{max} decreases, K_m remains unchanged compared to uninhibited.

Cell cycle phases

M (mitosis: prophase–metaphase–
    anaphase–telophase)
G_1 (growth)
S (synthesis of DNA)
G_2 (growth)
G_0 (quiescent G_1 phase)
G_1 and G_0 are of variable duration. Mitosis is usually
    shortest phase. Most cells are in G_0.
Rapidly dividing cells have a shorter G_1.

G stands for **G**ap or **G**rowth; **S**
for **S**ynthesis.

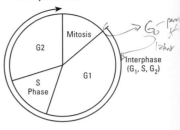

Plasma membrane composition

Plasma membranes contain cholesterol ($\approx$50%, promotes membrane stability),
    phospholipids ($\approx$50%), sphingolipids, glycolipids, and proteins. Only noncytoplasmic side
    of membrane contains glycosylated lipids or proteins (i.e., the plasma membrane is an
    asymmetric, fluid bilayer).

Phosphatidylcholine function

Phosphatidylcholine (lecithin) is a major component of RBC membranes, of myelin, of bile,
    and of surfactant (DPPC–dipalmitoyl phosphatidylcholine). Also used in esterification of
    cholesterol.

Keratin composition and function

Keratin is a protein with a high percentage of cysteine. It is found in intermediate filaments
    (nails and keratinized squamous epithelium).

Microtubule

Cylindrical structure 23 nm in diameter and of variable
    length. A helical array of polymerized dimers of α- and
    β-tubulin (13 per circumference). Each dimer has 2 GTP
    bound. Incorporated into flagella, cilia, mitotic spindles.
    Grows slowly, collapses quickly. Microtubules are also
    involved in slow axoplasmic transport in neurons.

Drugs that act on microtubules
    include colchicine (anti-gout),
    vinblastine/vincristine and
    taxol (anti-cancer), griseo-
    fulvin (anti-fungal), and
    mebendazole/thiabendazole
    (anti-helminthic). Colchicine
    inhibits microtubule polymer-
    ization. Vincristine and vin-
    blastine interact with tubulin
    to block assembly of mitotic
    spindle.

Collagen synthesis

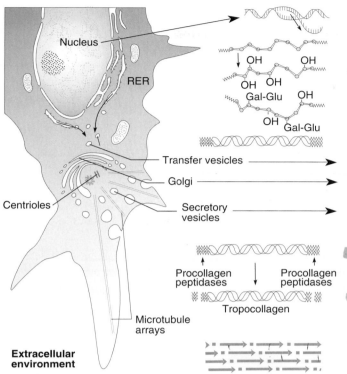

Formation of mRNA for alpha chains.

Synthesis of alpha chains of preprocollagen in the RER. Clipping of signal peptide.

Hydroxylation of specific prolyl and lysyl residues in the endoplasmic reticulum (requires vitamin C).

Attachment of galactosyl and glucosyl to specific hydroxylysyl residues.

Assembly of procollagen molecules (triple helix).

Transport of procollagen to Golgi apparatus.

Packaging of procollagen in secretory vesicles.

Secretory vesicles, assisted by microtubules and microfilaments, transport procollagen molecules to cell surface.

Exocytosis of procollagen molecules into extracellular space. Procollagen peptidases cleave terminal regions of procollagen, transforming procollagen into insoluble tropocollagen, which aggregates to form collagen fibrils.

Fibrillar structure is reinforced by the formation of covalent lysine-hydroxylysine cross-links between tropocollagen molecules.

Collagen structure	Collagen fibril = many staggered collagen molecules (linked by lysyl oxidase). Collagen molecule = 3 collagen α chains (usually X-Y-Gly, X and Y = proline, hydroxyproline, or hydroxylysine). Procollagen must be trimmed to collagen molecule.
Cholesterol lipoproteins	LDL and HDL carry most cholesterol. LDL transports cholesterol from liver to tissue; HDL tranports it from periphery to liver. **HDL** is **H**ealthy. **LDL** is **L**ousy.
Hemoglobin	Hemoglobin is composed of four polypeptide subunits (2α and 2β) and exists in two forms: 1. T (taut) form has low affinity for oxygen. 2. R (relaxed) form has high affinity for oxygen (300×). Hemoglobin exhibits positive cooperativity and negative allostery (accounts for the sigmoid-shaped O_2 dissociation curve for hemoglobin), unlike myoglobin. Carbon monoxide has a 200× greater affinity for hemoglobin than oxygen.

Hb structure regulation	Increased Cl^-, H^+, CO_2, DPG, and temperature favor T form over **R** form (shifts dissociation curve to right, leading to $\uparrow$ O_2 unloading). T form has low affinity for O_2.	When you're **R**elaxed, you do your job better (carry O_2).
CO_2 transport in blood	CO_2 binds to amino acids in globin chain (at N terminus) but not to heme. CO_2 binding favors T (taut) form of hemoglobin (and thus promotes O_2 unloading).	CO_2 must be transported from tissue to lungs, the reverse of O_2.
Hormonal effects on cAMP	Insulin reduces cAMP levels. Epinephrine, norepinephrine, and glucagon raise cAMP levels.	cAMP mobilizes resources (remember ATP $\rightarrow$ cAMP).
PIP_2 second messenger system	Involved in mast cell degranulation, α_1 receptor activation, and activation of some muscarinic receptors.	$PIP_2 \nearrow IP_3 \rightarrow \uparrow Ca^{2+}$ (from ER) $\searrow DAG \rightarrow$ protein kinase
Muscle activation: calcium	In skeletal muscle, calcium ions activate troponin, which moves tropomyosin, which exposes actin and allows actin-myosin interaction. In smooth muscle, Ca^{2+} activates contraction by binding to calmodulin (no troponins). $\rightarrow MLCK$	
Sodium pump	Na^+-K^+ATPase is located in the plasma membrane with ATP site on cytoplasmic side. For each ATP consumed, 3 Na^+ go out and 2 K^+ come in. During cycle, pump is phosphorylated (inhibited by vanadate). Ouabain inhibits by binding to K^+ site. Cardiac glycosides (digoxin, digitoxin) also inhibit the Na^+-K^+ATPase, causing increased cardiac contractility.	
Enzyme regulation methods	Enzyme concentration alteration (synthesis and/or destruction), covalent modification (e.g., phosphorylation), proteolytic modification (zymogen), allosteric regulation (e.g., feedback inhibition), and transcriptional regulation (e.g., steroid hormones). $\rightarrow$ sequestration	

Vitamins

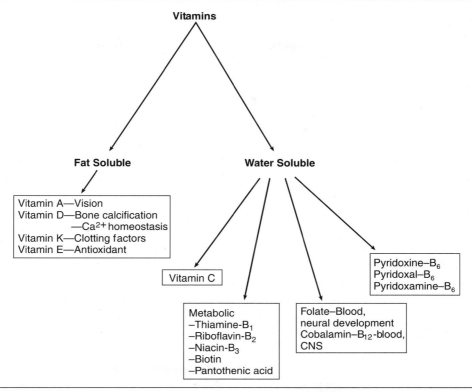

Vitamins: fat soluble	A, D, E, K. Absorption dependent on gut (ileum) and pancreas. Toxicity more common than for water-soluble vitamins, because these accumulate in fat.	Malabsorption syndromes (steatorrhea) such as cystic fibrosis and sprue can cause fat-soluble vitamin deficiencies. Mineral oil (laxative) can also cause malabsorption of fat-soluble vitamins.
Vitamins: water soluble	B_1 (thiamine: TPP) B_2 (riboflavin: FAD, FMN) B_3 (niacin: NAD^+) B_5 (pantothenate: CoA) B_6 (pyridoxine: PP) B_{12} (cobalamin) C (ascorbic acid) Biotin Folate	All wash out easily from body except B_{12} (stored in liver).

Vitamin A (retinol)

Deficiency	Night blindness and dry skin.	Retinol is vitamin A, so think Retin-A (used topically for wrinkles and acne).
Function	Constituent of visual pigments (retinal).	
Excess	Arthralgias, fatigue, headaches, skin changes, sore throat, alopecia	

Vitamin B$_1$ (thiamine)

Deficiency	Beriberi and Wernicke-Korsakoff syndrome. Seen in alcoholism and malnutrition.	Beriberi: characterized by polyneuritis, cardiac pathology, and edema. Spell beriberi as **Ber1Ber1**. Wet beriberi may lead to high output cardiac failure.
Function	In thiamine pyrophosphate, a cofactor for oxidative decarboxylation of α-keto acids (pyruvate, α-ketoglutarate) and a cofactor for transketolase.	

Vitamin B$_2$ (riboflavin)

Deficiency	Angular stomatitis.	**FAD** and **FMN** are derived from ribo**F**lavin (B$_2$ = **2** ATP).
Function	Cofactor in oxidation and reduction (e.g., FADH$_2$).	

Vitamin B$_3$ (niacin)

Deficiency	Pellagra can be caused by Hartnup disease, malignant carcinoid syndrome and INH.	Pellagra's symptoms are the **3 D's: D**iarrhea, **D**ermatitis, **D**ementia (also beefy glossitis). **N**AD derived from **N**iacin (B$_3$ = **3** ATP).
Function	Constituent of NAD$^+$, NADP$^+$ (used in redox reactions). Derived from tryptophan.	

Vitamin B$_5$ (pantothenate)

Deficiency	Dermatitis, enteritis, alopecia, adrenal insufficiency.	
Function	Constituent of CoA, part of fatty acid synthase. Cofactor for acyl transfers.	Pantothen-**A** is in Co-**A**.

Vitamin B$_6$ (pyridoxine)

Deficiency	Convulsions, hyperirritability (deficiency inducible by INH).
Function	Converted to pyridoxal phosphate, a cofactor used in transamination (e.g., ALT and AST), decarboxylation, and trans-sulfuration.

Biotin

Deficiency	Dermatitis, enteritis. Caused by antibiotic use, ingestion of raw eggs. *avidin*	"Buy-a-tin of CO$_2$" for carboxylations.
Function	Cofactor for carboxylations (pyruvate carboxylase, acetyl-CoA carboxylase, propionyl-CoA carboxylase) but not decarboxylations.	

Folic acid

Deficiency

Most common vitamin deficiency in US.
Macrocytic, megaloblastic anemia (often no neurologic symptoms), sprue.

Function

Coenzyme for one-carbon transfer; involved in methylation reactions.
Important for the synthesis of nitrogenous bases in DNA and RNA.

Eat green leaves (because folic acid is not stored very long). Supplemental folic acid in early pregnancy reduces neural tube defects.
PABA is the folic acid precursor in bacteria. Sulfa drugs and dapsone are PABA analogs.

Vitamin B_{12} (cobalamin)

Deficiency

Macrocytic, megaloblastic anemia; neurologic symptoms (optic neuropathy, subacute combined degeneration, paresthesia); glossitis.

Function

Cofactor for homocysteine methylation and methyl-malonyl-CoA handling.
Stored primarily in the liver.
Synthesized only by microorganisms. — *seen only in animal products*

Vit. B_{12} deficiency is usually caused by malabsorption (sprue, enteritis, *Diphyllobothrium latum*), no intrinsic factor (pernicious anemia), or no terminal ileum (Crohn's disease). *(ileostomy.*

Vitamin C (ascorbic acid)

Deficiency

Scurvy.

Function

Necessary for hydroxylation of proline and lysine in collagen synthesis.
Scurvy findings: swollen gums, bruising, anemia, poor wound healing. *perifollicular hemorrhage / subperiosteal hemorrhage*

Vitamin **C** **C**ross-links **C**ollagen.
British sailors carried limes to prevent scurvy (origin of the word "limey").

Vitamin D

D_2 = ergocalciferol, consumed in milk.
D_3 = cholecalciferol, formed in sun-exposed skin.

Deficiency

Rickets in children (bending bones), osteomalacia in adults (soft bones), and hypocalcemic tetany.

Function

Increases intestinal absorption of calcium and phosphate.

Excess

Hypercalcemia, loss of appetite, stupor. Seen in sarcoidosis, a disease where the epithelioid macrophages convert vit. D into its active form.

Remember that drinking milk (fortified with vitamin D) is good for bones.

Vitamin E

Deficiency

Increased fragility of erythrocytes.

Function

Antioxidant (protects erythrocytes from hemolysis).

Vitamin **E** is for **E**rythrocytes.

Vitamin K

Deficiency	Neonatal hemorrhage with ↑ PT, ↑ aPTT, but normal bleeding time.	**K** for **K**oagulation. Note that the vitamin K–dependent clotting factors are II, VII, IX, and X. Warfarin is a vitamin K antagonist.
Function	Catalyzes γ-carboxylation of glutamic acid residues on various proteins concerned with blood clotting. Synthesized by intestinal flora. Therefore, vit. K deficiency can occur after the prolonged use of broad-spectrum antibiotics.	

DNA/RNA/Protein

1. Molecular biology: tools and techniques (e.g., cloning, cDNA libraries, PCR, restriction fragment length polymorphism, restriction enzymes, sequencing).
2. Transcriptional regulation: the operon model (lac, trp operons) of transcription, eukaryotic transcription (e.g., TATA box, enhancers, effects of steroid hormones, transcription factors).
3. Protein synthesis: steps, regulation, energy (Which step requires ATP? GTP?), differences between prokaryotes and eukaryotes (N-formyl methionine), post-translational modification (targeting to organelles, secretion).
4. Acid base titration curve of amino acids, proteins.
5. SH2 domain: role.

Genetic Errors

1. Inherited hyperlipidemias: types, clinical manifestations, specific changes in serum lipids.
2. Glycogen and lysosomal storage diseases (e.g., type III glycogen storage disease), I cell disease.
3. Porphyrias: defects, clinical presentation, effect of barbiturates.
4. DNA repair defects (e.g., HNPCC, xeroderma pigmentosa).
5. Triplet repeat diseases (Huntington's chorea, Fragile X).
6. Inherited defects in amino acid metabolism.

Metabolism

1. Glycogen synthesis: regulation, inherited defects.
2. Oxygen consumption, carbon dioxide production, and ATP production for fats, proteins, and carbohydrates.
3. Amino acid degradation pathways (urea cycle, tricarboxylic acid cycle).
4. Effect of enzyme phosphorylation on metabolic pathways.
5. Rate limiting enzymes in different metabolic pathways (e.g., pyruvate decarboxylase).
6. Sites of different metabolic pathways (What organ? Where in the cell?).
7. Fed state versus fasting state: forms of energy used, direction of metabolic pathways.
8. Tyrosine kinases and their effects on metabolic pathways (insulin receptor, growth factor receptors).
9. Anti-insulin (gluconeogenic) hormones (e.g., glucagon, GH, cortisol).
10. Synthesis and metabolism of neurotransmitters (e.g., acetylcholine, epinephrine, norepinephrine, dopamine).
11. Purine/pyrimidine degradation.
12. Carnitine shuttle: function, inherited defects.
13. Cellular/organ effects of insulin secretion.
14. Effect of uncouplers on oxidative phosphorylation.

Microbiology

This high-yield material covers the basic concepts of microbiology and immunology. The emphasis in previous examinations has been approximately 40% bacteriology (20% basic, 20% quasi-clinical), 25% immunology, 25% virology (10% basic, 15% quasi-clinical), 5% parasitology, and 5% mycology. Learning the distinguishing characteristics, target organs, and method of spread of—as well as relevant laboratory tests for—major pathogens can improve your score substantially.

Many students preparing for this part of the boards make the mistake of studying bacteriology very well without devoting sufficient time to the other topics. For this reason, learning immunology and virology well is high yield. Learn the components and mechanistic details of the immune response, including T cells, B cells, and the structure and function of immunoglobulins. Also learn the major immunodeficiency diseases (e.g., AIDS, agammaglobulinemia, DiGeorge's syndrome). Knowledge of viral structures and genomes remains important.

Bugs

Viruses

Immunology

High-Yield Clinical Vignettes

High-Yield Glossy Material

High-Yield Topics

Auxotroph, autotroph, heterotroph

Auxotroph	Nutritionally deficient species. Require nutrients not needed by parental or prototype strain.	**Aux**otroph requires **Aux**iliary nourishment.
Heterotroph	Require carbon source, sugar, or amino acids.	All **h**uman pathogens are **h**eterotrophs.
Autotroph	Require only CO_2 and energy source.	

Obligate aerobes

Examples include *Pseudomonas aeruginosa* and *Mycobacterium tuberculosis*.
Mycobacterium tuberculosis has a predilection for the apices of the lung, which have the highest Po_2.

*P. **AER**uginosa* is an **AER**obe seen in burn wounds, nosocomial pneumonia, and pneumonias in cystic fibrosis patients.

Obligate anaerobes

Examples include *Clostridium* and *Bacteroides*. They lack catalase and/or superoxide dismutase and thus are susceptible to oxidative damage. They are generally foul-smelling (short-chain fatty acids), difficult to culture, and produce gas in tissue (CO_2 and H_2).

butyric acid : not so nice

Anaerobes are normal flora in GI tract, pathogenic elsewhere. Aminoglycosides are ineffective against anaerobes because these antibiotics require O_2 to enter into bacterial cell.

Bacterial growth curve

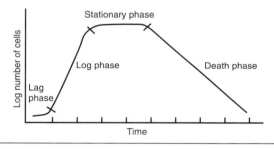

Bacterial structures

Structure	Function	Chemical composition
Peptidoglycan *CELL WALL*	Gives rigid support, protects against osmotic pressure	Sugar backbone with cross-linked peptide side chains
Cell wall/cell membrane (gram positives)	Major surface antigen *GM (+)*	Teichoic acid induces TNF and IL-1
Outer membrane (gram negatives)	Site of endotoxin (lipopolysaccharide) Major surface antigen	Lipid A induces TNF and IL-1 Polysaccharide
Plasma membrane	Site of oxidative and transport enzymes	Lipoprotein bilayer
Ribosome	Protein synthesis	RNA and protein in 50S and 30S subunits
Nucleoid	Genetic material	DNA
Mesosome	Participates in cell division	Invagination of plasma membrane
Periplasm	Space between the cytoplasmic membrane and outer membrane in gram-negative bacteria	Contains many hydrolytic enzymes, including β-lactamases
Capsule	Protects against phagocytosis	Polysaccharide (except *Bacillus anthracis,* which contains D-glutamate)
Pilus/fimbria	Mediates adherence of bacteria to cell surface and attachment to bacteria during conjugation	Glycoprotein
Flagellum	Motility	Protein
Spore	Provides resistance to dehydration, heat, and chemicals	Keratin-like coat Dipicolinic acid
Plasmid	Contains a variety of genes for antibiotic resistance, enzymes, and toxins	DNA
Glycocalyx	Mediates adherence to surfaces, especially foreign surfaces (e.g., indwelling catheters)	Polysaccharide

Cell walls

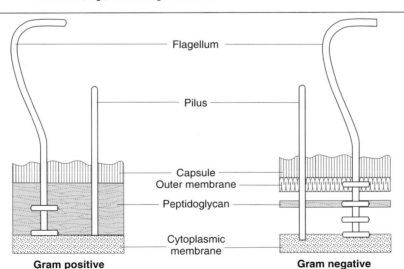

Gram positive   Gram negative

Component	Gram-positive cells	Gram-negative cells
Peptidoglycan	Thicker: multilayer	Thinner: single layer
Teichoic acids	Yes	No
Lipopolysaccharide (endotoxin)	No	Yes
Lipoprotein and phospholipid	No No	Yes Yes

Spores: bacterial	Only certain gram-positive rods form spores when nutrients are limited. Spores are highly resistant to destruction by heat and chemicals. Have dipicolinic acid in their core. Have no metabolic activity. Must autoclave to kill spores (as is done to surgical equipment).	Gram-positive soil bugs ≈ spore formers (*Bacillus anthracis, Clostridium perfringens, C. tetani*).
Spores: fungal	Most fungal spores are asexual. Both coccidioidomycosis and histoplasmosis are transmitted by inhalation of asexual spores. Ascospores from ascomycetes are sexual.	Conidia ≡ asexual fungal spores (e.g., blastoconidia, arthroconidia).
Antigenic variation	Classic examples: Bacteria: *Salmonella* (two flagellar variants), *Borrelia* (relapsing fever), *Neisseria gonorrhoeae* (pilus protein). Virus: influenza (major = shift, minor = drift). Parasites: trypanosomes (programmed rearrangement).	Some mechanisms for variation include DNA rearrangement and RNA segment rearrangement (e.g., influenza major shift).
Bacterial genetic transfer	Conjugation ≡ direct DNA transfer via sex (fertility, F) pilus. Transduction ≡ DNA transfer via bacteriophage vector. Transformation ≡ uptake of naked DNA (which is vulnerable to DNAse) from environment. Transposons ≡ "jumping genes," DNA sequences that jump from bacterium to bacterium or from bacterium to plasmid.	Conjugation = with joining. Transduction ≈ trans-**DUCK**-tion (imagine duck vector carrying DNA in bill). Transformation ≈ trans-**FROM**-ation (naked DNA **FROM** environment).
Exotoxins	Peptides that are excreted by both gram-positive and gram-negative bugs. They are highly antigenic and generally not associated with fever. They are relatively unstable to heat, are highly toxic, and have specific receptors. Usually encoded by lysogenic phage DNA.	**EX**otoxins are **EX**creted. Examples include tetanospasmin, botulinum toxin, and diphtheria toxin.

Bugs with exotoxins

Gram-positive bugs	Mode of action
Corynebacterium diphtheriae	Inactivates EF-2 by ADP ribosylation
Clostridium tetani	Blocks the release of the inhibitory neurotransmitter glycine
Clostridium botulinum	Blocks the release of acetylcholine: causes anticholinergic symptoms, CNS paralysis; spores found in canned food, honey (causes floppy baby)
Clostridium perfringens	Alpha toxin is a lecithinase in gas gangrene. Get double zone of hemolysis on blood agar
Bacillus anthracis	One of the toxins is an adenylate cyclase
Staphylococcus aureus	Toxin is a superantigen that binds to class II MHC protein and T-cell receptor, inducing IL-1 and IL-2 synthesis in toxic shock syndrome; also causes food poisoning
Streptococcus pyogenes	Erythrogenic toxin (causes rash of scarlet fever) and streptolysin O (antigen for ASO-antibody is found in rheumatic fever). Erythrogenic toxin is a superantigen; streptolysin O is a hemolysin
Gram-negative bugs	
Escherichia coli	Heat-labile toxin stimulates adenylate cyclase by ADP ribosylation of G protein Heat-stable toxin stimulates guanylate cyclase
Vibrio cholerae	Stimulates adenylate cyclase by ADP ribosylation of G protein; ↑ pumping of Cl⁻ and H_2O into gut
Bordetella pertussis	Stimulates adenylate cyclase by ADP ribosylation; causes whooping cough, lymphocytosis

Endotoxin

A lipopolysaccharide found only in cell wall of gram-negative bacteria.

N-dotoxin is an integral part of gram-**N**egative cell wall.
Endotoxin is heat stable.

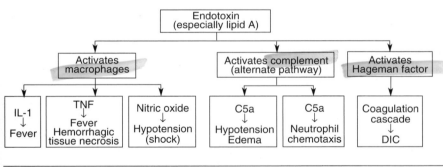

Endotoxins vs. exotoxins

	Exotoxin	Endotoxin
Source	Some gram-positive and gram-negative bacteria	Cell wall of most gram-negative bacteria
Secreted from cell	Yes	No
Composition	Polypeptide	Lipopolysaccharide (LPS)
Location of genes	Plasmid, bacteriophage, or bacterial chromosome	Bacterial chromosome
Clinical effects	Various effects	Fever, shock, DIC
Mode of action	Various modes	Induces TNF and IL-1 synthesis
Vaccines	Toxoids used as vaccines (highly antigenic)	No toxoids formed and no vaccine available (poorly antigenic)

Gram stain limitations	These bugs do not Gram stain well:	These Rascals May Microscopically Lack Color.
	Treponema (too thin to be visualized)	Treponemes—darkfield microscopy and fluorescent antibody staining.
	Rickettsia (intracellular parasite)	
	Mycobacteria (high-lipid-content cell wall requires acid-fast stain)	Mycobacteria—acid fast.
	Mycoplasma (no cell wall)	
	Legionella pneumophila (primarily intracellular)	*Legionella*—silver stain.
	Chlamydia (intracellular parasite)	
Fermentation patterns of *Neisseria*	The pathogenic *Neisseria* species are differentiated on the basis of sugar fermentation.	MeninGococci ferment Maltose and Glucose; Gonococci ferment Glucose.
Pigment-producing bacteria	*Staphylococcus aureus* produces a yellow pigment. *Pseudomonas aeruginosa* produces a blue-green pigment. *Serratia marcescens* produces a red pigment.	*Aureus* (Latin) = gold *Serratia marcescens* = maraschino cherries are red

IgA proteases

IgA proteases allow these organisms to colonize mucosal surfaces: *Streptococcus pneumoniae, Neisseria meningitidis, Neisseria gonorrhoeae, Haemophilus influenzae.*

Big players of meningitis save N. gonorrhea

- hence ability to cause meningitis: Nasopharyngeal colonization

Gram-positive lab algorithm

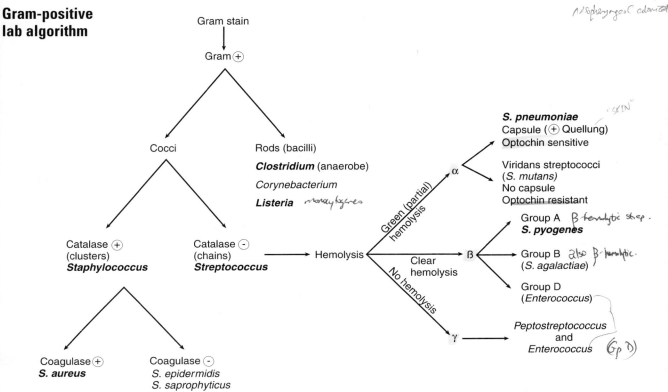

Important pathogens are in **bold type.**
Note: *Enterococcus* is Group D but it is not β-hemolytic; it is α- or γ-hemolytic.

Gram-negative lab algorithm

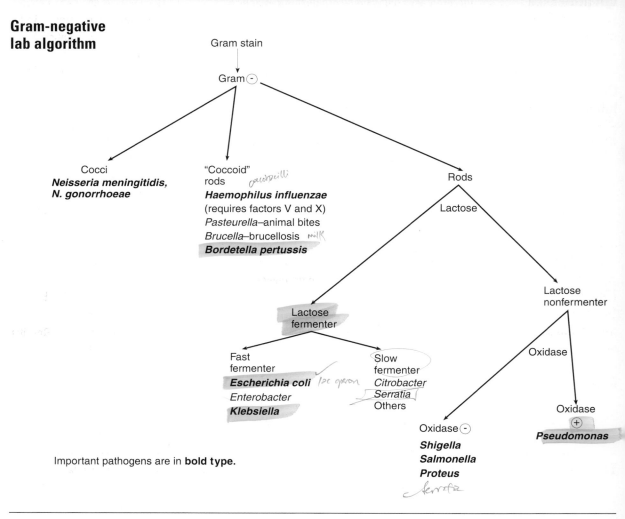

Important pathogens are in **bold type**.

α-hemolytic bacteria	Include the following organisms: 1. *Streptococcus pneumoniae* (catalase-negative and optochin-sensitive) 2. Viridans streptococci (catalase-negative and optochin-resistant)
β-hemolytic bacteria	Include the following organisms: 1. *Staphylococcus aureus* (catalase- and coagulase-positive) 2. *Streptococcus pyogenes* (catalase-negative and bacitracin-sensitive) 3. *Streptococcus agalactiae* (catalase-negative and bacitracin-resistant) 4. *Listeria monocytogenes* (tumbling motility, meningitis in newborns, unpasteurized milk)

Catalase/coagulase (gram-positive cocci)	Catalase degrades H_2O_2, an antimicrobial product of PMNs. Staphylococci make catalase, whereas streptococci do not. *S. aureus* makes coagulase, whereas *S. epidermidis* does not.	Staph make catalase because they have more "staff." Bad staph (*aureus*, because *epidermidis* is skin flora) make coagulase and toxins.
Staphylococcus aureus	Protein A (virulence factor) binds Fc-IgG, inhibiting complement fixation and phagocytosis. *Staphylococcus aureus* produces exfoliative toxin (scalded skin syndrome), TSST-1 (toxic shock syndrome: high fever, rash, shock), hemolysins, enterotoxins (rapid-onset/food poisoning), and coagulase.	TSST is a superantigen that binds to class II MHC and T-cell receptor, resulting in polyclonal T-cell activation. *S. aureus* food poisoning is due to ingestion of preformed toxin.
***Streptococcus pyogenes* (Group A β-hemolytic streptococci sequelae)**	Pharyngeal infection can lead to acute rheumatic fever (fever, polyarthritis, carditis, elevated ASO titer). Skin infection (also known as erysipelas or impetigo) can lead to acute glomerulonephritis (elevated ASO titer, low C3). Bacitracin sensitive. *Scarbr fevr*	Pharyngitis gives you rheumatic "phever." Rheumatic fever = **PECCS:** *St. Vitus's dance* **P**olyarthritis, **E**rythema marginatum, **C**horea, **C**arditis, **S**ubcutaneous nodules.
M protein	An antiphagocytic virulence factor on cell wall of ***S**treptococcus **p**yogenes* (strep group A). **A**ntibody to **M** protein enhances host defenses against *S. pyogenes*.	**SPAM**
Enterococci	Enterococci (*Enterococcus faecalis* and *E. faecium*) are penicillin G-resistant and cause UTI and subacute endocarditis. Lancefield group D includes the enterococci and the nonenterococcal group D streptococci. Lancefield grouping is based on differences in the C-carbohydrate on the bacterial cell wall.	*Entero* = intestine, *faecalis* = feces, *strepto* = twisted (chains), *coccus* = berry. Enterococci, hardier than nonenterococcal group D, can thus grow in 6.5% NaCl (lab test).

Diarrhea

Species	Typical findings	Fever/leukocytosis
Escherichia coli	Ferments lactose	No
Vibrio cholerae	Comma-shaped organisms	No
Salmonella	Does not ferment lactose, motile	Yes
Shigella	Does not ferment lactose, nonmotile, very low ID_{50}	Yes
Campylobacter jejuni	Comma- or S-shaped organisms; growth at 42°C	Yes
Vibrio parahaemolyticus	Transmitted by seafood	Yes
Yersinia enterocolitica	Usually transmitted from pet feces (e.g., puppies)	Yes

Viridans group streptococci

Viridans streptococci are α-hemolytic. They are normal flora of the oropharynx and cause dental caries (*Streptococcus mutans*) and bacterial endocarditis (*S. sanguis*). Resistant to optochin, differentiating them from *S. pneumoniae*, which is α-hemolytic but is optochin sensitive.

Sanguis (Latin) = blood. There is lots of blood in the heart (endocarditis). Viridans group strep live in the mouth because they are not afraid of-the-chin (op-to-chin resistant).

Clostridia (with exotoxins)

All gram-positive, spore-forming, anaerobic bacilli. *Clostridium tetani* produces an exotoxin causing tetanus.

C. botulinum produces a preformed, heat-labile toxin that inhibits ACh release, causing botulism.

C. perfringens produces α toxin, a hemolytic lecithinase that causes myonecrosis or gas gangrene.

C. difficile produces a cytotoxin, an exotoxin that kills enterocytes, causing pseudomembranous colitis. Often secondary to antibiotic use, especially clindamycin or ampicillin.

Tetanus is **tet**anic paralysis (blocks glycine, an inhibitory neurotransmitter).
***Bot**ulinum* is from bad **bot**tles of food (causes a flaccid paralysis).
***Perf**ringens* **perf**orates a gangrenous leg.
***Di**fficile* causes **di**arrhea. Treat with metronidazole. *or oral vancomycin.*

Diphtheria (and exotoxin)

Caused by *Corynebacterium diphtheriae* via exotoxin encoded by β-prophage. Potent exotoxin inhibits protein synthesis via ADP-ribosylation of EF-2. Symptoms include pseudomembranous pharyngitis (grayish-white membrane) with lymphadenopathy. Lab diagnosis based on gram-positive rods with metachromatic granules.

Coryne = club shaped. Grows on tellurite agar.
ABCDEFG:
Adenopathy
Beta-prophage
Corynebacterium
Diphtheriae
Elongation Factor 2
Granules (*metachromatic*)

Actinomycetes

Actinomycetes are bacteria (prokaryotes) that form filaments resembling hyphae of fungi (eukaryotes).

Actino = ray, radiating (as in the filaments they form).

Actinomyces versus *Nocardia*

Actinomyces israelii, a gram-positive anaerobe, causes oral/facial abscesses with "sulfur granules" that may drain through sinus tracts in skin. Normal oral flora.
Nocardia asteroides, a gram-positive and also a weakly acid-fast aerobe in soil, causes pulmonary infection in immunocompromised patients.

A. israelii forms "sulfur" granules in sinus tracts.
Nocardia has **no car**, so it walks fast on acid (acid fast) and on soil but gets out of breath (pulmonary infection).

Penicillin and gram-negative bugs

Gram-negative bugs are resistant to benzyl penicillin G but may be susceptible to penicillin derivatives like ampicillin. The gram-negative outer membrane layer inhibits entry of penicillin G and vancomycin.

Bugs causing food poisoning	*Vibrio parahaemolyticus* and *Vibrio vulnificus* in contaminated seafood. *Bacillus cereus* in reheated rice. *Staphylococcus aureus* in meats, mayonnaise, custard. *Clostridium perfringens* in reheated meat dishes.	**V**omit **B**ig **S**melly **C**hunks. *Staphylococcus aureus* food poisoning starts quickly, ends quickly. "Food poisoning from reheated rice? Be serious!" (*B. cereus*)
Enterobacteriaceae	All species have somatic (O) antigen (which is the polysaccharide of endotoxin). The capsular (K) antigen is related to the virulence of the bug. The flagellar (H) antigen is found in motile species. All ferment glucose and are oxidase negative.	Think **KOH**: **K**apsular s**O**matic flag**H**ellar (or think flagella spin like **H**elicopter blades).
Haemophilus influenzae	Causes meningitis, otitis media, pneumonia, epiglottitis. Small gram-negative (coccobacillary) rod. Aerosol transmission. Most invasive disease caused by capsular type b. Produces IgA protease. Culture on chocolate agar, requires factors V (NAD) and X (hemin) for growth. Treat meningitis with ceftriaxone. Rifampin prophylaxis in close contacts. Does not cause the flu (influenza virus does).	When a child has "flu," mom goes to five (V) and dime (X) store to buy some chocolate. Vaccine contains type b capsular polysaccharide conjugated to diphtheria toxoid or other protein. Given between 2 and 18 months of age.
Legionella pneumophila	Legionnaire's disease ("atypical" pneumonia). Gram-negative rod. Gram stains poorly—use silver stain. Grow on charcoal yeast extract culture with iron and cysteine. Aerosol transmission from environmental water source habitat. No person-to-person transmission. Treat with erythromycin.	Think of a French legionnaire (soldier) with his **silver** helmet, sitting around a campfire (**charcoal**) with his **iron** dagger—he is no sissy (**cysteine**).
Pseudomonas aeruginosa	Causes wound and burn infections, UTI, pneumonia (especially in cystic fibrosis), sepsis (black lesions on skin), external otitis (swimmer's ear), hot tub folliculitis. Aerobic gram-negative rod. Non–lactose fermenting, oxidase positive. Produces pyocyanin (blue-green) pigment. Water source. Produces endotoxin (fever, shock) and exotoxin A (inactivates EF-2). Treat with aminoglycoside plus extended-spectrum penicillin (e.g., piperacillin, ticarcillin).	**AER**uginosa—**AER**obic Think water connection and blue-green pigment. *oxidase ⊕*

Helicobacter pylori

Causes gastritis and up to 90% of duodenal ulcers. Risk factor for peptic ulcer and gastric carcinoma. Gram-negative rod. Urease positive (e.g., urease breath test). Creates alkaline environment. Treat with triple therapy: bismuth (Pepto-Bismol), metronidazole, and either tetracycline or amoxicillin.

Pylori—think pyloris of stomach. *Proteus* and *H. pylori* are both urease positive (cleave urea to ammonia).

Lactose-fermenting enteric bacteria

These bacteria grow pink colonies on MacConkey's agar. Examples include *Citrobacter*, *E. coli*, *Enterobacter*, and *Klebsiella*.

They **"CEEK"** (seek) lactose.

Salmonella versus *Shigella*

typhoid May

Both are non–lactose fermenters; both invade intestinal mucosa and can cause bloody diarrhea. Only *Salmonella* is **m**otile and can invade further and disseminate hematogenously. Symptoms of salmonellosis may be prolonged with antibiotic treatments. *Shigella* is more virulent (10^1 organisms) than *Salmonella* (10^5 organisms).

Salmon swim (motile and disseminate). *Salmonella* has an animal reservoir; *Shigella* does not and is transmitted via "food, fingers, feces, and flies."

Bugs causing watery diarrhea

Include *Vibrio cholerae* (associated with rice-water stools), enterotoxigenic *E. coli*, viruses (e.g., rotaviruses), and protozoans (e.g., *Cryptosporidium* and *Giardia*).

Bugs causing bloody diarrhea

Include *Salmonella, Shigella, Campylobacter jejuni*, enterohemorrhagic/enteroinvasive *E. coli*, *Yersinia enterocolitica*, and *Entamoeba histolytica* (a protozoan). *Amoebiasis ← flask-shaped ulcers*

Cholera and pertussis toxins

Vibrio cholerae toxin permanently activates G_s, causing rice-water diarrhea.

Pertussis toxin permanently disables G_i, causing whooping cough.

Both toxins act via ADP ribosylation that permanently activates adenyl cyclase (resulting in ↑ cAMP).

Cholera turns the "on" on. Pertussis turns the "off" off. Pertussis toxin also promotes lymphocytosis.

Zoonotic bacteria

Species	Disease	Transmission and source	
Borrelia burgdorferi	Lyme disease	Tick bite; *Ixodes* ticks that live on deer and mice	**B**ugs
Francisella tularensis	Tularemia	Tick bite; rabbits, deer	**F**rom
Yersinia pestis	Plague	Flea bite; rodents, especially prairie dogs	**Y**our
Pasteurella multocida	Cellulitis	Animal bite; cats, dogs	**P**et

Undulant fever/ brucellosis

Caused by ingestion of unpasteurized dairy products contaminated with *Brucella abortus* (cattle) or *B. melitensis* (goats) or contact with animals (goats, cattle, pigs). *Brucella* can replicate within macrophages. Undulant fever is an occupational hazard for butchers and meat handlers. Treat with tetracycline.

Picture ungulates (hoofed mammals) "hoofing it up" in your macrophages— **un**gulates give you **un**dulant fever.

Intracellular bugs

Obligate intracellular   *Rickettsia, Chlamydia*. Can't make own ATP.

Facultative intracellular *Mycobacterium, Brucella, Francisella, Listeria*

Stay inside (cells) when it is **R**eally **C**old.

1° and 2° tuberculosis

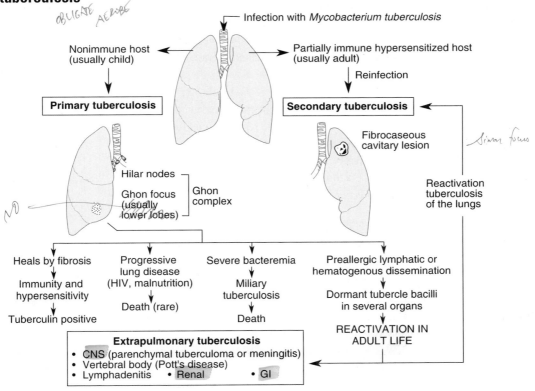

OBLIGATE AEROBE

Infection with *Mycobacterium tuberculosis*

Nonimmune host (usually child) ← → Partially immune hypersensitized host (usually adult)

Reinfection

Primary tuberculosis   **Secondary tuberculosis**

Fibrocaseous cavitary lesion

Simon focus

Hilar nodes
Ghon focus (usually lower lobes) } Ghon complex

Reactivation tuberculosis of the lungs

Heals by fibrosis   Progressive lung disease (HIV, malnutrition)   Severe bacteremia   Preallergic lymphatic or hematogenous dissemination

Immunity and hypersensitivity   Death (rare)   Miliary tuberculosis   Dormant tubercle bacilli in several organs

Tuberculin positive   Death   REACTIVATION IN ADULT LIFE

Extrapulmonary tuberculosis
- CNS (parenchymal tuberculoma or meningitis)
- Vertebral body (Pott's disease)
- Lymphadenitis   • Renal   • GI

Mycobacteria

Mycobacterium tuberculosis (TB)
M. kansasii (pulmonary TB-like symptoms).
M. scrofulaceum (cervical lymphadenitis in kids).
M. avium–intracellulare (often resistant to multiple drugs; causes disseminated disease in AIDS).
All mycobacteria are acid-fast organisms.

high lipid content of cell walls.

TB symptoms include fever, night sweats, weight loss, hemoptysis.

weakly gram (+)

Leprosy (Hansen's disease)

Caused by *Mycobacterium leprae,* an acid-fast bacillus that likes cool temperatures (infects skin and superficial nerves), and cannot be grown in vitro. Reservoir in US: armadillos.   PABA analog

Treatment: long-term oral dapsone; toxicity is hemolysis and metHb.

Alternate treatments include rifampin and combination of clofazimine and dapsone.

Hansen's disease has two forms: lepromatous and tuberculoid; lepromatous is worse (failed cell-mediated immunity), tuberculoid is self-limited.

LEpromatous = **LE**thal

Rickettsiae

Rickettsiae are obligate intracellular parasites (except *R. quintana*) and need CoA and NAD. All except *Coxiella* are transmitted by an arthropod vector and cause headache, fever, and rash; *Coxiella* is an atypical rickettsia, because it is transmitted by aerosol.

Tetracycline is the treatment of choice for most rickettsial infections.

Classic triad: headache, fever, rash (vasculitis)

Lyme disease

Classic symptom is erythema chronicum migrans, an expanding "bull's eye" red rash with central clearing. Also affects joints, CNS, and heart.

Caused by *Borrelia burgdorferi,* which is transmitted by the tick *Ixodes.*

Mice are important reservoirs. Deer required for tick life cycle.

Treat with tetracycline.

Named after Lyme, Connecticut; disease is common in northeastern US.

3 stages of Lyme disease:
Stage 1: Erythema chronicum migrans, flu-like symptoms
Stage 2: Neurologic and cardiac manifestations
Stage 3: Autoimmune migratory polyarthritis

Rickettsial diseases and vectors

Rocky Mountain spotted fever (tick): *Rickettsia rickettsii*
Endemic typhus (fleas): *R. typhi*
Epidemic typhus (human body louse): *R. prowazekii*
Q fever (inhaled aerosols): *Coxiella burnetii*
Treatment for all: tetracycline.

Ty**PH**us has centri**PH**ugal (outward) spread of rash, s**P**otted fever is centri**P**etal (inward). **Q** fever is **Q**ueer because it has no rash, has no vector, has negative Weil-Felix, and its causative organism can survive outside for a long time and does not have *Rickettsia* as its genus name.

Rocky Mountain spotted fever

Caused by *Rickettsia rickettsii.*
Symptoms: rash on palms and soles (migrating to wrists, ankles, then trunk), headache, fever.
Endemic to East Coast (in spite of name).

Palm and sole rash is seen in Rocky Mountain spotted fever, syphilis, and coxsackievirus infection (hand, foot, and mouth disease).

Chlamydiae

Chlamydiae are obligate intracellular parasites that cause mucosal infections. Two forms:
1. Elementary body (small, dense), which Enters cell via endocytosis
2. Initial or Reticular body, which Replicates in cell by fission

Chlamydiae cause arthritis, conjunctivitis, pneumonia, and nongonococcal urethritis. The peptidoglycan wall is unusual in that it lacks muramic acid.

Treatment: erythromycin or tetracycline.

Chlamys = cloak (intracellular).
Chlamydia psittaci notable for an avian reservoir.
C. trachomatis infects only humans.
Lab diagnosis: cytoplasmic inclusions seen on Giemsa or fluorescent-antibody stained smear.

Chlamydia trachomatis serotypes

Types A, B, and C: chronic infection, causes blindness in Africa.

Types D–K: urethritis/PID, neonatal pneumonia, or neonatal conjunctivitis.

Types L1, L2, and L3: lymphogranuloma venereum (acute lymphadenitis: positive Frei test).

TWAR = new strain, pneumonia. Now called C. pneumoniae.

ABC = Africa/Blindness/Chronic infection.
L1–3 = Lymphogranuloma venereum.
D–K = everything else.

Neonatal disease acquired by passage through infected birth canal.

Spirochetes

The spirochetes are spiral-shaped bacteria with axial filaments and include Borrelia (big size), Leptospira, and Treponema. Only Borrelia can be visualized using aniline dyes (Wright's stain or Giemsa stain).

BLT. B is Big. L is Lean (thin spiral).
Leptospira = thin spiral.
"light spiral"

Treponemal disease

Treponemes are spirochetes.
Treponema pallidum causes syphilis.
T. pertenue causes yaws (a tropical infection that is not an STD although VDRL test is positive).

Syphilis
1° syphilis
2° syphilis
3° syphilis

Caused by spirochete Treponema pallidum.
Presents with painless chancre.
Constitutional symptoms, maculopapular rash. plantar (spreads inward)
Gummas, aortitis, neurosyphilis.

Treat with penicillin G.

VDRL versus FTA-ABS

FTA-ABS is specific for treponemes, turns positive earliest in disease, and remains positive longest during disease. VDRL is less specific.

FTA-ABS = Find The Antibody-ABSolutely:
1. Most specific
2. Earliest positive
3. Remains positive the longest

VDRL false positives

VDRL detects nonspecific Ab that reacts with beef cardiolipin. Used for diagnosis of syphilis, but many biologic false positives, including viral infection (mononucleosis, hepatitis), some drugs, rheumatic fever, rheumatoid arthritis, SLE, and leprosy.

VDRL = Venereal Disease (also Very Doubtful) Research Laboratory. The 3 A's of false positives: Aged, Addiction, Autoimmune.

lupus + leprosy

Mycoplasma pneumoniae

Mycoplasma pneumoniae is classic cause of atypical "walking" pneumonia (insidious onset, headache, nonproductive cough). X-ray looks worse than patient. High titer of cold agglutinins. Grown on Eaton's agar.
Treatment: tetracycline or erythromycin (bugs are penicillin resistant because they have no cell wall).

No cell wall.
Only bacterial membrane containing cholesterol.
Mycoplasma pneumonia is less frequent in patients older than age 30.
Frequent outbreaks in military recruits and prisons.

Candida albicans

Systemic or superficial fungal infection (budding yeast with pseudohyphae, germ tube formation at 37°C).
Thrush in throat with immunocompromised patients (neonates, steroids, diabetes, AIDS), endocarditis in IV drug users, vaginitis (post-antibiotic), diaper rash.
Treatment: nystatin for superficial infection; amphotericin B for serious systemic infection.

Alba = white.

not necessarily!

Systemic mycoses

Disease	Endemic location	Notes
Coccidioidomycosis	Southwestern US, California.	San Joaquin Valley or desert (desert bumps)
Histoplasmosis	Mississippi and Ohio river valleys	Bird or bat droppings; intracellular
Paracoccidioidomy-cosis	Rural Latin America	"Captain's wheel" appearance
Blastomycosis	States east of Mississippi River and Central America	**B**ig, **B**road-**B**ased **B**udding

Broad-based budding

All of the above are dimorphic fungi, which are mold in soil (at lower temperature) and yeast in tissue (at higher/body temperature: 37°C) except coccidioidomycosis, which is a spherule in tissue.

Cold = Mold.
Culture on Sabouraud's agar.

8.9
13.95
13.5
18
36.0
91.15 → 93.15 93.75
31/35 70/75 85/95 108/120 92
88.57 93 90 90
8.857 14 13.42 18 = 54.3 90.5
91.5
93.5
~56.1 37.6
93.7
.16

Opportunistic fungal infections

Candida albicans — Thrush in immunocompromised (neonates, steroids, diabetes, AIDS), vulvovaginitis (high pH, diabetes, use of antibiotics), disseminated candidiasis (to any organ), chronic mucocutaneous candidiasis.

Aspergillus fumigatus — Ear fungus, lung cavity aspergilloma ("fungus ball"), invasive aspergillosis. **Mold** with septate hyphae that branch at a V-shaped (45°) angle. Not dimorphic.

Cryptococcus neoformans — Cryptococcal meningitis, cryptococcosis. Heavily encapsulated **yeast.** Not dimorphic. Found in soil, pigeon droppings. Culture of Sabouraud's agar. Stains with India ink. Latex agglutination test detects polysaccharide capsular antigen. Cryptographer uses India ink.

Mucor and Rhizopus species — Mucormycosis. **Mold** with irregular nonseptate hyphae branching at wide angles (≥ 90°). Disease mostly in ketoacidotic diabetic and leukemic patients.

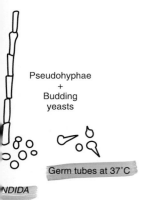

Pseudohyphae + Budding yeasts

Germ tubes at 37°C

NDIDA

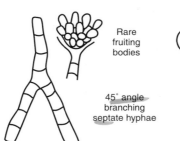

Rare fruiting bodies

45° angle branching septate hyphae

ASPERGILLUS

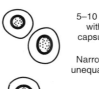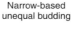

5–10 μ yeasts with wide capsular halo

Narrow-based unequal budding

CRYPTOCOCCUS

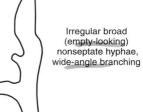

Irregular broad (empty-looking) nonseptate hyphae, wide-angle branching

MUCOR

Pneumocystis carinii

Causes pneumonia (PCP). Yeast (originally classified as protozoan). Inhaled. Most infections asymptomatic. Immunosuppression (e.g., AIDS) predisposes to disease. Silver stain of lung tissue. Treat with TMP-SMX, pentamidine.

Sporothrix schenckii

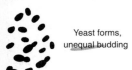

Yeast forms, unequal budding

Sporotrichosis. Dimorphic fungus that lives on vegetation. When traumatically introduced into the skin, typically by a thorn ("rose gardener's" disease), causes local pustule or ulcer with nodules along draining lymphatics. Little systemic illness. Cigar-shaped budding cells visible in pus.

Encapsulated bacteria

SKIN

Examples are *Streptococcus pneumoniae* (also known as pneumococcus), *Haemophilus influenzae* (especially b serotype), *Neisseria meningitidis* (also known as meningococcus), and *Klebsiella pneumoniae*.
Polysaccharide capsule is an antiphagocytic virulence factor.
Positive **Quellung** reaction: if encapsulated bug is present, capsule **swells** when specific anticapsular antisera are added.

IgG_2 necessary for immune response. Capsule serves as antigen in vaccines (Pneumovax, *H. influenzae* b, meningococcal vaccines).
Quellung = capsular "swelling."
Pneumococcus associated with "rusty" sputum, sepsis in sickle cell anemia.

Normal flora: dominant

Skin–*S. epidermidis*
Nose–*S. aureus*
Oropharynx–Viridans streptococci
Dental plaque–*S. mutans*
Colon–*B. fragilis* > *E. coli*
Vagina–*Lactobacillus, E. coli*, group B strep

chondromatitis, pneumonia

hence "baby" infections.

Neonates delivered by cesarean section have no flora, but are rapidly colonized after birth.

Common causes of pneumonia

Children (6 wk–18 y) →	Adults (18–40 y) →	Adults (40–65 y) →	Elderly
Viruses (RSV)	*Mycoplasma*	*S. pneumoniae*	*S. pneumoniae*
Mycoplasma	*C. pneumoniae*	*H. influenzae*	Anaerobes
Chlamydia pneumoniae	*S. pneumoniae*	Anaerobes	*H. influenzae*
S. pneumoniae		Viruses	Gram-negative rods
		Mycoplasma	**Viruses**

Special Groups

Nosocomial (hospital acquired)	*Staphylococcus*, gram-negative rods
Immunocompromised	*Staphylococcus*, gram-negative rods, **fungi**, viruses, ***Pneumocystis carinii*—with HIV**
Aspiration	Anaerobes
Alcoholic/IV drug user	*S. pneumoniae, Klebsiella, Staphylococcus*
Postviral	*Staphylococcus, H. influenzae*
Neonate	Group B streptococci, *E. coli*
Atypical	*Mycoplasma, Legionella, Chlamydia*

Causes of meningitis

Newborn (0–6 mo) →	Children (6 mo–6 y) →	6 y–60 y →	60 y +
Group B streptococci	*H. influenzae* B	Enteroviruses	*S. pneumoniae*
E. coli	*S. pneumoniae*	*N. meningitidis*	Gram-negative rods
Listeria	*N. meningitidis*	*S. pneumoniae*	Listeria
	Enteroviruses	HSV	

HIV—*Cryptococcus*, CMV, toxoplasmosis (brain abscess), JC virus (PML)

Note: Incidence of *H. influenzae* meningitis has ↓ greatly with introduction of *H. influenzae* vaccine in last 10–15 years.

CSF findings in meningitis

Bacterial: pressure ↑, polys ↑, proteins ↑, sugar ↓.
Viral: pressure normal/↑, lymphs ↑, proteins **normal,** sugar **normal.**
TB/fungal: pressure ↑, lymphs ↑, proteins ↑, sugar ↓.

Osteomyelitis

Most people: *S. aureus*
Sexually active: *N. gonorrhoeae* (rare: septic arthritis more common)
Drug addicts: *Pseudomonas aeruginosa*
Sickle cell: *Salmonella*
Hip replacement: *S. aureus* and *S. epidermidis*

Assume *S. aureus* if no other information.

Most osteomyelitis occurs in children. Elevated ESR.

Urinary tract infections

Ambulatory: *E. coli* (50–80%), *Klebsiella* (8–10%). *Staphylococcus saprophyticus* (10–30%) is the second most common cause of UTI in young ambulatory women.

Hospital: *E. coli, Proteus, Klebsiella, Serratia, Pseudomonas.*

Epidemiology: women to men = 30 to 1 (short urethra colonized by fecal flora).

UTIs mostly caused by ascending infections. In males: babies with congenital defects; elderly with enlarged prostates.

UTI: dysuria, frequency, urgency, suprapubic pain.

Pyelonephritis: fever, chills and flank pain.

UTI bugs

Species	Features of the organism	Ferments lactose
Serratia marcescens	Some strains produce a red pigment; often nosocomial and drug-resistant	No (slow)
Escherichia coli	Colonies show metallic sheen on EMB agar	Yes
Enterobacter cloacae	Often nosocomial and drug-resistant	Yes
Klebsiella pneumoniae	Large mucoid capsule and viscous colonies	Yes
Proteus mirabilis	Motility causes "swarming" on agar; produces urease; associated with Struvite stones MgAl(PO₄)	No
Pseudomonas aeruginosa	Blue-green pigment and fruity odor; usually nosocomial and drug-resistant	No

SEEK PP S- Saprophyticus

Sexually transmitted diseases

Disease	Clinical features	Organism
Gonorrhea	Urethritis, cervicitis, PID, prostatitis, epididymitis, arthritis rarely creeches Telos	*Neisseria gonorrhoeae*
Primary syphilis	Chancre	*Treponema pallidum*
Secondary syphilis	Fever, lymphadenopathy, skin rashes, condylomata lata	
Tertiary syphilis	Gummas, tabes dorsalis, general paresis, aortitis	
Genital herpes	Penile, vulvar, or cervical ulcers	HSV-2
Chlamydial urethritis/ cervicitis	Conjunctivitis, Reiter's syndrome, PID	*Chlamydia trachomatis* (D-K)
Lymphogranuloma venereum	Ulcers, lymphadenopathy, rectal strictures bubues	*Chlamydia trachomatis* (L1-L3)
Trichomoniasis	Vaginitis	*Trichomonas vaginalis*
AIDS	Opportunistic infections, Kaposi's sarcoma, lymphoma	HIV
Condylomata acuminata	Cervical cancer	HPV
Hepatitis B	Jaundice	HBV

Pelvic inflammatory disease

Top bugs: *Chlamydia trachomatis* (subacute, often undiagnosed), *N. gonorrhoeae* (acute, high fever). *C. trachomatis* is the most common STD in the US (3–4 million cases per year). Cervical motion tenderness, purulent cervical discharge. PID may include salpingitis, endometritis, hydrosalpinx, and tubo-ovarian abscess.

Salpingitis is a risk factor for ectopic pregnancy, infertility, chronic pelvic pain, and adhesions.

Other STDs include *Gardnerella* (clue cells) and *Trichomonas* (motile on wet prep).

Nosocomial infections

By risk factor:
Newborn nursery: CMV, RSV
Urinary catheterization: *E. coli, Proteus mirabilis*

Respiratory therapy equipment: *P. aeruginosa*
Work in renal dialysis unit: HBV
Hyperalimentation: *Candida albicans*
Water aerosols: *Legionella*

The two most common causes of nosocomial infections are *E. coli* (UTI) and *S. aureus* (wound infection).
Presume *Pseudomonas air-uginosa* when **air** or burns are involved.
Legionella when water source is involved.

Bug hints (if all else fails)

Pus, empyema, abscess: *S. aureus*
Pediatric infection: *H. influenzae* (including epiglottitis)
Aerobic infection: *P. aeruginosa* (pneumonia in CF, burn infections)
Branching rods in oral infection: *Actinomyces israelii*
Traumatic open wound: *C. perfringens*
Surgical wound: *S. aureus, E. coli, Klebsiella*
Dog or cat bite: *Pasteurella multocida*

Weil-Felix reaction

Weil-Felix reaction assays for antirickettsial antibodies, which cross-react with *Proteus* antigen. Weil-Felix is usually positive for typhus and Rocky Mountain spotted fever but negative for Q fever.

Special culture requirements

Bug	Media used for isolation
H. influenzae	Chocolate agar with factors V (NAD) and X (hematin)
N. gonorrhoeae	Thayer–Martin media
B. pertussis Bordet - ella	Bordet–Gengou (potato) agar
C. diphtheriae	Tellurite agar
M. tuberculosis	Löwenstein–Jensen agar
S. aureus	Mannitol–salt agar
M. pneumoniae	Eaton's agar
Lactose-fermenting enterics (e.g., *Escherichia, Klebsiella,* and *Enterobacter*)	Pink colonies on MacConkey's agar
Legionella pneumophila	Charcoal yeast extract agar buffered with ↑ iron and cysteine
Fungi	Sabouraud's agar

Medically important protozoa

Organism	Disease	Endemic to US?	Mode of Transmission	Diagnosis	Treatment
Entamoeba histolytica	Amebiasis Bloody diarrhea Liver abscess	Yes	Cysts in food	Serology and/or trophozoites or cysts in stool	Metronidazole and iodoquinol
Giardia lamblia	Giardiasis Bloating Flatulence Diarrhea	Yes	Cysts in food	Trophozoites or cysts in stool	Metronidazole
Cryptosporidium	Severe diarrhea in AIDS Mild disease in non-HIV	Yes	Cysts in food	Cysts on acid-fast stain	None
Toxoplasma	Brain abscess in HIV Birth defects FUO "Mono" symptoms	Yes	Cysts in meat or cat feces	Serology, biopsy	Sulfonamide + pyrimethamine
Pneumocystis carinii (is called a fungus, currently)	Pneumonia in HIV	Yes	Inhalation	Lung biopsy or lavage; methenamine silver stain	TMP-SMX or pentamidine
Plasmodium *vivax* *ovale* *malariae*	Malaria	No (rare)	Mosquito (*Anopheles*)	Blood smear	Chloroquine (primaquine for *vivax*, *ovale*)
falciparum	Malaria—severe (cerebral)	No (only travelers)	Mosquito (*Anopheles*)	Blood smear	Chloroquine Mefloquine Quinine
Trichomonas vaginalis	Vaginitis	Yes	Sexual	Trophozoites on wet mount	Metronidazole

Latin parvo = small

DNA viral strands	All DNA viruses except the Parvoviridae are dsDNA. All are linear except papovaviruses and hepadnaviruses (circular).	All are dsDNA (like our cells) except "part-of-a-virus" (parvovirus) is ssDNA.
RNA viral strands	All RNA viruses except Reoviridae are ssRNA.	All are ssRNA (like our mRNA), except "**re**peat**o**-virus" (**reo**virus) is dsRNA.
Naked viral genome infectivity	Naked nucleic acids of most dsDNA (except poxviruses and HBV) and (+) strand ssRNA (≈mRNA) viruses are infectious. Naked nucleic acids of (–) strand ssRNA and dsRNA viruses are not infectious. **Naked** (nonenveloped) RNA viruses include **C**alicivirus, **P**icornavirus, and **R**eovirus.	Viral nucleic acids with the same structure as host nucleic acids are infective alone; others require special enzymes (contained in intact virion). **Naked CPR.**
Enveloped viruses	Generally, enveloped viruses acquire their envelopes from plasma membrane when they exit from cell. Exceptions are herpesviruses, which acquire envelopes from nuclear membrane.	
Virus ploidy	All viruses are haploid (with one copy of DNA or RNA) except retroviruses, which have two identical ssRNA molecules (≈diploid).	
Viral vaccines	Live attenuated: measles, mumps, rubella, Sabin polio, VZV. Killed: rabies, influenza, hepatitis A, and Salk polio vaccines. Recombinant: HBV (antigen = recombinant HBsAg).	MMR = measles, mumps, rubella. sal**K** = **K**illed.

Viral replication

DNA viruses	All replicate in the nucleus (except poxvirus).
RNA viruses	All replicate in the cytoplasm (except influenza virus and retroviruses).

Viral genetics

Recombination	Exchange of genes between 2 chromosomes by crossing over within regions of significant base sequence homology.
Reassortment	When viruses with segmented genomes (e.g., influenza virus) exchange segments. High-frequency recombination.
Complementation	When one of 2 viruses that infects the cell has a mutation that results in a nonfunctional protein. The nonmutated virus "complements" the mutated one by making a functional protein that serves both viruses.
Phenotypic mixing	Genome of virus A can be coated with the surface proteins of virus B. Type B protein coat determines the infectivity of the phenotypically mixed virus. However, the progeny from this infection has a type A coat and is encoded by its type A genetic material.

Viral vaccines: dead or alive

Live attenuated vaccines induce humoral and cell-mediated immunity, but have reverted to virulence on rare occasion. Killed vaccines induce only humoral immunity but are stable.

Dangerous to give live vaccines to immunocompromised patients or their close contacts.

Viral pathogens

Structure	Viruses
DNA enveloped viruses	Herpesviruses (herpes simplex virus types 1 and 2, varicella-zoster virus, cytomegalovirus, Epstein-Barr virus), hepatitis B virus, smallpox virus
DNA nucleocapsid viruses	Adenovirus, papillomaviruses, *parvovirus*
RNA enveloped viruses	Influenza virus, parainfluenza virus, respiratory syncytial virus, measles virus, mumps virus, rubella virus, rabies virus, human T-cell leukemia virus, human immunodeficiency virus
RNA nucleocapsid viruses	Enteroviruses (poliovirus, coxsackievirus, echovirus, hepatitis A virus), rhinovirus, reovirus *Picornaviruses* *Calicivirus*

Prions

Infectious agents that do not contain RNA or DNA (consist only of proteins); diseases include Creutzfeldt-Jakob disease (CJD: rapid progressive dementia), kuru, scrapie (sheep), and "mad cow disease." *BSE*

Latent virus infections

Virus exists in patient for months to years before it manifests as clinical disease. SSPE (late sequela of measles), PML (reactivation of JC virus) in immuno-compromised patients.

Hepatitis transmission

HAV (RNA virus) is transmitted primarily by fecal–oral route. Short incubation (3 wk). No carriers.

Hep **A: A**symptomatic (usually)

HBV (DNA virus) is transmitted primarily by parenteral, sexual, and maternal–fetal routes. Long incubation (3 mo). Carriers. Reverse transcription occurs; however, the virion enzyme is a DNA-dependent DNA polymerase.

Hep **B: B**lood-borne
also → CA

HCV is transmitted primarily via blood and resembles HBV in its course and severity. Carriers. Common cause of posttransfusion and IV drug use hepatitis in the United States.

Hep **C: C**hronic, **C**irrhosis, **C**arcinoma, **C**arriers

HDV (delta agent) is a defective virus that requires HBsAg as its envelope. Carriers.

Hep **D: D**efective, **D**ependent on HBV

HEV is transmitted enterically and causes water-borne epidemics. Resembles HAV in course, severity, incubation. High mortality rate in pregnant women.

Hep **E: E**nteric

Both HBV and HCV predispose a patient to hepato-cellular carcinoma.

DNA viruses

Viral family	Envelope?	DNA structure	Medical importance
Parvovirus	No	SS-linear	B19 virus—aplastic crises in sickle cell disease —"slapped cheeks" rash—erythema infectiosum
Papovavirus	No	DS-circular	AAV—adeno-assisted virus HPV—warts, CIN, cervical cancer JC—progressive multifocal leukoencephalopathy in HIV BK—in kidney transplant patients *"BK fucks up your kidneys"*
Adenovirus	No	DS-linear	Possible gene therapy vector Febrile pharyngitis—sore throat Pneumonia Conjunctivitis—"pink eye"

Hepadnavirus	Yes	DS-partial circular	Hepatitis B virus
			  Acute or chronic hepatitis
			  Vaccine available—use has ↑ tremendously
			  Not a retrovirus but has reverse transcriptase

Herpesviruses	Yes	DS-linear	HSV 1—oral (and some genital) lesions HSV 2—genital (and some oral) lesions Varicella-zoster virus—chickenpox, zoster, shingles Epstein-Barr virus—mononucleosis, Burkitt's lymphoma, *nasopharyngeal* Cytomegalovirus—infection in immunosuppressed patients, esp. transplant recipients HHV 6 HHV 7—monkey bites (fatal in humans) HHV 8 (KSHV)—Kaposi's sarcoma–associated herpesvirus
Poxvirus	Yes	DS-linear	Smallpox eradication Vaccinia—cowpox ("milkmaid's blisters")

RNA viruses

Viral family	Envelope?	RNA structure	Capsid symmetry	Medical importance
Picornaviruses	No	SS + linear	Icosahedral	**P**oliovirus—polio-Salk/Sabin vaccines KPV/OPV **E**chovirus—aseptic meningitis **R**hinovirus—"common cold" **C**oxsackievirus—aseptic meningitis 　Herpangina—febrile pharyngitis 　"Hand, foot, and mouth" disease 　Myocarditis **H**epatitis A—acute viral hepatitis
Caliciviruses	No	SS + linear	Icosahedral	Hepatitis E Norwalk virus—viral gastroenteritis
Reoviruses	No	DS linear Segmented	Icosahedral (double)	Reovirus—Colorado tick fever Rotavirus—#1 cause of fatal diarrhea in children
Flaviviruses	Yes	SS + linear	Icosahedral	Hepatitis C Yellow fever Dengue
Togaviruses	Yes	SS + linear	Icosahedral	Rubella (German measles) Congenital heart defects
Retroviruses	Yes	SS + linear	Icosahedral	Have reverse transcriptase HIV—AIDS HTLV—T-cell leukemia
Orthomyxoviruses	Yes	SS − linear Segmented (8)	Helical	Influenza virus
Paramyxoviruses	Yes	SS − linear Nonsegmented	Helical	Measles Mumps Parainfluenza—croup RSV—bronchiolitis in babies; Rx−ribavirin
Rhabdoviruses	Yes	SS − linear	Helical	Rabies
Filoviruses	Yes	SS − linear	Helical	Ebola/Marburg Hemorrhagic fever—often fatal!
Coronaviruses	Yes	SS + linear	Helical	Coronavirus—"common cold"
Arenaviruses	Yes	SS − circular	Helical	LCV—lymphocytic choriomeningitis 　Meningitis—spread by mice
Bunyaviruses	Yes	SS − circular	Helical	California encephalitis Sandfly/Rift Valley fevers Crimea-Congo hemorrhagic fever Hantavirus—hemorrhagic fever, pneumonia

SS, single-stranded; DS, double-stranded; +, + polarity; −, − polarity

"PERCH"

Hepatitis serologic markers

	Description
IgM HAVAb	IgM antibody to HAV; best test to detect active hepatitis A.
HBsAg	Antigen found on surface of HBV; continued presence indicates carrier state.
HBsAb	Antibody to HBsAg; provides immunity to hepatitis B.
HBcAg	Antigen associated with core of HBV.
HBcAb	Antibody to HBcAg; positive during window phase. IgM HBcAb is an indicator of recent disease.
HBeAg	A second, different antigenic determinant in the HBV core. Important indicator of transmissibility.
HBeAb	Antibody to e antigen; indicates low transmissibility.

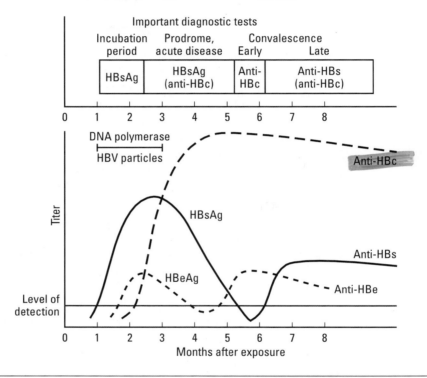

Segmented viruses	All are RNA viruses. They include arenaviruses, reoviruses, bunyaviruses, and orthomyxoviruses (influenza viruses). Influenza virus consists of 8 segments of negative-stranded RNA. These segments can undergo reassortment, causing worldwide epidemics of the flu.	Arena = "grains of sand" (due to ribosomes in the viral capsid as seen on electron microscopy). **Reo** = **re**peat**o** = segmented.
Picornavirus	Includes poliovirus, rhinovirus, coxsackievirus, echovirus, hepatitis A virus. RNA is translated into one large polypeptide that is cleaved by proteases into many small proteins. Can cause aseptic meningitis (except rhinovirus and hep A virus).	The discovery of **polio,** on a **rhino** in **Coxsackie**, NY, was **echo**ed around the world. Pico**RNA**virus = small **RNA** virus.
Rhinovirus	Nonenveloped RNA virus. Cause of common cold: more than 100 serologic types.	**Rhino** has a runny nose.
Rotavirus	Rotavirus, the most important global cause of infantile gastroenteritis, is a segmented dsRNA virus (a reovirus). Major cause of acute diarrhea in US during winter.	**ROTA** = **R**ight **O**ut **T**he **A**nus.
Paramyxoviruses	Paramyxoviruses include those that cause parainfluenza (croup), mumps, and measles as well as RSV, which causes respiratory tract infection (bronchiolitis, pneumonia) in infants. Paramyxoviruses cause disease in children. All paramyxoviruses have 1 serotype except parainfluenza virus, which has 4.	
Mumps virus	A paramyxovirus with one serotype. Symptoms: parotitis, orchitis (inflammation of testes), and aseptic meningitis. Can cause sterility (especially after puberty).	**M**umps gives you **b**umps (parotitis).
Measles virus	A paramyxovirus that causes measles. Koplik spots (bluish-gray spots on buccal mucosa) are diagnostic. SSPE, encephalitis (1 in 2000), or giant cell pneumonia (rarely, in immunosuppressed) are possible sequelae. _Maculopapular rash_	**3 C**'s of measles: **C**ough **C**oryza **C**onjunctivitis Also look for **K**oplik spots.
Influenza viruses _Orthomyxovindae_ Genetic shift Genetic drift	(*) Enveloped, single-stranded RNA viruses with segmented genome. Contain hemagglutinin and neuraminidase antigens. Responsible for worldwide influenza epidemics; patients at risk for fatal bacterial superinfection. Rapid genetic changes. Reassortment of viral genome (such as when human flu virus recombines with swine flu virus). Minor changes based on random mutation.	Killed viral vaccine is major mode of protection; reformulated vaccine offered each fall to elderly, health-care workers, etc. Amantadine and rimantadine are approved for use against influenza A (especially prophylaxis), but are not useful against influenza B or C.

Rabies virus

Negri bodies are characteristic cytoplasmic inclusions in neurons infected by rabies virus. Has bullet-shaped capsid. Rabies has long incubation period (weeks to 3 mo). Causes fatal encephalitis with seizures and hydrophobia.

More commonly from bat, raccoon, and skunk bites than from dog bites.

Travels to the CNS by migrating in a retrograde fashion up nerve axons.

Arboviruses

Transmitted by arthropods (mosquitoes, ticks). Classic examples are dengue fever (also known as break-bone fever) and yellow fever. A variant of dengue fever in Southeast Asia is hemorrhagic shock syndrome.

Arbo virus = **Ar**thropod = **bo**rne virus

Yellow fever

Caused by flavivirus, an arbovirus transmitted by *Aedes* mosquitos. Virus has a monkey or human reservoir.
Symptoms: high fever, black vomitus, and jaundice. Councilman bodies (acidophilic inclusions) may be seen in liver.

Flavi = yellow.

Herpesviruses

	Diseases	Route of transmission
HSV-1	Gingivostomatitis, temporal lobe encephalitis, herpes labialis	Respiratory secretions, saliva
HSV-2	Herpes genitalis, neonatal herpes	Sexual contact, perinatal
VZV	Varicella zoster (shingles), encephalitis, pneumonia	Respiratory secretions
EBV	Infectious mononucleosis, Burkitt's lymphoma	Respiratory secretions, saliva
CMV	Congenital infection, mononucleosis, pneumonia	Congenital, transfusion, sexual contact, saliva, urine, transplant
KSAV	Kaposi's sarcoma (HIV patients)	Sexual contact

Mononucleosis

Caused by EBV, a herpesvirus. Characterized by fever, hepatosplenomegaly, pharyngitis, and lymphadenopathy (especially posterior auricular nodes).
Peak incidence 15–20 y old. Positive heterophil Ab test. Abnormal circulating cytotoxic T cells (atypical lymphocytes).

Most common during peak kissing years ("kissing disease").

Tzanck test

A smear of an opened skin vesicle to detect multi-nucleated giant cells. Used to assay for herpesvirus.

Tzanck heavens I do not have herpes.

HIV diagnosis

Presumptive diagnosis made with ELISA; positive results are then confirmed with Western blot assay.
HIV PCR/viral load tests are increasing in popularity; they allow physician to monitor the effect of drug therapy on viral load.

ELISA/Western blot tests look for antibodies to viral proteins; these tests are often falsely negative in the first 1–2 months of HIV infection.

Time course of HIV infection

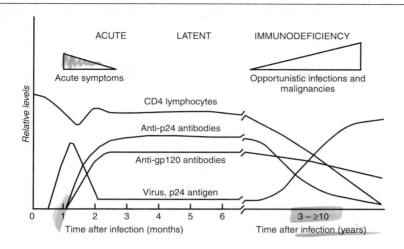

Opportunistic infections in AIDS

Bacterial	Tuberculosis, *M. avium-intracellulare* complex.	Alphabet soup: TB, MAC, HSV,
Viral	Herpes simplex, varicella-zoster virus, cytomegalovirus, progressive multifocal leukoencephalopathy (JC virus).	VZV, CMV, PCP. JC
Fungal	Thrush (*Candida albicans*), cryptococcosis (cryptococcal meningitis), histoplasmosis, pneumocystis pneumonia.	
Protozoal	Toxoplasmosis, cryptosporidiosis.	

Antibody structure   Variable part of L and H chains recognizes antigens. Constant part of H chain of IgM and IgG fixes complement. Heavy chain contributes to Fc and Fab fractions. Light chain contributes only to Fab fraction.

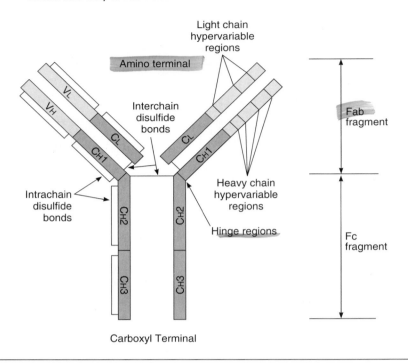

Carboxyl Terminal

Immunoglobulins

IgG   Opsonizes bacteria, fixes complement, neutralizes bacterial toxins and viruses, crosses the placenta.

IgA   Prevents attachment of bacteria and viruses to mucous membranes, does not fix complement. Monomer or dimer. Found in secretions. Picks up secretory component from epithelial cells before secretion.

IgM   Produced in the primary response to an antigen. Fixes complement but does not cross the placenta. Antigen receptor on the surface of B cells. Monomer or pentamer.

IgD   Unclear function. Found on the surface of many B cells and in serum.

IgE   Mediates immediate (type I) hypersensitivity by inducing the release of mediators from mast cells and basophils when exposed to allergen. Mediates immunity to worms.

Ig epitopes   Allotype = Ig epitope common to some members of a species.

Isotype = Ig epitope common to a single class of Ig (five classes, determined by heavy chain).

Idiotype = Ig epitope determined by antigen-binding site.

Isotype = Iso (same). Common to same class.

Idiotype = Idio (unique). Hypervariable region is unique.

Components of immune response

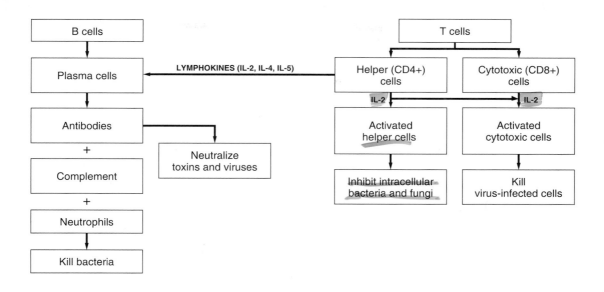

Adjuvant definition	Adjuvants are nonspecific stimulators of the immune response but are not immunogenic by themselves. Adjuvants are given with a weak immunogen to enhance response.

Adjuvant = that which aids another.

MHC I and II	MHC = major histocompatibility complex. Consists of 3 class I genes (A, B, C) and 3 class II genes (DP, DQ, DR). All nucleated cells have class I MHC proteins. Antigen-presenting cells (e.g., macrophages) also have class II MHC proteins. Class II are the main determinants of organ rejection. MHC I Ag loading occurs in rER (viral antigens). MHC II Ag loading occurs in acidified endosome.

Class I = 1 polypeptide, with β_2-microglobulin.
Class II = 2 polypeptides, an α and a β chain.

T-cell glycoproteins Helper T cells have CD4, which binds to class II MHC on antigen-presenting cells. Cytotoxic T cells have CD8, which binds to class I MHC on virus-infected cells.

Product of CD and MHC = 8. (CD4 × MHC II = 8 = CD8 × MHC I).

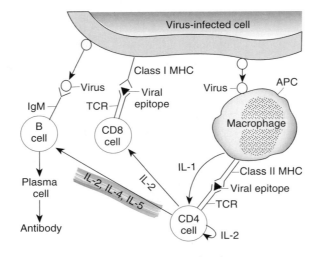

CD3 complex Cluster of polypeptides associated with a T-cell receptor. Consists of γ, ε, δ, and two zeta chains. Important in signal transduction.

Precipitin curve

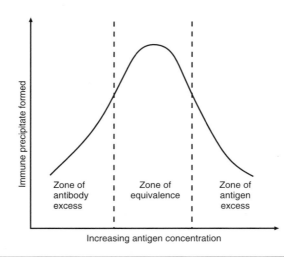

In the presence of a constant amount of antibody, the amount of immune precipitate formed is plotted as a function of increasing amounts of antigen.

Prozone phenomenon: a suboptimal precipitate of Ab-Ag complexes due to antibody excess.

Important cytokines

IL-1	Secreted by macrophages. Stimulates T cells, B cells, neutrophils, fibroblasts, epithelial cells to grow, differentiate, or synthesize specific products. Is an endogenous pyrogen.	**"Hot T-bone stEAk".** IL-1: fever (**hot**) IL-2: stimulates **T** cells IL-3: stimulates **bone** marrow
IL-2	Secreted by helper T cells. Stimulates growth of helper and cytotoxic T cells. _+ MONOCYTES_	IL-4: stimulates Ig**E** production
IL-3	Secreted by activated T cells. Supports the growth and differentiation of bone marrow stem cells. Has a function similar to GM-CSF. _promotes myeloid differentiation._	IL-5: stimulates Ig**A** production
IL-4	Secreted by helper T cells. Promotes growth of B cells. Enhances the synthesis of IgE and IgG.	
IL-5	Secreted by helper T cells. Promotes differentiation of B cells. Enhances the synthesis of IgA. Stimulates production and activation of eosinophils.	
Gamma interferon	Secreted by helper T cells. Stimulates macrophages.	_"Macrophage-activating factor"_
TNF-α	Secreted by macrophages. ↑ IL-2 receptor synthesis by helper T cells. ↑ B-cell proliferation. Attracts and activates neutrophils.	
TNF-β	Secreted by activated T lymphocytes. Functions similar to those of TNF-α.	

Actions of IL-1 and TNF

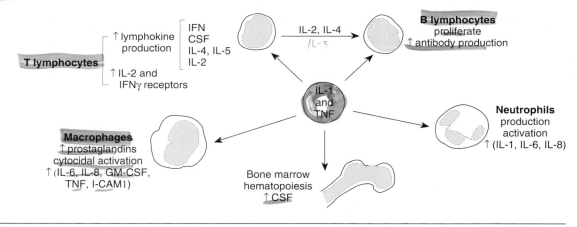

183

Complement

Complement defends against gram-negative bacteria. *en encapsulated organisms* Activated by Ig**G** or Ig**M** in the **classic** pathway, and activated by toxins (including endotoxin), aggregated IgA, or other conditions in the alternate pathway.

GM makes **classic** cars.
C1, C2, C3, C4: viral neutralization.
C3b: opsonization.
C3a, C5a: anaphylaxis.
C5a: neutrophil chemotaxis.
C5b-9: cytolysis by **M**embrane **A**ttack **C**omplex **(MAC)** (deficiency in *Neisseria* sepsis). *SKIN*

Deficiency of C1 esterase inhibitor leads to angioedema (overactive complement).

Alternative

Microbial surfaces (nonspecific activators) → C3(H₂O) + B + D → C̄3̄b̄,̄B̄b̄ (C3 convertase)

→ C3 → C̄3̄b̄,̄B̄b̄,̄C̄3̄b̄ + C3a (C5 convertase)

Target cell membrane (M)

C5 → C5a + MC5b → MC5b,6,7 → MC5b,6,7,8,9 (membrane attack complex) → LYSIS, CYTOTOXICITY

C7, C9 ; C6, C8

C3a + C̄4̄b̄,̄2̄b̄,̄3̄b̄ (C5 convertase)

Classic

Antigen-antibody complexes → C1 → C̄1̄ → C2, C4 → C̄4̄b̄,̄2̄b̄ (C3 convertase)

Interferon mechanism

Interferons (α, β) are proteins that place uninfected cells in an antiviral state. Interferons induce the production of a second protein that inhibits viral protein synthesis by degrading viral mRNA (but not host mRNA).

Interferes with viral protein synthesis.

Hypersensitivity

Type I

Mast cell or basophil

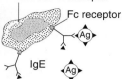

Fc receptor

Ag

IgE

Ag

Anaphylactic and atopic: Ag cross-links IgE on presensitized mast cells and basophils, triggering release of vasoactive amines. Reaction develops rapidly after Ag exposure due to preformed Ab. Possible manifestations include anaphylaxis, asthma, or local wheal and flare.

First and **Fast** (anaphylaxis). I, II, and III are all antibody mediated.

Type II

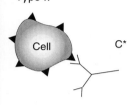

Cell   C*

Cytotoxic: IgM, IgG bind to Ag on "enemy" cell, leading to lysis (by complement) or phagocytosis. Examples include autoimmune hemolytic anemia, Rh disease (erythroblastosis fetalis), Goodpasture's syndrome.

Cy-2-toxic.
Antibody and complement mediated.

Type III

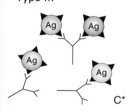

Ag   Ag

Ag

Ag

C*

Immune complex: Ag-Ab complexes activate complement, which attracts neutrophils; neutrophils release lysosomal enzymes (e.g., PAN, immune complex GN).

Serum sickness: an immune complex disease (type III) in which Abs to the foreign proteins are produced (takes 5 days). Immune complexes form and are deposited in membranes, where they fix complement (leads to tissue damage). More common than Arthus reaction.

Arthus reaction: a local subacute Ab-mediated hypersensitivity (type III) reaction. Intradermal injection of Ag induces antibodies, which form Ag-Ab complexes in the skin. Characterized by edema, necrosis, and activation of complement.

Imagine an immune complex as **three** things stuck together: Ag–Ab–complement.

Most serum sickness is now caused by drugs (not serum). Fever, urticaria, arthralgias, proteinuria lymphadenopathy 5–10 days after Ag exposure.

Ag-Ab complexes cause the Arthus reaction.

Type IV

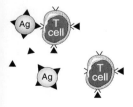

Ag   T cell

Ag   T cell

Delayed (cell-mediated) type: Sensitized T lymphocytes encounter antigen and then release lymphokines (leads to macrophage activation). Examples include TB skin test, transplant rejection, contact dermatitis.

4th and last = delayed.
Cell mediated; therefore, it is not transferable by serum.
ACID =
Anaphylactic and **A**topic (type I)
Cytotoxic (type II)
Immune complex (type III)
Delayed (cell-mediated) (type IV)

C* = complement

Passive versus active immunity

Active	Induced after exposure to foreign antigens. Slow onset. Long-lasting protection (memory).	After exposure to **T**etanus toxin, **B**otulinum toxin, **H**BV, or **R**abies, patients are given preformed antibodies (passive)—**To Be Healed Rapidly.**
Passive	Based on receiving preformed antibodies from another host. Rapid onset. Short life span of antibodies.	

Immune deficiencies

Thymic aplasia (DiGeorge's syndrome)	**T**-cell deficiency. Thymus and parathyroids fail to develop owing to failure of development of the 3rd and 4th pharyngeal pouches. Presents with tetany owing to hypocalcemia.
Chronic mucocutaneous candidiasis	T-cell dysfunction specifically against *Candida albicans*.
Bruton's agammaglobulinemia	**B**-cell deficiency. X-linked recessive defect in a tyrosine-kinase gene associated with low levels of all classes of immunoglobulins. Associated with recurrent bacterial infections after 6 months of age, when levels of maternal IgG antibody decline.
Selective immunoglobulin deficiency	Deficiency in a specific class of immunoglobulins. Possibly due to a defect in isotype switching. Selective IgA deficiency is the most common selective immunoglobulin deficiency.
Severe combined immunodeficiency	B- and T-cell deficiency. Defect in early stem-cell differentiation. Presents with recurrent viral, bacterial, fungal, and protozoal infections. May have multiple causes (e.g., failure to synthesize class II MHC antigens, defective IL-2 receptors, or adenosine deaminase deficiency).
Wiskott–Aldrich syndrome	B- and T-cell deficiency. Defect in the ability to mount an IgM response to capsular polysaccharides of bacteria. Associated with elevated IgA levels, normal IgE levels, and low IgM levels. Triad of symptoms includes recurrent pyogenic infections, eczema, and thrombocytopenia.
Ataxia–telangiectasia	B- and T-cell deficiency, with associated IgA deficiency. Presents with cerebellar problems (ataxia) and spider angiomas (telangiectasia).
Chronic granulomatous disease	Phagocyte deficiency. Defect in phagocytosis of neutrophils owing to lack of NADPH oxidase activity or similar enzymes. Presents with marked susceptibility to opportunistic infections with bacteria, especially *S. aureus* and *E. coli*, and *Aspergillus*.
Chédiak–Higashi disease	Autosomal recessive defect in phagocytosis that results from microtubular and lysosomal defects of phagocytic cells. Presents with recurrent pyogenic infections by staphylococci and streptococci.
Job's syndrome	Neutrophils fail to respond to chemotactic stimuli. Associated with high levels of IgE. Presents with recurrent cold staphylococcal abscesses.

Transplant rejection

Hyperacute rejection—Antibody mediated due to the presence of preformed anti-donor antibodies in the transplant recipient. Occurs within minutes after transplantation.

Acute rejection—Cell mediated due to cytotoxic T lymphocytes reacting against foreign MHCs. Occurs weeks after transplantation. Reversible with immunosuppressants such as cyclosporin and OKT3.

Chronic rejection—Antibody-mediated vascular damage (fibrinoid necrosis); occurs months to years after transplantation. Irreversible.

These abstracted case vignettes are designed to demonstrate the thought processes necessary to answer multistep clinical reasoning questions.

- Urinalysis of patient shows WBC casts → what is the diagnosis? → pyelonephritis.
- Patient presents with tetany and candidiasis → hypocalcemia and immunosuppression are found → what cell is deficient? → DiGeorge's = T-cell deficiency.
- Patient presents with rose gardener's scenario (thorn prick with ulcers along lymphatic drainage) → what is the infectious bug? → *Sporothrix schenckii.*
- 25-year-old medical student from the Midwest has a queasy feeling in his gut after meals → biopsy of gastric mucosa shows gram-negative rods → what is the likely organism? → *H. pylori.*
- 32-year-old male has cauliflower lesions on calf after traveling to South America → what is the likely organism? → *Blastomyces.*
- Breast-feeding woman suddenly develops redness and swelling of her right breast → on examination, it is found to be a fluctuant mass → what is the diagnosis? → mastitis caused by *S. aureus.*
- Child with SCID has recurrent lung infections and granulomatous lesions → what is the defect in neutrophils? → NADPH oxidase.
- Kid presents with hacking dry cough with fever → what is the diagnosis? → ?mycoplasma. *aproductive cough, pneumonia*
- 20-year-old college student with lymphadenopathy, fever, and hepatosplenomegaly → a double-stranded DNA virus is implicated → what cell is infected? → B cell.
- One hour after eating custard at a picnic, whole family began to vomit. After 10 hours, they were all right → what is the organism? → *S. aureus.*
- Woman becomes flaccid after eating home-canned green beans → Gram stain shows gram-positive rods → *Clostridium botulinum* → what is the mechanism of action? → inhibited release of acetylcholine.
- Man with squamous cell carcinoma of penis had exposure to what virus? → HPV.

1. Patient who visited Mexico presents with bloody diarrhea → what infectious form is found in the stool? → erythrocyte-ingesting trophozoite → *Entamoeba histolytica.*
2. Glossy photograph of cardiac valve with cauliflower growth → diagnosis? → bacterial endocarditis.
3. Adolescent with sore throat and rusty sputum → what does Gram stain of sputum show? → gram-positive diplococci. *Pneumococcus*
4. HIV-positive patient with CSF showing 75/mm³ lymphocytes suddenly dies. Picture of yeast in meninges → diagnosis? → cryptococcal meningitis.

Microbiology

1. Principles and interpretation of bacteriologic lab tests (culture, incubation time, drug sensitivity, specific growth requirements).
2. Dermatologic manifestations of bacterial and viral infections (e.g., syphilis, Rocky Mountain spotted fever, meningococcemia, herpes zoster, coxsackievirus infection).
3. Common sexually transmitted diseases (e.g., syphilis, AIDS, HSV, gonorrhea, chlamydia).
4. Viral gastroenteritis in the pediatric and adult populations.
5. Common causes of community acquired and nosocomial pneumonia.
6. Infections that cause congenital/neonatal complications (ToRCHeS: toxoplasmosis, rubella, CMV, HSV, syphilis).
7. Protozoa that frequently cause disease in the U.S. (e.g., *Entamoeba histolytica, Giardia*).
8. Parasites (protozoa, helminthes) that more commonly cause disease outside the U.S. (e.g., malaria, Chagas' disease, elephantiasis).
9. Herpes simplex encephalitis (medial temporal lobe lesion, mental status changes, treat with acyclovir).
10. Tests available for diagnosis of viral infections (e.g., plaque assay, PCR).
11. Microscopic appearance of organisms.
12. Fever patterns associated with specific diseases.

Immunology

1. Principles and interpretation of immunologic tests (e.g., ELISA, complement-fixation tests, direct and indirect Coombs' test, Ouchterlony reactions).
2. Immune complex diseases (e.g., Goodpasture's syndrome, systemic lupus erythematosus, serum sickness).
3. Genetics of immunoglobulin variety and specificity (class switching, VDJ recombination, affinity maturation).
4. Mechanisms of antigenic variation and immune system evasion employed by bacteria, fungi, protozoa, and viruses.
5. How different types of immune deficiencies lead to different susceptibilities to infection (e.g., T-cell defects and viral/fungal infection; splenectomy and encapsulated organisms).
6. MHC/HLA serotypes: transplant compatibility, disease associations, familial inheritance.
7. Allergies: common antigens, antigen-IgE-mast cell complex, presumed mechanism of immunotherapy (blocking antibodies).
8. Granulomas: role of macrophages, foreign body versus immune granulomas, caseating (TB) versus noncaseating (sarcoid) granulomas, common causes (e.g., TB, sarcoid, fungi).
9. Components of vaccines and how they produce immunity.
10. Characteristics and functions of macrophage and NK (natural killer) cells.

Pathology

Questions dealing with this discipline are difficult to prepare for because of the sheer volume of material. Review the basic principles and hallmark characteristics of each key disease. Given the clinical orientation of the Step 1, it is no longer enough to know the "trigger words" or key associations of certain diseases (e.g., café au lait macules and neurofibromatosis); you must also know the clinical descriptions of these trigger words.

With the increasingly clinical slant of the USMLE Step 1, it is also important to review the classic presenting signs and symptoms of diseases as well as their associated laboratory findings. Delve deeply into the signs, symptoms, and pathophysiology of the major diseases having a high prevalence in the US (e.g., alcoholism, diabetes, hypertension, heart failure, ischemic heart disease, infectious diseases). Be prepared to think one step beyond the simple diagnosis.

The examination includes a number of color photomicrographs and photographs of gross specimens, which are presented in the setting of a brief clinical history. However, read the question and the choices carefully before looking at the illustration, because the history will help you identify the pathologic process. Flip through your illustrated pathology textbook, color atlases, and appropriate web sites in order to look at the pictures in the days before the exam. Pay attention to potential clues such as age, sex, ethnicity, occupation, specialized lab tests, and activity.

Congenital

Neoplastic

Gastrointestinal

Neurologic

Rheumatic/
Autoimmune

Vascular/Cardiac

Other

Findings

Photomicrographs

High-Yield Clinical
Vignettes

High-Yield Glossy
Material

High-Yield Topics

Vascular
Inflammatory
Neoplastic
D
I
Congenital
A
Trauma
E
Psychiatric

| **Common congenital malformations** | 1. Heart defects (congenital rubella)
 2. Hypospadias
 3. Cleft lip with or without cleft palate
 4. Congenital hip dislocation
 5. Spina bifida
 6. Anencephaly
 7. Pyloric stenosis (associated with polyhydramnios); projectile vomiting | Neural tube defects (spina bifida and anencephaly) are associated with increased levels of AFP (in the amniotic fluid and maternal serum). Their incidence is decreased with maternal folate ingestion during pregnancy. |

Congenital heart disease

| R-to-L shunts
 (early cyanosis)
 "blue babies" | 1. **T**etralogy of Fallot (most common cause of early cyanosis)
 2. **T**ransposition of great vessels
 3. **T**runcus arteriosus
 4. **T**ricuspid atresia
 5. **T**otal anomalous pulmonary return | The **5 T's:**
 Tetralogy
 Transposition
 Truncus
 Tricuspid
 Total |
| L-to-R shunts
 (late cyanosis)
 "blue kids" | 1. VSD (most common congenital cardiac anomaly)
 2. ASD
 3. PDA (close with indomethacin) | Frequency: VSD > ASD > PDA.
 ↑ pulmonary resistance due to arteriolar thickening
 → progressive pulmonary hypertension |

| **Tetralogy of Fallot**
 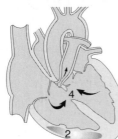 | 1. **P**ulmonary stenosis
 2. **R**VH
 3. **O**verriding aorta (overrides the VSD)
 4. **V**SD
 This leads to **e**arly cyanosis from a R-to-L shunt across the VSD. On x-ray, boot-shaped heart due to RVH. Patients suffer "cyanotic spells."
 The cause of tetralogy of Fallot is anterosuperior displacement of the infundibular septum. _overgrowth of conus muscle_ | _Tetra_ = **4**
 PROVe |

| **Transposition of great vessels**
 high blood [glc] may predispose? | Aorta leaves RV (anterior) and pulmonary trunk leaves LV (posterior) → separation of systemic and pulmonary circulations. Not compatible with life unless a shunt is present to allow adequate mixing of blood (e.g., VSD, PDA, or patent foramen ovale). | Without surgical correction, most infants die within the first months of life. Common in offspring of diabetic mothers. |

| **Coarctation of aorta**
 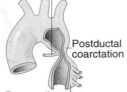 | Infantile type: aortic stenosis proximal to insertion of ductus arteriosus (preductal).

 Adult type: stenosis is distal to ductus arteriosus (postductal). Associated with notching of the ribs, hypertension in upper extremities, weak pulses in lower extremities. | Affects males:females 3:1.
 Check femoral pulses on physical exam.
 INfantile: **IN** close to the heart. (Associated with Turner's syndrome.) AD**ult:** **D**istal to **D**uctus. |

Patent ductus arteriosus

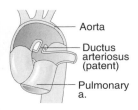

- Aorta
- Ductus arteriosus (patent)
- Pulmonary a.

In fetal period, shunt is R-to-L (normal). In neonatal period, lung resistance decreases and shunt becomes L-to-R with subsequent RV hypertrophy and failure (abnormal). Associated with a continuous, "machine-like" murmur. Patency is maintained by PGE synthesis and low oxygen tension.

Indomethacin is used to close a PDA. PGE is used to keep a PDA open, which may be necessary to sustain life in conditions such as transposition of the great vessels.

Eisenmenger's syndrome

Uncorrected VSD, ASD, or PDA leads to progressive pulmonary hypertension. As pulmonary resistance increases, the shunt changes from L → R to R → L, which causes late cyanosis (clubbing and polycythemia).

Autosomal trisomies

Down's syndrome (trisomy 21), 1:700

Most common chromosomal disorder and cause of congenital mental retardation. *of hands*
Findings: mental retardation, flat facial profile, prominent epicanthal folds, simian crease, duodenal atresia (double bubble sign on x-ray), congenital heart disease (most common malformation is endocardial cushion defect), Alzheimer's disease in affected individuals > 35 years old, associated with an increased risk of ALL. Ninety-five percent of cases are due to meiotic nondisjunction of homologous chromosomes, 4% of cases are due to Robertsonian translocation, and 1% of cases are due to Down mosaicism. Associated with advanced maternal age (from 1:1500 in women under 20 to 1:25 in women over 45).

Edwards' syndrome (trisomy 18), 1:8000

Findings: severe mental retardation, rocker bottom feet, low-set ears, micrognathia, congenital heart disease, clenched hands (flexion of fingers), prominent occiput. Death usually occurs within 1 year of birth.

Patau's syndrome (trisomy 13), 1:6000

Findings: severe mental retardation, microphthalmia, microcephaly, cleft lip/palate, abnormal forebrain structures, polydactyly, congenital heart disease. Death usually occurs within 1 year of birth.

Genetic gender disorders

Klinefelter's syndrome [male] (XXY), 1:850

Testicular atrophy, eunuchoid body shape, tall, long extremities, gynecomastia, female hair distribution. Presence of inactivated X chromosome (Barr body).

One of the most common causes of hypogonadism in males.

Turner's syndrome [female] (XO), 1:3000

Short stature, ovarian dysgenesis, webbing of neck secondary to cystic hygroma, coarctation of the aorta.

Imagine turning into a circle (XO). No Barr body.

Double Y males [male] (XYY), 1:1000

Phenotypically normal, very tall, severe acne, antisocial behavior (seen in 1–2% of XYY males).

Observed with increased frequency among inmates of penal institutions.

this is lower than nl! (3%)

Pseudohermaphroditism

	Disagreement between the phenotypic (external genitalia) and gonadal (testes versus ovaries) sex.	Gender identity is based on external genitalia and sex of upbringing.
Female pseudo-hermaphrodite (XX)	Ovaries present, but external genitalia are virilized or ambiguous. Due to excessive and inappropriate exposure to androgenic steroids during early gestation (i.e., congenital adrenal hyperplasia or exogenous administration of androgens during pregnancy).	
Male pseudo-hermaphrodite (XY)	Testes present, but external genitalia are female or ambiguous. Most common form is testicular feminization (androgen insensitivity), which results from a mutation in the androgen receptor gene (X-linked recessive).	

Cri-du-chat syndrome	Congenital deletion of short arm of chromosome 5 (46 XX or XY, 5p–). ~~5, 9 translocation?~~ Findings: microcephaly, severe mental retardation, high-pitched crying/mewing, epicanthal folds, cardiac abnormalities. ~~lethal.~~	*Cri-du-chat* = cry of the cat.
Fragile X syndrome	X-linked defect affecting the methylation and expression of the *FMR 1* gene. It is the second most common cause of genetic mental retardation (the most common cause is Down's syndrome). Associated with macro-orchidism (enlarged testes), long face with a large jaw, large everted ears, and autism.	Triplet repeat disorder (CGG_n) that may show genetic anticipation.
DiGeorge's syndrome	Due to failure of development of 3rd + 4th pharyngeal pouches and associated with: 1. Total absence of cell-mediated immune responses (lack of thymus/T cells) 2. Tetany (lack of parathyroids and hence hypocalcemia) 3. Congenital defects of heart and great vessels	Think "deep gorge" where thymus should have been. Recurrent viral and fungal infections because of defect in cellular immunity.
Duchenne's muscular dystrophy	An X-linked recessive muscular disease featuring a deleted dystrophin gene, leading to accelerated muscle breakdown. Onset before 5 years of age. Weakness begins in pelvic girdle muscles and progresses superiorly. Pseudohypertrophy of calf muscles due to fibro-fatty replacement of muscle; cardiac myopathy. The use of Gower's maneuver, requiring assistance of the upper extremities to stand up, is characteristic but not specific (indicates proximal lower limb weakness). Becker's muscular dystrophy is due to dystrophin gene mutations (not deletions) and is less severe.	

Handwritten notes near DiGeorge's: "Chromo 22 abnormalities" "Ti George" "Twenty-Two" "Tetany" "T cell ↓m" "Thymic absence"

Handwritten notes near Duchenne's: "others say proximal extremity m.m."

| **Cystic fibrosis** | Autosomal recessive defect in CFTR gene on chromosome 7. Defective Cl⁻ channel → secretion of abnormally thick mucus that plugs lungs, pancreas, salivary glands, and liver → recurrent pulmonary infections (*Pseudomonas* species and *Staphylococcus aureus*), chronic bronchitis, bronchiectasis, pancreatic insufficiency (malabsorption and steatorrhea), meconium ileus in newborns. Increased concentration of Cl⁻ ions in sweat test is diagnostic. | Infertility in males. Fat-soluble vitamin deficiencies (A, D, K). *& E.* Can present as failure to thrive in infancy. |

impaired abs. of fat-sol. vitamins.
delayed postnatal defecation.

| **Juvenile polycystic kidney disease** | Autosomal recessive bilateral enlargement of kidneys, with numerous small cysts of collecting ducts at right angles to the cortical surface. Associated with multiple liver cysts, congenital hepatic fibrosis, and proliferation of bile ducts. *Liver problems.* |

Autosomal dominant diseases

Adult polycystic kidney disease	Bilateral massive enlargement of kidneys due to multiple large cysts. Patients present with pain, hematuria, hypertension, progressive renal failure. Ninety percent of cases are due to mutation in APKD1 (chromosome 16). Associated with polycystic liver disease, berry aneurysms, mitral valve prolapse.
Familial hypercholesterolemia	Elevated LDL owing to defective or absent LDL receptor. Heterozygotes (1 in 500) have cholesterol ≈ 300 mg/dL. Homozygotes (very rare) have cholesterol ≈ 700+ mg/dL, severe atherosclerotic disease early in life and tendon xanthomas (classically in the Achilles tendon). Myocardial infarction may develop before age 20.
Marfan's syndrome	Fibrillin gene mutation → connective tissue disorders.
	Skeletal abnormalities: tall with long extremities, hyperextensive joints, and long, tapering fingers and toes *arachnodactyly*
	Cardiovascular: cystic medial necrosis of aorta → aortic incompetence and dissecting aortic aneurysms. Floppy mitral valve.
	Ocular: subluxation of lenses. *lenticular dislocation as well.*
← 17 letters → Von Recklinghausen's disease (NFT1)	Findings: café au lait spots, neural tumors, Lisch nodules (pigmented iris hamartomas). On long arm of chromosome 17; 17 letters in von Recklinghausen.
Von Hippel-Lindau disease	Findings: hemangioblastomas of retina/cerebellum/medulla; about half of affected individuals develop multiple bilateral renal cell carcinomas and other tumors. Associated with deletion of VHL gene (tumor suppressor) on chromosome 3 (3p).
Huntington's disease	Findings: depression, *suicide* progressive dementia, choreiform movements, caudate atrophy and decreased levels of GABA and acetylcholine in the brain. Symptoms manifest in affected individuals between the ages of 20 and 50. Gene located on chromosome 4; triplet repeat disorder.
Familial adenomatous polyposis	Colon becomes covered with adenomatous polyps after puberty; unless the colon is removed, the risk of cancer is 100%. Deletion of APC (tumor suppressor) gene on chromosome 5.

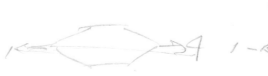

Neural tube defects Associated with low folic acid intake during pregnancy. Spina bifida occulta: failure of bony spinal canal to close but no structural herniation. Usually seen at lower vertebral levels.
Meningocele: meninges herniate through spinal canal defect.
Meningomyelocele: meninges and spinal cord herniate through spinal canal defect.

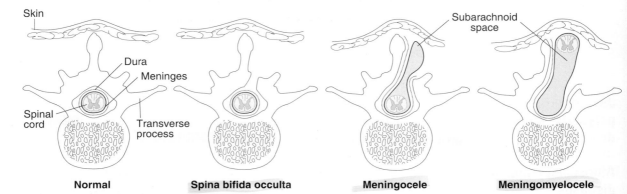

Skin
Dura
Meninges
Spinal cord
Transverse process
Subarachnoid space

Normal   **Spina bifida occulta**   **Meningocele**   **Meningomyelocele**

Teratogens Examples include actinomycin D (preimplantation), x-rays, iodine, thalidomide, aminopterin, DES, alcohol, warfarin, phenytoin, retinoic acid (Accutane).
Most susceptible in 3rd–8th week of pregnancy.
Alcohol is the number 1 known cause of congenital malformations in U.S.

Note that teratogens can act before pregnancy is discovered. Fetal infections can also cause congenital malformations.

Blood dyscrasias

Sickle cell anemia
Hb^S mutation is a single amino acid replacement in β-chain (substitution of normal glutamic acid with valine). Low O_2 or dehydration precipitates sickling. Heterozygotes are relatively malaria resistant (balanced polymorphism). Complications in homozygotes (Hb^{SS}) include aplastic crisis (due to B19 parvovirus infection), autosplenectomy, ↑ risk of encapsulated organism infection, *Salmonella* osteomyelitis, painful crisis (vaso-occlusive), and splenic sequestration crisis.
Hb^c defect is a different β chain mutation; patients with Hb^{cc} or Hb^{sc} (1 of each mutant gene) have milder disease than Hb^{ss} patients. New therapies for sickle cell anemia include hydroxyurea (↑ Hb^F) and bone marrow transplantation.

Eight percent of African-Americans carry the Hb^S trait. 0.2% have the disease.
Sickled cells are crescent-shaped RBCs.

α-thalassemia
There are four α-globin genes. In α-thalassemia, the α-globin chain is underproduced (as a function of number of bad genes, one to four). There is no compensatory increase of any other chains. HbH (β$_4$-tetramers, lacks three α-globin genes). Hb Barts (γ$_4$-tetramers, lacks all four α-globin genes) results in hydrops fetalis and intrauterine fetal death.

Thalassemia is prevalent in Mediterranean populations (*thalassa* = sea). Think of thala**SEA**mia.

β-thalassemia
In β-minor thalassemia (heterozygote), the β-chain is underproduced; in β-major (homozygote), the β-chain is absent. In both cases, fetal hemoglobin production is compensatorily increased but is inadequate. Hb^s/β-thalassemia heterozygote has mild to moderate disease.

β-thalassemia major results in severe anemia requiring blood transfusions. Cardiac failure due to secondary hemochromatosis.

HLA associations

	Disease ✓	
HLA-B27	**P**soriasis, **A**nkylosing spondylitis, **I**nflammatory bowel disease, **R**eiter's syndrome	**PAIR**
HLA-DR4 *(diabetes type I.)*	Rheumatoid arthritis	
HLA-DR3	Sjögren's syndrome; chronic active hepatitis	
HLA-DR2, HLA-DR3	Systemic lupus erythematosus	*DR5, B5 : Hashimoto's*
HLA-A3	Primary hemochromatosis	
HLA-DR3, HLA-DR4	Type I diabetes mellitus (IDDM)	

PATHOLOGY—NEOPLASTIC

-plasia definitions
Hyperplasia = Increase in number of cells (reversible).
Metaplasia = One adult cell type is replaced by another (reversible). Often secondary to irritation and/or environmental exposure (e.g., squamous metaplasia in trachea and bronchi of smokers).
Dysplasia = Abnormal growth with loss of cellular orientation, shape, and size in comparison to normal tissue maturation, commonly preneoplastic (reversible).
Anaplasia = Abnormal cells lacking differentiation; like primitive cells of same tissue, often equated with undifferentiated malignant neoplasms. Tumor giant cells may be formed.
Neoplasia = A clonal proliferation of cells that is uncontrolled and excessive.

Neoplastic progression

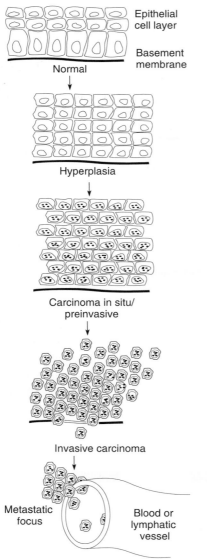

- Normal cells with basal → apical differentiation

- Cells have ↑ in number - **hyperplasia**
- Abnormal proliferation of cells with loss of size, shape, and orientation - **dysplasia**

- **In situ carcinoma**
- Cells are severely dysplastic but have not invaded basement membrane
- High nuclear/cytoplasmic ratio and clumped chromatin

- Cells have invaded basement membrane using **collagenases** and **hydrolases**
- Will metastasize if they reach a blood or lymphatic vessel

Metastasis - spread to distant organ
- Must survive immune attack
- "Seed and soil" theory of metastasis
  - Seed = tumor embolus
  - Soil = target organ - liver, lungs, bone, brain...

Tumor nomenclature

Cell type	Benign	Malignant
Epithelium	Adenoma, papilloma	Adenocarcinoma, papillary carcinoma
Mesenchyme		
Blood cells		Leukemia, lymphoma
Blood vessels	Hemangioma	Angiosarcoma
Smooth muscle	Leiomyoma	Leiomyosarcoma
Skeletal muscle	Rhabdomyoma	Rhabdomyosarcoma
More than one cell type	Mature teratoma	Immature teratoma

Precancerous conditions and associated neoplasms

Condition	Neoplasm
1. Down's syndrome → ALL → Alzheimer's	1. Acute lymphoblastic leukemia
2. Xeroderma pigmentosum	2. Squamous cell and basal cell carcinomas of skin *nt melanoma per se*
3. Chronic atrophic gastritis, pernicious anemia, postsurgical gastric remnants	3. Gastric adenocarcinoma
4. Tuberous sclerosis (facial angiofibroma, seizures, mental retardation)	4. Astrocytoma and cardiac rhabdomyoma *renal angiomyolipoma*
5. Café au lait skin patches	5. Neurofibromatosis
6. Actinic keratosis	6. Squamous cell carcinoma of skin
7. Barrett's esophagus (chronic GI reflux)	7. Esophageal adenocarcinoma
8. Plummer–Vinson syndrome (atrophic glossitis, esophageal webs, plus anemia; all due to iron deficiency)	8. Squamous cell carcinoma of esophagus
9. Cirrhosis (alcoholic, hepatitis B/C)	9. Hepatocellular carcinoma
10. Ulcerative colitis *(Crohn's to a small degree)*	10. Colonic adenocarcinoma
11. Paget's disease of bone	11. Secondary osteosarcoma and fibrosarcoma
12. Immunodeficiency states	12. Malignant lymphomas
13. AIDS	13. Aggressive malignant lymphomas and Kaposi's sarcoma
14. Autoimmune diseases (e.g., Hashimoto's thyroiditis, myasthenia gravis)	14. Malignant thymomas, benign thymomas, thymic hyperplasia *migrating thrombophlebitis*
15. Acanthosis nigricans (hyperpigmentation and epidermal thickening)	15. Visceral malignancy → (stomach, lung, breast, uterus)

Oncogenes

(har-2-new i breast CA)

Oncogene	Associated tumor
c-myc	Burkitt's lymphoma
N-myc	Neuroblastoma
L-myc	Small cell carcinoma of lung
bcl-2	Follicular and undifferentiated lymphomas (inhibits apoptosis) – *bax promotes.*
erb-B2	Breast, ovarian, and gastric carcinomas
ret	Multiple endocrine neoplasia (II, III)

Tumor suppressor genes

Gene	Chromosome	Associated tumor
VHL	3p	Renal cell carcinoma, von Hippel–Lindau disease
APC	5q	Colorectal carcinoma, familial adenomatous polyposis coli
WT-1	11p	Wilms' tumor
Rb	13q	Retinoblastoma, osteosarcoma
BRCA-2	13q	Breast cancer
p53	17p	Most human cancers, Li–Fraumeni syndrome
NF-1	17q	Neurofibromatosis type I
BRCA-1	17q	Breast cancer, ovarian cancer
DCC	18q	Carcinomas of colon and stomach
DPC	18q	Pancreatic cancer
NF-**2**	**22**q	Neurofibromatosis type **II** (**bi**lateral acoustic neuroma)

Tumor markers

PSA, prostatic acid phosphatase	Prostatic carcinoma	Tumor markers should not be used as the primary tool for cancer diagnosis. They may be used to confirm diagnosis, to monitor for tumor recurrence, and to monitor response to therapy.
CEA	Carcinoembryonic antigen. Very nonspecific but produced by ~70% of colorectal and pancreatic cancers; also by gastric and breast carcinomas.	
α-fetoprotein	Normally made by fetus. Hepatocellular carcinomas. Nonseminomatous germ cell tumors of the testis (e.g., yolk sac tumor).	
β-**hCG**	**H**ydatidiform moles, **C**horiocarcinomas, and **G**estational trophoblastic tumors.	
α$_1$-antitrypsin	Liver and yolk sac tumors.	
CA-125	Ovarian tumors.	
S-100	Melanoma, neural tumors, astrocytomas. *neural crest/neural origin.*	
Bombesin	Neuroblastoma, small cell carcinomas, gastric and pancreatic carcinomas.	

Oncogenic viruses

Virus	Associated cancer
HTLV-1	Adult T-cell leukemia
HBV	Hepatocellular carcinoma
EBV	Burkitt's lymphoma, nasopharyngeal carcinoma
HPV	Cervical carcinoma, penile/anal carcinoma
HHV 8 (Kaposi's sarcoma–associated herpesvirus)	Kaposi's sarcoma

Tumor grade versus stage

Grade	Histologic appearance of tumor. Usually graded I–IV based on degree of differentiation and number of mitoses per high-power field.	Stage has more prognostic value than grade. –Save NHL. TNM staging system:
Stage	Based on site and size of primary lesion, spread to regional lymph nodes, presence of metastases.	**T** = size of **T**umor **N** = regional **N**ode involvement **M** = **M**etastases

Brain tumors

Adult	Seventy percent above tentorium (e.g., cerebral hemispheres). Incidence: **metastases** > astrocytoma (including glioblastoma) > meningioma > pituitary tumor.	Adults are taller than kids; therefore their tumors are supratentorial. Glioblastoma multiforme: necrosis,
Childhood	Seventy percent below tentorium (e.g., cerebellum). Incidence: **medulloblastoma** > astrocytoma > ependymoma.	hemorrhage, and pseudo-palisading; "butterfly" glioma; very poor prognosis.

Cardiac tumors

Myxomas are the most common 1° cardiac tumor in adults. Ninety percent occur in the atria (mostly LA). Myxomas are usually described as a "ball-valve" obstruction in the LA. Rhabdomyomas are the most frequent 1° cardiac tumor in children. *Tuberous sclerosis*

Skin cancer

Squamous cell carcinoma	Very common. Associated with excessive exposure to sunlight. Commonly appear on hands and face. Locally invasive but rarely metastasizes. *ulcerate*	Actinic keratosis is a precursor to squamous cell carcinoma. Keratin "pearls." Arsenic exposure.
Basal cell carcinoma	Most common in sun-exposed areas of body. Locally invasive but almost never metastasizes. Gross pathology: pearly papules.	Basal cell tumors have "palisading" nuclei.
Melanoma	Common tumor with significant risk of metastasis. Associated with sunlight exposure. Incidence increasing. Depth of tumor correlates with risk of metastasis.	Increased risk in fair-skinned persons. Dysplastic nevus is a precursor to melanoma.

Colorectal cancer risk factors

Risk factors for carcinoma of colon: colorectal villous adenomas, chronic inflammatory bowel disease, low-fiber diet, increasing age, familial adenomatous polyposis (FAP), hereditary nonpolyposis colorectal cancer (HNPCC), personal and family history of colon cancer. Screen patients > 50 years old with stool occult blood test.

Barrett's esophagus

Glandular (columnar epithelial) metaplasia—replacement of stratified squamous epithelium with gastric (columnar) epithelium in the distal esophagus. Predisposes to esophageal adenocarcinoma; usually secondary to gastroesophageal reflux.

Multiple endocrine neoplasias (MEN)

MEN type I (Wermer's syndrome)—pancreas (e.g., ZE syndrome, insulinomas, VIPomas), parathyroid and pituitary tumors. "3 P's"

MEN type II (Sipple's syndrome)—medullary carcinoma of the thyroid, pheochromocytoma, parathyroid tumor or adenoma.

MEN type III (formerly MEN IIb)—medullary carcinoma of the thyroid, pheochromocytoma, and oral and intestinal ganglioneuromatosis (mucosal neuromas).

All MEN syndromes are auto-somal dominantly inherited.

MEN I = 3 "P" organs (**P**ancreas, **P**ituitary, and **P**arathyroid).

Most common leukemias by age group

Age < 15	15–39	40–59	60+
ALL (acute lymphocytic leukemia)	AML (acute myelocytic leukemia)	AML and **CML** (chronic myelocytic leukemia)	CLL (chronic lymphocytic leukemia)

"acute mid life"

(**ML** = **m**id**l**ife)

smudge cells

Chromosomal translocations

t(9, 22), or the Philadelphia chromosome, is associated with CML (*abl-bcr* hybrid). bcr-abl

t(8, 14) is associated with Burkitt's lymphoma (c-*myc* activation).

t(14, 18) is associated with follicular lymphomas (*bcl*-2 activation).

Zollinger–Ellison syndrome

Gastrin-secreting tumor that is usually located in the pancreas. Causes recurrent ulcers. May be associated with MEN syndrome type I.

Multiple myeloma

Osteoclast activating factor

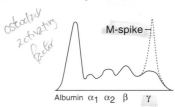

Monoclonal plasma cell ("fried-egg" appearance) cancer that arises in the marrow and produces large amounts of IgG (55%) or IgA (25%). Most common 1° tumor arising within bone in adults. Destructive bone lesions and consequent hypercalcemia. Renal insufficiency, ↑ susceptibility to infection, and anemia. Ig light chains in urine (Bence Jones protein). Associated with primary amyloidosis and punched-out lytic bone lesions on x-ray. Characterized by monoclonal immunoglobulin spike (M protein) on serum protein electrophoresis. Blood smear shows RBCs stacked like poker chips (rouleau formation).

Prostatic adenocarcinoma

Common in men over age 50. Arises most often from the peripheral lobe (posterior zone) of the prostate gland and is most frequently diagnosed by digital rectal examination (hard nodule) and prostate biopsy. Prostatic acid phosphatase and prostate-specific antigen (PSA) are useful tumor markers. Osteoblastic metastases in bone may develop in late stages, as indicated by an increase in serum alkaline phosphatase and PSA.

Tumors of the adrenal medulla

Pheochromocytoma is the most common tumor of the adrenal medulla in adults.

Neuroblastoma is the most common tumor of the adrenal medulla in children, but it can occur anywhere along the sympathetic chain.

Pheochromocytomas may be associated with neurofibromatosis, MEN type II and MEN type III.

Pheochromocytoma

Most of these neoplasms secrete a combination of norepinephrine and epinephrine. Urinary VMA levels and plasma catecholamines are elevated. Associated with MEN type II and type III. Have a dusky color on gross pathology. Treated with α antagonists, especially phenoxybenzamine, a nonselective, **irreversible** α blocker.

Episodic hypercholinergic symptoms **(5 P's):**
- **P**ressure (elevated blood pressure)
- **P**ain (headache)
- **P**erspiration
- **P**alpitations
- **P**allor/diaphoresis

Rule of 10s:
- **10%** malignant
- **10%** bilateral
- **10%** extraadrenal
- **10%** calcify
- **10%** kids
- **10%** familial

Also discussed **10**-fold more often than actually seen!

Lung cancer

Bronchogenic carcinoma

Tumors that arise **centrally:**
1. **S**quamous cell carcinoma—clear link to smoking
2. **S**mall-cell carcinoma—clear link to smoking. Associated with ectopic hormone production.

Tumors that arise peripherally:
1. Adenocarcinoma
2. Bronchioalveolar carcinoma (thought not to be related to smoking)
3. Large cell carcinoma—undifferentiated

Carcinoid tumor — Can cause carcinoid syndrome 5-HT especially

Metastases — Very common. Brain (epilepsy), bone (pathologic fracture), and liver (jaundice, hepatomegaly)

Lung cancer is the leading cause of cancer death.
Presentation: cough, hemoptysis, bronchial obstruction, wheezing, pneumonic **"coin"** lesion on x-ray.
Other clinical features:
1. Hoarseness
2. SVC syndrome
3. Pleural effusion
4. Paraneoplastic syndromes
5. Chylothorax
6. Pericardial effusion

Pancoast's tumor

Carcinoma that occurs in apex of lung and may affect cervical sympathetic plexus, causing Horner's syndrome. may cause hoarseness → recurrent laryngeal nerve obstruct traitez

Horner's syndrome: ptosis, miosis, anhidrosis. ↳ lack of sweating

---

Carcinoid syndrome

Rare syndrome caused by carcinoid tumors, especially those of the small bowel; the tumors secrete high levels of serotonin (5HT) that does not get metabolized by the liver due to liver metastases. Results in recurrent diarrhea, cutaneous flushing, asthmatic wheezing, and carcinoid heart disease. ↑ 5-HIAA in urine. right-sided.

Rule of 1/3s:
- **1/3** metastasize
- **1/3** present with second malignancy
- **1/3** multiple

Treat with methysergide (5HT antagonist)

Metastasis to bone

These primary tumors metastasize to bone: **B**reast, **L**ung, **T**hyroid, **T**estes, **K**idney, **P**rostate.
Metastasis from breast and prostate are most common.
Metastatic bone tumors are far more common than 1° bone tumors.

BLT[2] with a **K**osher **P**ickle
Lung = **L**ytic
Prostate = blastic
Breast = **B**oth lytic and blastic

Metastasis to brain   Primary tumors that metastasize to brain: lung (bronchogenic carcinoma) > breast > skin (melanoma) > kidney (renal cell carcinoma) > GI tract. Overall, approximately 50% of brain tumors are from metastases.

Metastasis to liver   The liver and lung are the most common sites of metastasis after the regional lymph nodes. Primary tumors that metastasize to the liver: **C**olon (42%), **S**tomach (23%), **P**ancreas (21%), **B**reast (14%), and **L**ung (13%).

Metastases >> 1° liver tumors. **C**ancer **S**ometimes **P**enetrates **B**enign **L**iver.

Hepatocellular carcinoma   Also called hepatoma. Most common primary malignant tumor of the liver in adults. Increased incidence of hepatocellular carcinoma is associated with hepatitis B/C, Wilson's disease, hemochromatosis, α_1-antitrypsin deficiency, alcoholic cirrhosis, and carcinogens (e.g., aflatoxin B1).

Hepatocellular carcinoma, like renal cell carcinoma, commonly spread by hematogenous dissemination.

Local effects of tumors

Local effect	Cause
Mass	Tissue lump or tumor.
Nonhealing ulcer	Destruction of epithelial surfaces (e.g., stomach, colon, mouth, bronchus).
Hemorrhage	From ulcerated area or eroded vessel.
Pain	Any site with sensory nerve endings. Tumors in brain are initially painless.
Seizures	Tumor mass in brain.
Obstruction	Of bronchus → pneumonia. Of biliary tree → jaundice. Of left colon → constipation.
Perforation	Of ulcer in viscera → peritonitis, free air.
Bone destruction	Pathologic fracture, collapse of bone.
Inflammation	Of serosal surface → pleural effusion, pericardial effusion, ascites.
Space-occupying lesion	Raised intracranial pressure with brain neoplasms. Anemia due to bone marrow replacement.
Localized loss of sensory or motor function	Compression or destruction of nerve (e.g., recurrent laryngeal nerve by lung or thyroid cancer, with hoarseness).
Edema	Venous or lymphatic obstruction.

Paraneoplastic and distant effects of tumors

Effect	Causes	Associated neoplasm
Cushing's syndrome	ACTH or ACTH-like peptide.	Small cell lung carcinoma.
SIADH	ADH or ANP.	Small cell lung carcinoma and intracranial neoplasms.
Hypercalcemia	PTH-related peptide, TGF-α, TNF-α, IL-2. *PTHrP*	Squamous cell lung carcinoma, renal carcinoma, breast carcinoma, multiple myeloma, and bone metastasis (lysed bone).
Polycythemia	Erythropoietin.	Renal cell carcinoma (hypernephroma).
Myasthenia gravis	Unclear.	Thymoma, bronchogenic carcinoma.
Hyperviscosity syndrome, Waldenström's macroglobulinemia, Raynaud's phenomenon	Monoclonal immunoglobulin (usually IgM).	Lymphoma, myeloma.
Purpura	Decreased platelets due to bone marrow involvement. Effects of chemotherapy.	
Gout	Hyperuricemia due to excess nucleic acid turnover (i.e., cytotoxic therapy).	
Clubbing (of fingers)	Unknown.	Lung cancer and other intrathoracic neoplasms.
Cachexia, hypoalbuminemia, fever	Possibly autoimmune, toxic, or nutritional factors. TNF-α. *cachectin*	Advanced cancer.

Cancer epidemiology

	Male	Female	
Incidence	Prostate (32%)	Breast (32%)	Deaths from lung cancer have plateaued in males, but deaths continue to increase in females.
	Lung (16%)	Lung (13%)	
	Colon and rectum (12%)	Colon and rectum (13%)	
Mortality	Lung (33%)	Lung (23%)	Cancer is the second leading cause of death in the U.S. (heart disease is first).
	Prostate (13%)	Breast (18%)	

Achalasia

Failure of relaxation of lower esophageal sphincter due to loss of myenteric (Auerbach's) plexus. Causes progressive dysphagia. Barium swallow shows dilated esophagus with an area of distal stenosis. Associated with an increased risk of esophageal carcinoma.

A-chalasia = absence of relaxation.
2° achalasia may arise from Chagas' disease.
"Bird beak" on barium swallow.

Hirschsprung's disease

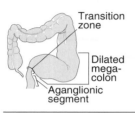
Transition zone
Dilated mega-colon
Aganglionic segment

Congenital megacolon characterized by absence of parasympathetic ganglion cells (Auerbach's and Meissner's plexuses) on intestinal biopsy. Due to failure of neural crest cell migration. Presents as chronic constipation early in life. Dilated portion of the colon proximal to the aganglionic segment, resulting in a "transition zone."

Think of a giant spring that **sprung** in the colon.

Whipple's disease

Caused by *Tropheryma whippelii* and treated with antibiotics.
Multisystem, affects mainly small bowel. Can also affect skin, joints, CNS, heart, liver, spleen. Small intestine infiltrated by PAS-positive macrophages containing rod-shaped bacilli.
Symptoms: diarrhea, weight loss, polyarthritis, and lymphadenopathy.
Affects mostly white adult males.

Mr. Whipple has diarrhea and can't squeeze the Charmin (arthritis).
Surgical resection of terminal ileum can lead to vitamin B$_{12}$ deficiency.

Gastritis

Type A
Autoimmune disorder characterized by **A**utoantibodies to parietal cells, pernicious **A**nemia, and **A**chlorhydria.

Type B
Caused by *H. pylori* infection

Type **A** = 4 **A**'s

Type **B** = a **B**ug, *H pylori*

Peptic ulcer disease

Gastric ulcer
Pain worse with meals
Weight loss
H. pylori infection in 70%; NSAID use also implicated
Due to ↓ mucosal protection against gastric acid

Duodenal ulcer
Pain lessens with meals
Almost 100% have *H. pylori* infection
Due to ↑ gastric acid secretion or ↓ mucosal protection
No ↑ risk of malignancy

Potential complications include bleeding, penetration, perforation, and obstruction.
   H. pylori infection can be treated with "triple therapy" (metronidazole, bismuth salicylate, and either amoxicillin or tetracycline) or new "double therapy" (omeprazole plus clarithromycin).
Smoking cessation is second-best treatment.

Crohn's disease

Inflammation mainly in the terminal ileum and cecum but can be anywhere along GI tract. Segmental involvement (skip lesions); transmural involvement; cobblestone mucosa; bowel wall thickening ("string sign" on x-ray); lymphoid infiltrates; noncaseating granulomas; linear ulcers, fissures, fistulas. Migratory arthritis, erythema nodosum.

Also called regional enteritis or ileitis. Transmural and skip lesions are key.
Surgical resection of terminal ileum can lead to vitamin B_{12} deficiency.

Ulcerative colitis

Begins in rectum and extends proximally. Continuous involvement; microabscesses (crypt abscesses) and ulcers; pseudopolyps (inflamed mucosal tags). Inflammatory cell infiltration confined to mucosa and submucosa, not transmural. Pyoderma gangrenosum, sclerosing cholangitis.

Colitis = colon inflammation.
Key is continuous cephalad progression; not transmural.
Associated with increased risk of colorectal carcinoma and toxic megacolon.

Diverticular disease

Diverticulum — Blind pouch leading off the alimentary tract, lined by mucosa, muscularis, and serosa, that communicates with the lumen of the gut. Most diverticula (esophagus, stomach, duodenum, colon) are acquired and are termed "false" in that they lack or have an attenuated muscularis propria.

Diverticulosis — The prevalence of diverticulosis (many diverticula) in patients over age 60 approaches 50%. Caused by increased intraluminal pressure and focal weakness in the colonic wall. Most frequently involves the sigmoid colon. Associated with low-fiber diets. Most often asymptomatic or associated with vague discomfort.

Diverticulitis — Inflammation of diverticula classically causing LLQ pain. May be complicated by perforation, peritonitis, abscess formation, or bowel stenosis.

Cirrhosis/ portal hypertension

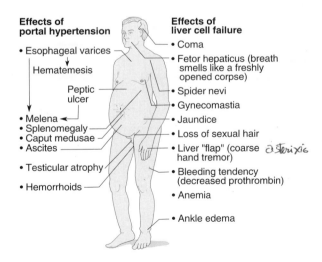

Effects of portal hypertension
- Esophageal varices
  ↓
  Hematemesis
- Peptic ulcer
- Melena ←
- Splenomegaly
- Caput medusae
- Ascites
- Testicular atrophy
- Hemorrhoids

Effects of liver cell failure
- Coma
- Fetor hepaticus (breath smells like a freshly opened corpse)
- Spider nevi
- Gynecomastia
- Jaundice
- Loss of sexual hair
- Liver "flap" (coarse hand tremor)
- Bleeding tendency (decreased prothrombin)
- Anemia
- Ankle edema

Cirrho (Greek) = tawny yellow.
Diffuse fibrosis of liver, destroys normal architecture.
Nodular regeneration.
Micronodular: nodules < 3 mm, uniform size.
Macronodular: nodules > 3 mm, varied size.
Micronodular cirrhosis is due to metabolic insult (e.g., alcohol), whereas macronodular is usually due to significant liver injury leading to hepatic necrosis (e.g., postinfectious or drug-induced hepatitis).
Increased risk of hepatocellular carcinoma.

Alcoholic hepatitis	Swollen and necrotic hepatocytes, neutrophil infiltration, Mallory bodies (hyaline), fatty change, and fibrosis around central vein. SGOT (AST) to SGPT (ALT) ratio is usually greater than 1.5.	
Wilson's disease	Due to failure of copper to enter circulation in the form of ceruloplasmin. Leads to copper accumulation, especially in liver, brain, cornea. Also known as hepatolenticular degeneration. Cirrhosis (micronodular to macronodular), Mallory bodies in liver. Neuronal degeneration in basal ganglia (especially putamen). Associated with dementia, asterixis (flapping tremor), and an increased risk of hepatocellular carcinoma.	↓ serum ceruloplasmin. Kayser–Fleischer rings (copper deposits in Descemet's membrane of the cornea). Treat with penicillamine.
Hemochromatosis	Increased iron deposition in many organs. Classic triad of micronodular pigment cirrhosis, "bronze" diabetes, skin pigmentation. Results in CHF and an increased risk of hepatocellular carcinoma. Disease may be a primary (autosomal recessive) disorder or secondary to chronic transfusion therapy. ↑ ferritin, ↑ transferrin saturation.	Total body iron may reach 50 g, enough to set off the metal detectors at airports. Treat with repeated phlebotomy, deferoxamine.

Hereditary hyperbilirubinemias

Crigler–Najjar syndrome, type I	Absent UDP-glucuronyl transferase. Presents early in life; patients die within a few years. Findings: jaundice, kernicterus (bilirubin deposition in brain), ↑ unconjugated bilirubin. Treatment: plasmapheresis and phototherapy.	Crigler–Najjar type I is a severe disease.
Gilbert's syndrome	Mildly ↓ UDP-glucuronyl transferase. Asymptomatic, but unconjugated bilirubin is elevated without overt hemolysis. Associated with stress.	Gilbert's may represent a milder form.
Dubin–Johnson syndrome	Conjugated hyperbilirubinemia due to defective liver excretion. Grossly black liver.	Rotor's syndrome is similar but less severe and does not cause black liver.

Gallstones

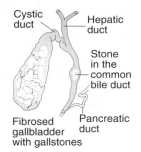

Cystic duct

Hepatic duct

Stone in the common bile duct

Pancreatic duct

Fibrosed gallbladder with gallstones

Form when solubilizing bile acids and lecithin are overwhelmed by increased cholesterol and/or bilirubin. Three types of stones:

1. Cholesterol stones: Associated with obesity, Crohn's disease, cystic fibrosis, advanced age, clofibrate, estrogens, multiparity, rapid weight loss, and Native American origin.
2. Mixed stones: Have both cholesterol and pigment components.
3. Pigment stones: Seen in patients with chronic RBC hemolysis, alcoholic cirrhosis, advanced age, and biliary infection.

Diagnose with ultrasound. Treat with cholecystectomy.

Risk factors (5 F's):
1. Female
2. Fat
3. Fertile
4. Forty
5. Flatulent

Epigastric/RUQ pain, fever, nausea/emesis.

Acute pancreatitis

Abdominal pain: epigastric, radiates to the back.
Elevated amylase, lipase.
Can lead to DIC, ARDS, diffuse fat necrosis, and hypocalcemia.

Alcoholism
Gallstones
Trauma (children)
Chronic pancreatitis is strongly associated with alcoholism.

PATHOLOGY—NEUROLOGIC

Degenerative diseases

Cerebral cortex	**Alzheimer's disease:** Most common cause of dementia in the elderly. Associated with senile plaques (β amyloid core) and neurofibrillary tangles (abnormally phosphorylated tau protein). Familial form (10%) associated with genes on chromosomes 1, 11, 19 (Apo-E4 allele), and 21 (p-App gene).	Multi-infarct dementia is the second most common cause of dementia in the elderly.
	Pick's disease: Associated with Pick bodies and is specific for the frontal and temporal lobes.	
Basal ganglia and brainstem	**Huntington's disease:** Autosomal dominant inheritance, chorea, dementia. Lesion in caudate nucleus.	
	Parkinson's disease: Associated with Lewy bodies and depigmentation of the substantia nigra. Rare cases have been linked to exposure to MPTP, a contaminant in illicit street drugs.	Parkinsonian symptoms **(RAFT):** Cogwheel **R**igidity, **A**kinesia, **F**lat facies, and **T**remor (at rest).
Spinocerebellar	**Olivopontocerebellar atrophy** **Friedreich's ataxia**	
Motor neuron	**Amyotrophic lateral sclerosis (ALS)**	ALS is associated with both lower and upper motor neuron signs. Commonly known as Lou Gehrig's disease (for famous New York Yankee baseball player who died of ALS).
	Werdnig–Hoffmann disease: Presents at birth as a "floppy baby"; tongue fasciculations.	
	Polio: Lower motor neuron signs.	

Demyelinating and dysmyelinating diseases

1. Multiple sclerosis (MS)—Higher prevalence in northern latitudes; periventricular plaques, preservation of axons, loss of oligodendrocytes, reactive astrocytic gliosis; ↑ protein (IgG) in CSF. Many patients have a relapsing–remitting course. Patients can present with optic neuritis (loss of vision), MLF syndrome (internuclear ophthalmoplegia), hemiparesis, hemisensory symptoms, or bladder/bowel incontinence.
2. Progressive multifocal leukoencephalopathy (PML)—Associated with JC virus and seen in 2–4% of AIDS patients (reactivation of latent viral infection).
3. Postinfectious encephalomyelitis
4. Metachromatic leukodystrophy (a sphingolipidosis)
5. Guillain-Barré syndrome—Inflammation and demyelination of peripheral nerves; ascending muscle weakness and paralysis beginning in distal lower extremities. In some cases it follows herpesvirus or *C. jejuni* infection. CSF shows ↑ protein and normal cells.

peripheral MS

Guillain-Barré syndrome (acute idiopathic polyneuritis)

Sensory and motor neuron loss at the level of the peripheral nerves and motor fibers of the ventral roots (sensory effect less severe than motor), causing symmetric weakness with variable paresthesia or dysesthesia. Facial diplegia in 50% of cases. Autonomic function may be severe (e.g., cardiac irregularities, hypertension, or hypotension).

Findings: elevated CSF protein with normal cell count.

Associated with viral infections, inoculations, and stress, but no definitive link to pathogens.

Mycoplasma pneumoniae

Poliomyelitis

Caused by poliovirus, which is transmitted by the fecal-oral route. Replicates in the oropharynx and small intestine before spreading through the bloodstream to the CNS, where it leads to the destruction of cells in the anterior horn of the spinal cord, leading in turn to LMN destruction.

Symptoms: malaise, headache, fever, nausea, abdominal pain, sore throat. Signs of LMN lesions: muscle weakness and atrophy, fasciculations, fibrillation, and hyporeflexia.

Findings: CSF with lymphocytic pleocytosis with slight elevation of protein. Virus recovered from stool or throat.

Seizures

Partial seizures: one area of the brain.
1. Simple partial (awareness intact): motor, sensory, autonomic, psychic.
2. Complex partial (impaired awareness).

Generalized seizures: diffuse.
1. Absence: blank stare (petit mal).
2. Myoclonic: quick, repetitive jerks.
3. Tonic-clonic: alternating stiffening and movement (grand mal).
4. Tonic: stiffening.
5. Atonic: "drop" seizures.

Epilepsy is a disorder of recurrent seizures.
Partial seizures can secondarily generalize.
Causes of seizures by age:
Children: genetic, infection, trauma, congenital, metabolic.
Adults: tumors, trauma, stroke, infection.
Elderly: stroke, tumor, trauma, metabolic, infection.
Febrile seizures are not epilepsy.

NYSTAGMUS

Wernicke–Korsakoff syndrome	Caused by vitamin B$_1$ (thiamine) deficiency in alcoholics. Classically may present with triad of psychosis, ophthalmoplegia, and ataxia (Wernicke's encephalopathy). May progress to memory loss, confabulation, confusion (Korsakoff's syndrome; irreversible). Associated with periventricular hemorrhage/necrosis, especially in mamillary bodies. Treatment: IV vitamin B$_1$ (thiamine).

Broca's versus Wernicke's aphasia

Broca's is nonfluent aphasia with intact comprehension (expressive aphasia). Wernicke's is fluent aphasia with impaired comprehension (receptive aphasia).

Broca's area = inferior frontal gyrus. — *i.e., motor cortex ass'd*
Wernicke's area = superior temporal gyrus. — *closer to somatosensory.*

BROca's is **BRO**ken speech; **W**ernicke's is **W**ordy but makes no sense. ↳ *"word salad"*

Horner's syndrome

Sympathectomy of face:
1. Ptosis (slight drooping of eyelid)
2. Miosis (pupil constriction)
3. Anhidrosis (absence of sweating) and flushing (rubor) of affected side of face

Associated with Pancoast's tumor.

Arnold–Chiari malformation ↙

Congenital protrusion of cerebellum and medulla through foramen magnum. Associated with lumbar meningomyelocele and obstructive hydrocephalus.

Duret's hemorrhage
major ass'n w/ syringomyelia

Syringomyelia ↳ *Spinothalamic*

Softening and cavitation around central canal of spinal cord. Crossing fibers of spinothalamic tract are damaged. Bilateral loss of pain and temperature sensation in upper extremities with preservation of touch sensation. — *may produce significant pain.*

Syrinx (Greek) = tube as in syringe.
Often presents in patients with Arnold-Chiari malformation.

Tabes dorsalis

Degeneration of dorsal columns and dorsal roots due to 3° syphilis, resulting in impaired proprioception and locomotor ataxia. Associated with Charcot joints, shooting (lightning) pain, Argyll-Robertson pupils, and absence of deep tendon reflexes.

Tabes (Latin) = wasting away.

Osteoarthritis

Destruction of articular cartilage (primarily weight-bearing joints), Heberden's nodes, eburnation, subchondral bone formation, sclerosis, osteophytes. Caused by wear and tear of joints. Classically hurts in evening after joint use, improves with rest. Commonly in older patients. No systemic symptoms.

Bouchard's, also

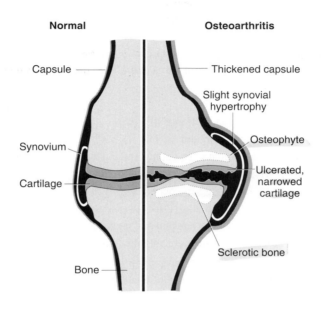

Normal | Osteoarthritis

Capsule — Thickened capsule

Slight synovial hypertrophy

Osteophyte

Synovium

Cartilage — Ulcerated, narrowed cartilage

Sclerotic bone

Bone

Rheumatoid arthritis

Pannus formation in joints (metacarpophalangeal, proximal interphalangeal); ulnar deviation, subluxation; subcutaneous rheumatoid nodules at pressure points (e.g., elbows); morning stiffness (decreased pain with use); symmetric involvement; 80% have positive rheumatoid factor (anti-IgG antibody). More common in females and is associated with HLA-DR4. Associated with systemic symptoms: fever, fatigue, pleuritis, pericarditis.

Gout

Precipitation of monosodium urate crystals into joints due to hyperuricemia. Asymmetric joint distribution. Favored manifestation is painful MTP joint in the big toe (podagra). Crystals are needle-shaped and negatively birefringent. Tophus formation (often on external ear). Hyperuricemia can be caused by Lesch-Nyhan disease, PRPP excess, decreased excretion of uric acid, or G6P deficiency. Treatment is allopurinol, probenecid, colchicine, and NSAIDs. Gout is associated with the use of thiazide diuretics, because they competitively inhibit the secretion of uric acid. More common in men.

Pseudogout

positive birefringence (handwritten)

Caused by deposition of calcium pyrophosphate crystals within the joint space. Forms basophilic, rhomboid crystals (as opposed to the birefringent, needle-shaped crystals in gout). Usually affects large joints (classically the knee). >50 years old; both sexes affected equally. No treatment.

Systemic lupus erythematosus

HLA-D2,D3 (handwritten)

90% are female, most between ages 14 and 45. Fever, fatigue, weight loss. Joint pain, malar rash, pleuritis, pericarditis, nonbacterial verrucous endocarditis, Raynaud's phenomenon. **Wire loop** lesions in kidney with immune complex deposition (with nephrotic syndrome); death from renal failure and infections. False positives on syphilis tests (RPR/VDRL). Lab tests detect presence of: *bpo blo* (handwritten)

1. Antinuclear antibodies (ANA): sensitive, but not specific for SLE
2. Antibodies to double-stranded DNA (anti-ds DNA): very specific
3. Anti-Smith antibodies (anti-Sm): very specific

Lupus (Latin) = wolf, a reference to the malar rash (on cheeks) causing wolflike facies. Also, **wire loopus** erythematosus.

Most common and severe in black females.

Drugs (procainamide, INH, hydralazine) can produce an SLE-like syndrome that is commonly reversible.

Sarcoidosis

Associated with restrictive lung disease, bilateral hilar lymphadenopathy, erythema nodosum, Bell's palsy, epithelial granulomas containing microscopic Schaumann and asteroid bodies, uveoparotitis, and hypercalcemia (due to elevated conversion of vit. D to its active form in epithelioid macrophages). Also associated with immune-mediated, widespread noncaseating granulomas and elevated serum ACE levels. Common in black females.

Sarko (Greek) = flesh, describing exuberant noncaseating granulomas.
GRUELING:
Granulomas
Rheumatoid arthritis
Uveitis
Erythema nodosum
Lymphadenopathy
Interstitial fibrosis
Negative TB test *lymphocyte "consumption"* (handwritten)
Gammaglobulinemia

Scleroderma (progressive systemic sclerosis–PSS)

Excessive fibrosis and collagen deposition throughout the body. 75% female. Commonly sclerosis of skin but also of cardiovascular and GI systems, kidney. Two major categories:

1. Diffuse scleroderma: widespread skin involvement, rapid progression, early visceral involvement. Associated with anti-Scl-70 antibody.
2. **CREST** syndrome: **C**alcinosis, **R**aynaud's phenomenon, **E**sophageal dysmotility, **S**clerodactyly, and **T**elangiectasia. Limited skin involvement, often confined to fingers and face. More benign clinical course. Associated with anticentromere antibody.

Goodpasture's syndrome

Findings: pulmonary hemorrhages, renal lesions, hemoptysis, hematuria, anemia, proliferative glomerulonephritis, crescents.
Anti-glomerular basement membrane antibodies produce linear staining on immunofluorescence.

There are **two G**ood **P**astures for this disease: **G**lomerulus and **P**ulmonary. Also, a type **II** hypersensitivity disease.
Most common in men 20–40 yo.

Reiter's syndrome	A seronegative spondyloarthropathy. Strong HLA-B27 link. Classic triad: 1. Urethritis 2. Conjunctivitis and anterior uveitis 3. Arthritis Has a strong predilection for males.	"Can't see (anterior uveitis/conjunctivitis), can't pee (urethritis), can't climb a tree (arthritis)."
Sjögren's syndrome	Classic triad: dry eyes (conjunctivitis, xerophthalmia), dry mouth (dysphagia, xerostomia), arthritis. Parotid enlargement, ↑ risk of B-cell lymphoma. Predominantly affects females between 40 and 60 years of age.	Associated with rheumatoid arthritis. HLA-DR3 Sicca: dry eyes, dry mouth, nasal and vaginal dryness, chronic bronchitis, reflux esophagitis.
Reye's syndrome	Rare, often fatal childhood hepatoencephalopathy. Findings: fatty liver (microvesicular fatty change), hypoglycemia, coma. Associated with viral infection (especially VZV and influenza B) and salicylates; thus aspirin is no longer recommended for children (use acetaminophen, with caution).	Encephalopathy and liver failure. "Don't give your baby a baby aspirin."

PATHOLOGY—VASCULAR/CARDIAC

Intracranial hemorrhage

Epidural hematoma	Rupture of middle meningeal artery, often 2° to fracture of temporal bone.
Subdural hematoma	Rupture of bridging veins. Venous bleeding (less pressure) with delayed onset of symptoms. Seen in elderly individuals, alcoholics, blunt trauma.
Subarachnoid hemorrhage	Rupture of an aneurysm (usually berry aneurysm) or an AVM. Patients complain of "worst headache ever." Bloody or xanthochromic spinal tap.
Parenchymal hematoma	Caused by hypertension, amyloid angiopathy, diabetes mellitus and tumor.

| **Berry aneurysms** | Berry aneurysms occur at the bifurcations in the circle of Willis. Most common site is bifurcation of the anterior communicating artery. Rupture (most common complication) leads to hemorrhagic stroke. Associated with adult polycystic kidney disease. → *Mitral valve prolapse* | Red **b**erries at **b**ifurcations **b**ulge and **b**low out. |

(handwritten: dK (cl ant. comm))

| **Infarcts: red versus pale** | Red (hemorrhagic) infarcts occur in loose tissues with collaterals, such as lungs, intestine, or brain, or following reperfusion. Pale infarcts occur in solid tissues with single blood supply, such as heart, kidney, and spleen. | **RE**d = **RE**perfusion. |

| **Atherosclerosis** | Disease of elastic arteries and large and medium-sized muscular arteries. Risk factors: smoking, hypertension, diabetes mellitus, hyperlipidemia. *(handwritten: ↓HDL, ↑TAG's)* Progression: fatty streaks → proliferative plaque → complex atheromas. Complications: aneurysms, ischemia, infarcts, peripheral vascular disease, thrombus, emboli. Location: abdominal aorta > coronary artery > popliteal artery > carotid artery. Symptoms: angina, claudication, but can be asymptomatic. | |

| **Ischemic heart disease** *(handwritten: IHD)* | Possible manifestations: 1. Angina: Stable: mostly 2° to atherosclerosis (retrosternal chest pain with exertion) Prinzmetal's variant: occurs at rest, 2° to coronary artery spasm Unstable/crescendo: thrombosis in a branch (worsening chest pain) 2. Myocardial infarction—most often occurs in CAD involving the left anterior descending artery 3. Sudden cardiac death—death from cardiac causes within 1 hour of onset of symptoms, most commonly due to a lethal arrhythmia *(handwritten: w/in several hrs)* 4. Chronic ischemic heart disease—progressive onset of congestive heart failure over many years due to chronic ischemic myocardial damage | |

Pregnancy-induced hypertension (preeclampsia-eclampsia)	Preeclampsia is the triad of hypertension, proteinuria, and edema; eclampsia is the addition of seizures to the triad. Affects 7% of pregnant women from 20 weeks' gestation to 6 weeks postpartum. Increased incidence in patients with preexisting hypertension, diabetes, chronic renal disease, and autoimmune disorders.	
Clinical features	Headache, blurred vision, abdominal pain, altered mentation, hyperreflexia; lab findings may include thrombocytopenia, hyperuricemia. *(handwritten: HELLP → Hyperreflexia elevated liver enz... low platelets)*	
Treatment	Delivery of fetus as soon as is viable. Otherwise bed rest, salt restriction, and monitoring and treatment of hypertension. For eclampsia, a medical emergency, IV magnesium sulfate and diazepam.	

Evolution of MI

Coronary artery occlusion: LAD > RCA > circumflex.

Symptoms: severe retrosternal pain, pain in left arm and/or jaw, shortness of breath, fatigue, adrenergic symptoms.

A. First day

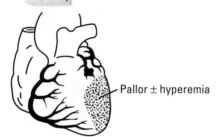

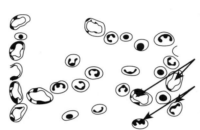

Coagulative necrosis leads to release of contents of necrotic cells into bloodstream

Muscle shows minimal changes

Occluded artery

Infarct

Pallor

B. 2 to 4 days

Pallor ± hyperemia

Tissue surrounding infarct shows acute inflammation

Dilated vessels (hyperemia)

Neutrophil emigration

Muscle shows microscopic changes of coagulative necrosis

C. 5 to 10 days

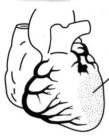

Hyperemic border; central yellow-brown softening— maximally yellow and soft by 10 days

Outer zone (ingrowth of granulation tissue)

Macrophage zone

Neutrophil zone

D. 7 weeks

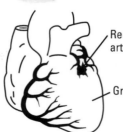

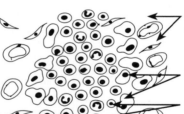

Recanalized artery

Gray-white

Contracted scar complete

Diagnosis of MI

Troponin is used within the first 8 hours.
CK-MB is test of choice in the first 24 hours post-MI.
LDH_1 is test of choice from 2 to 7 days post-MI.
AST is nonspecific and can be found in cardiac, liver,
and skeletal muscle cells. EKG changes can include
ST elevation (transmural ischemia) and Q waves
(transmural infarct).

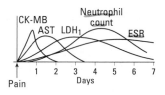

MI complications

1. Cardiac arrhythmia (90%)
2. LV failure and pulmonary edema (60%)
3. Thromboembolism: mural thrombus
4. Cardiogenic shock (large infarct: high risk of mortality)
5. Rupture of ventricular free wall, interventricular septum, papillary muscle (4–10 days post-MI), cardiac tamponade
6. Fibrinous pericarditis: friction rub (3–5 days post-MI)
7. Dressler's syndrome: autoimmune phenomenon resulting in fibrinous pericarditis (several weeks post-MI)

Cardiomyopathies

Dilated (congestive) cardiomyopathy

Most common cardiomyopathy (90% of cases). Etiologies include chronic **A**lcohol abuse, **B**eriberi, postviral myocarditis by **C**oxsackievirus B, chronic **C**ocaine use, **D**oxorubicin toxicity, peripartum cardiomyopathy. Heart dilates and looks like a balloon on chest x-ray.

Systolic dysfunction ensues.
Alcohol
Beriberi
Coxsackievirus B, **C**ocaine
Doxorubicin

Hypertrophic cardiomyopathy

Hypertrophy often asymmetric and involving the intraventricular septum. 50% of cases are familial and are inherited as an AD trait. Cause of sudden death in young athletes. Walls of LV are thickened and chamber becomes banana-shaped on echocardiogram.

Also referred to as IHSS, or idiopathic hypertrophic subaortic stenosis. Diastolic dysfunction ensues.

Restrictive/obliterative cardiomyopathy

Major causes include sarcoidosis, amyloidosis, endocardial fibroelastosis, and endomyocardial fibrosis (Löffler's).

Valvular heart disease

Aortic stenosis	Crescendo-decrescendo systolic ejection murmur, with LV >> aortic pressure during systole.
Aortic regurgitation	High-pitched "blowing" diastolic murmur. → Austin Flint murmur
Mitral stenosis	Rumbling late diastolic murmurs. LA >> LV pressure during diastole.
Mitral regurgitation	High-pitched "blowing" systolic murmur.

CHF

Abnormality	Cause
Ankle, sacral edema	RV failure → increased venous pressure → fluid transudation.
Hepatomegaly	Increased central venous pressure → increased resistance to portal flow. Rarely leads to "cardiac cirrhosis."
Pulmonary congestion	LV failure → increased pulmonary venous pressure → pulmonary venous distention and transudation of fluid. Presence of hemosiderin-laden macrophages ("heart failure" cells).
Dyspnea on exertion	Failure of left ventricular output to increase during exercise.
Paroxysmal nocturnal dyspnea, pulmonary edema	Failure of left heart output to keep up with right heart output → acute rise in pulmonary venous and capillary pressure → transudation of fluid.
Orthopnea (shortness of breath when supine)	Pooling of blood in lungs in supine position adds volume to congested pulmonary vascular system; increased venous return not put out by left ventricle.
Cardiac dilation	Greater ventricular end-diastolic volume.

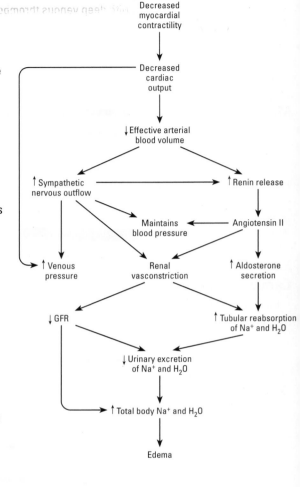

Embolus types

Fat, Air, Thrombus, Bacteria, Amniotic fluid, Tumor. Fat emboli are associated with long bone fractures and liposuction. Amniotic fluid emboli can lead to DIC, especially postpartum. Pulmonary embolus: chest pain, tachypnea, dyspnea.

An embolus moves like a **FAT BAT**. Approximately 95% of pulmonary emboli arise from deep leg veins.

Bacterial endocarditis

New murmur, anemia, fever, Osler nodes (tender raised lesions on finger or toe pads), Roth's spots (round white spots on retina surrounded by hemorrhage), Janeway lesions (small erythematous lesions on palm or sole). Multiple blood cultures necessary for diagnosis (continuous bacteremia).
  1. Acute: *Staphylococcus aureus* (high virulence). Large vegetations on previously normal valves. Rapid onset.
  2. Subacute: *Streptococcus viridans* (low virulence). Smaller vegetations on congenitally abnormal or diseased valves. More insidious onset.

Mitral valve is most frequently involved. Tricuspid valve endocarditis is associated with IV drug abuse.

Marantic/ thrombotic endocarditis (nonbacterial)	Fibrin precipitation on valve leaflets, 2° to metastasis, renal failure, or sepsis. Vegetations are small and sterile but can produce emboli and infarctions. Often occurs in patients with deep venous thromboses and/or pulmonary emboli.	
Rheumatic fever/ rheumatic heart disease	Rheumatic fever is a consequence of pharyngeal infection with group A, β-hemolytic streptococci. Multiple episodes can cause rheumatic heart disease, which affects heart valves: mitral > aortic >> tricuspid. Associated with Aschoff bodies, migratory polyarthritis, erythema marginatum, elevated ASO titers. Due to cross-reactivity, not direct effect of bacteria or toxin.	**PH**ever follows **PH**aryngeal infection. High-pressure valves are affected most. **PECCS:** **P**olyarthritis (migratory) **E**rythema marginatum **C**arditis **C**horea **S**ubcutaneous nodules
Pericarditis	Causes: infection (viruses, TB, pyogenic bacteria, often by direct spread from lung or mediastinal lymph nodes), ischemic heart disease, chronic renal failure → uremia, and connective tissue disease. Effusions are usually serous; hemorrhagic effusions are associated with TB and malignancy. Renal failure causes serous or fibrinous effusions. *(uremia)* Findings: pericardial pain, friction rub, EKG changes, pulsus paradoxus. Can resolve without scarring or lead to chronic adhesive or chronic constrictive pericarditis.	
Pancytopenia	Pancytopenia is associated with the following pathologic conditions: 1. AML *acute myelogenous leukemia (Auer rods)* 2. Recurrent ovarian cancer 3. Aplastic anemia 4. Drug reactions *folate deficiency* *B_{12} deficiency*	
Diagnosis of congenital hematologic defects	*crystallized Hgb* Heinz bodies are seen in G6PD deficiency. *aggregated oxidized Hgb.* Ham's test is used to diagnose paroxysmal nocturnal hemoglobinuria (PNH). *complement hyperactivity* Osmotic fragility test is used to diagnose hereditary spherocytosis (treat with splenectomy).	
Syphilitic heart disease *syphilitic aortitis*	Tertiary syphilis disrupts the vasa vasorum of aorta via endarteritis obliterans and disrupts elastica (with consequent dilation of aorta and valve ring). Often affects the aortic root and ascending aorta. Associated with a tree-bark appearance of the aorta.	Can result in aneurysm of ascending aorta or aortic arch and aortic valve incompetence.
Buerger's disease	Known as smoker's disease and thromboangiitis obliterans; idiopathic, segmental, thrombosing vasculitis of intermediate and small peripheral arteries and veins. Findings: intermittent claudication, superficial nodular phlebitis, cold sensitivity (Raynaud's phenomenon), severe pain in affected part; may lead to gangrene. Treatment: quit smoking.	

Takayasu's arteritis	Known as "pulseless disease": thickening of aortic arch and/or proximal great vessels, causing weak pulses in upper extremities and ocular disturbances. Associated with an elevated ESR. Primarily affects young Asian females. Fever, night sweats, myalgia, arthritis, skin nodules.	Affects medium and large arteries.
Temporal arteritis	Most common vasculitis that affects medium and small arteries, usually branches of carotid artery. Findings include unilateral headache, jaw claudication, impaired vision (occlusion of ophthalmic artery, which can lead to blindness). Half of patients have systemic involvement and syndrome of polymyalgia rheumatica. Associated with elevated ESR.	**Tem**poral = signs near **Tem**ples. ESR is markedly elevated. Also known as giant cell arteritis. Affects elderly females.

Polyarteritis nodosa   Characterized by necrotizing immune complex inflammation of small or medium-sized muscular arteries, typically involving renal and visceral vessels.   **PAN** = P-ANca

Symptoms	Fever, weight loss, malaise, abdominal pain, headache, myalgia, hypertension.
Findings	Cotton-wool spots, microaneurysms, pericarditis, myocarditis, palpable purpura. Increased ESR. Associated with hepatitis B infection in 30% of patients. **P-AN**CA (perinuclear pattern of antineutrophil cytoplasmic antibodies) is often present in the serum and correlates with disease activity, primarily in small vessel disease.
Treatment	Corticosteroids, azathioprine, and/or cyclophosphamide. *antiimmune Rx.*

Budd–Chiari syndrome	Occlusion of IVC or hepatic veins with centrilobular congestion and necrosis, leading to congestive liver disease (hepatomegaly, ascites, abdominal pain, and eventual liver failure). Associated with polycythemia vera, pregnancy, hepatocellular carcinoma.

Wegener's granulomatosis   Characterized by focal necrotizing vasculitis and necrotizing granulomas in the lung and upper airway and by necrotizing glomerulonephritis.

Symptoms	Perforation of nasal septum, chronic sinusitis, otitis media, mastoiditis, cough, dyspnea, hemoptysis.
Findings	C-ANCA is a strong marker of disease; CXR may reveal large nodular densities; hematuria and red cell casts.
Treatment	Cyclophosphamide, corticosteroids, and/or methotrexate. *also antiimmune Rx.*

Glomerular pathology

Nephritic syndrome: Hematuria, hypertension, oliguria.

1. Acute poststreptococcal glomerulonephritis
   LM: glomeruli enlarged and hypercellular;
   neutrophils; "lumpy-bumpy." EM: subepithelial
   humps. IF: granular pattern.

   Most frequently seen in children. Peripheral, periorbital edema. Resolves spontaneously.

2. Rapidly progressive (crescentic) glomerulonephritis
   LM and IF: crescent-moon shape.

   Rapid course to renal failure from one of many causes.

3. Goodpasture's syndrome
   IF: linear pattern; anti-GBM.   *crescents*

   Hemoptysis, hematuria.

4. Membranoproliferative glomerulonephritis
   EM: subendothelial humps; "tram track."

   Slowly progresses to renal failure.

5. IgA nephropathy (Berger's disease)
   IF and EM: mesangial deposits of IgA.

   Mild disease.

[handwritten: 5% poststreptococcal]

Nephrotic syndrome: Massive proteinuria, hypoalbuminemia, generalized edema, hyperlipidemia.

1. Membranous glomerulonephritis
   LM: diffuse capillary thickening. IF: granular pattern.

   Most common cause of adult nephrotic syndrome.

2. Minimal change disease (lipoid nephrosis)
   LM: normal glomeruli. EM: foot process effacement (fusion).

   Most common cause of childhood nephrotic syndrome.

3. Focal segmental glomerular sclerosis with hyalinosis
   LM: segmental sclerosis and hyalinosis.

   More severe disease in HIV patients.

4. Diabetic nephropathy
   LM: Kimmelstiel-Wilson lesions.   *[handwritten: linear IF?]*

(LM = light microscopy; EM = electron microscopy; IF = immunofluorescence)

Kidney stones

Can lead to severe complications such as hydronephrosis and pyelonephritis.
Four major types:

Calcium

Comprises the majority of kidney stones (80-85%). Calcium oxalate or calcium phosphate or both. Stones are radiopaque. Disorders or conditions that cause hypercalcemia (e.g., cancer, increased PTH, increased vitamin D, milk-alkali syndrome) can all lead to hypercalciuria and stones.

Ammonium magnesium phosphate

Second most common kidney stone. Radiolucent and formed in alkaline urine by urease-positive bugs such as *Proteus vulgaris* or *Staphylococcus*. Can form large struvite calculi that can be a nidus for UTIs.

Uric acid

Strong association with hyperuricemia (e.g., gout). Often seen as a result of diseases with increased cell proliferation and turnover, such as leukemia and myeloproliferative disorders.

Cystine

Most often secondary to cystinuria.

Electrolytes

Electrolyte	Functions	Causes and signs of deficiency	Causes and signs of toxicity
Ca^{2+}	Muscle contraction Neurotransmitter release Bones, teeth	Kids—rickets Adults—osteomalacia Contributes to osteoporosis Tetany	Excess vitamin D Hyperparathyroidism Sarcoid*osis* (↑ Vit D *Pancreatitis* *from mem*)
PO_4^{3-}	ATP Nucleic acids Phosphorylation Bones, teeth	Kids—rickets Adults—osteomalacia	Low serum Ca^{2+} Can cause bone loss
Na^+	Extracellular fluid Maintains plasma volume Nerve/muscle function	2° to injury or illness	Hypertension if salt sensitive

K^+	Intracellular fluid
	Nerve/muscle function
		2° to injury, illness, or
		  diuretics
		Causes weakness, paralysis,
		  confusion
			Cardiac arrest , *arrhythmia*
			Small bowel ulcers

Cl^-	Fluid/electrolyte balance
	Gastric acid
	HCO_3^-/Cl^- shift in RBC *chloride shift.*
		2° to emesis, diuretics,
		  renal disease
			None that are
			  clinically significant

Mg^{2+}	Bones, teeth Enzyme cofactor	2° to malabsorption Diarrhea, alcoholism	↓ Reflexes ↓ Respiration *potentiates hypokalemia* *via ↑ Ca^{2+} channel fxn* *(I think)*

Acidosis/alkalosis

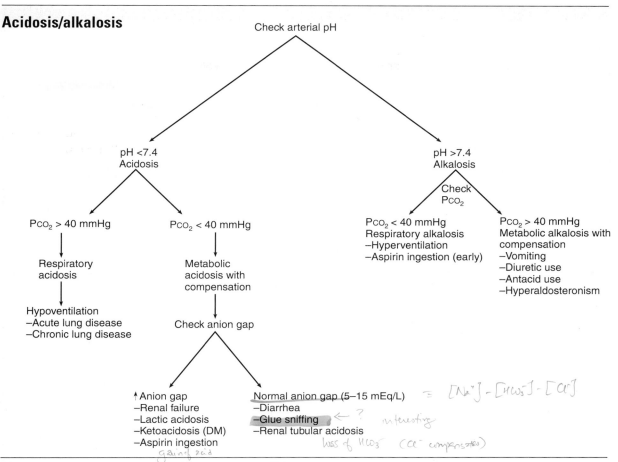

Check arterial pH

pH <7.4 Acidosis

- PCO₂ > 40 mmHg → Respiratory acidosis → Hypoventilation
  - Acute lung disease
  - Chronic lung disease
- PCO₂ < 40 mmHg → Metabolic acidosis with compensation → Check anion gap
  - ↑ Anion gap
    - Renal failure
    - Lactic acidosis
    - Ketoacidosis (DM)
    - Aspirin ingestion
    - *gain of acid*
  - Normal anion gap (5–15 mEq/L) = $[Na^+] - [HCO_3^-] - [Cl^-]$
    - Diarrhea
    - Glue sniffing ← ? *interesting*
    - Renal tubular acidosis
    - *loss of HCO_3^- (Cl^- compensates)*

pH >7.4 Alkalosis → Check PCO₂

- PCO₂ < 40 mmHg Respiratory alkalosis
  - Hyperventilation
  - Aspirin ingestion (early)
- PCO₂ > 40 mmHg Metabolic alkalosis with compensation
  - Vomiting
  - Diuretic use
  - Antacid use
  - Hyperaldosteronism

Benign prostatic hypertrophy	Common in men over age 50. May be due to an age-related increase in estradiol with possible sensitization of the prostate to the growth-promoting effects of DHT. *dihydrotestosterone* Characterized by a nodular enlargement of the periurethral (lateral and middle) lobes of the prostate gland, compressing the urethra into a vertical slit. Often presents with increased frequency of urination, nocturia, difficulty starting and stopping the stream of urine, and dysuria. May lead to distention and hypertrophy of the bladder, hydronephrosis, and urinary tract infections. Not considered a premalignant lesion.
Cretinism	Endemic cretinism occurs wherever endemic goiter is prevalent (lack of dietary iodine); sporadic cretinism is caused by defect in T4 formation or developmental failure in thyroid formation. Findings: pot-bellied, pale, puffy-faced child with protruding umbilicus and protuberant tongue. Cretin means Christ-like (French *chrétien*). Those affected were considered so mentally retarded as to be incapable of sinning. Still common in China.
Hydatidiform mole	A pathologic ovum ("empty egg"—ovum with no DNA) resulting in cystic swelling of chorionic villi and proliferation of chorionic epithelium (trophoblast). Most common precursor of choriocarcinoma. High β-HCG. "Honeycombed uterus," "cluster of grapes" appearance. Genotype of a complete mole is 46,XX and is purely paternal in origin (no maternal chromosomes). Partial mole is commonly triploid or tetraploid. *"snowstorm" on ultrasound*

Asbestosis	Diffuse pulmonary interstitial fibrosis caused by inhaled asbestos fibers. Increased risk of pleural mesothelioma and bronchogenic carcinoma. Long latency. Ferruginous bodies in lung (asbestos fibers coated with hemosiderin). Ivory-white pleural plaques.	Smokers have synergistically higher risk of cancer. Seen in ship builders and plumbers.

Neonatal respiratory distress syndrome	Surfactant deficiency leading to ↑ surface tension, resulting in alveolar collapse. Surfactant is made by type II cells most abundantly after 35th wk gestation. The lecithin-to-sphingomyelin ratio in the amniotic fluid, a measure of lung maturity, is usually less than 1.5 in neonatal respiratory distress syndrome. Surfactant: dipalmitoyl phosphatidylcholine lecithin. Prevention: maternal steroids before birth; artificial surfactant for infant.

Bleeding disorders

Platelet abnormalities (microhemorrhage)	Mucous membrane bleeding Petechiae Purpura Prolonged bleeding time	Causes include ITP, TTP, drugs, and DIC (↑ fibrin split products)
Coagulation factor defects (macrohemorrhage)	Hemarthroses (bleeding into joints) Easy bruising Prolonged PT and/or aPTT	Coagulopathies include hemophilia A (factor VIII deficiency), hemophilia B (factor IX deficiency), and von Willebrand's disease (nasal, sinus, GI bleeds).

Hypothyroidism and hyperthyroidism

Hypothyroidism	Cold intolerance, hypoactivity, weight gain, fatigue, lethargy, ↓ appetite, constipation, weakness, ↓ reflexes, myxedema (facial/periorbital), dry, cool skin, and coarse, brittle hair.	↑ TSH (sensitive test for 1° hypothyroidism), ↓ total T4, ↓ free T4, ↓ T3 uptake
Hyperthyroidism	Heat intolerance, hyperactivity, weight loss, chest pain/palpitations, arrhythmias, diarrhea, ↑ reflexes, warm, dry skin, and fine hair.	↓ TSH (if 1°), ↑ total T4, ↑ free T4, ↑ T3 uptake
Graves' disease	Ophthalmopathy (proptosis, EOM swelling), pretibial myxedema, diffuse goiter.	An autoimmune hyperthyroidism with thyroid stimulating/TSH receptor antibodies

Osteoporosis	Reduction of bone mass in spite of normal bone mineralization.	Affects whites > blacks > Asians.
Type I	Postmenopausal (10–15 years after menopause); ↑ bone resorption due to ↓ estrogen levels. Treated with estrogen replacement.	Vertebal crush fractures: acute back pain, loss of height, kyphosis.
Type II	Senile osteoporosis—affects men and women > 70 years.	Distal wrist (Colles') fractures, vertebral wedge fractures.

Alcoholism

Physiologic tolerance and dependence with symptoms of withdrawal (tremor, tachycardia, hypertension, malaise, nausea, delirium tremens) when intake is interrupted. Continued drinking despite medical and social contraindications and life disruptions.

Treatment: disulfiram to condition the patient negatively against alcohol use. Supportive treatment of other systemic manifestations. Alcoholics Anonymous and other peer support groups are most successful in sustaining abstinence.

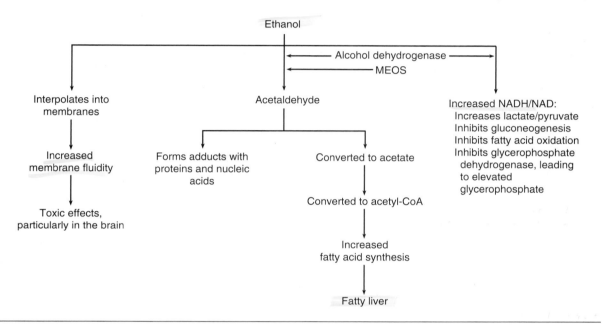

Ethanol

Alcohol dehydrogenase
MEOS

Interpolates into membranes → Increased membrane fluidity → Toxic effects, particularly in the brain

Acetaldehyde → Forms adducts with proteins and nucleic acids / Converted to acetate → Converted to acetyl-CoA → Increased fatty acid synthesis → Fatty liver

Increased NADH/NAD:
Increases lactate/pyruvate
Inhibits gluconeogenesis
Inhibits fatty acid oxidation
Inhibits glycerophosphate dehydrogenase, leading to elevated glycerophosphate

Long-term consequences of alcohol use

Alcoholic hepatitis and cirrhosis, pancreatitis, dilated cardiomyopathy, peripheral neuropathy, cerebellar degeneration, Wernicke-Korsakoff syndrome, testicular atrophy and hyperestrinism, and Mallory-Weiss syndrome.

Alcoholic cirrhosis
Long-term alcohol use leads to micronodular cirrhosis with accompanying symptoms of jaundice, hypoalbuminemia, coagulation factor deficiencies, and portal hypertension, leading to peripheral edema and ascites, encephalopathy, and neurologic manifestations (e.g., asterixis, flapping tremor of the hands).

Wernicke-Korsakoff syndrome
Caused by severe malnutrition and thiamine (Vitamin B_1) deficiency due to alcohol use. Causes lesions in the mamillary bodies characterized by anterograde amnesia and confabulations.

Mallory-Weiss syndrome
Longitudinal lacerations at the gastroesophageal junction caused by excessive vomiting with failure of LES relaxation that could lead to fatal hematemesis.

Boerhaave's Syndrome - complete esophageal rupture
Etotism, pregnancy, bulimia

Diabetes mellitus

Acute manifestations   Polydipsia, polyuria, polyphagia, weight loss, DKA (IDDM), hyperosmolar coma (NIDDM), unopposed secretion of GH and epinephrine (exacerbating hyperglycemia).

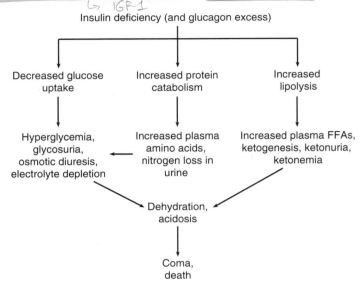

↳ IGF-1

Insulin deficiency (and glucagon excess)

| Decreased glucose uptake | Increased protein catabolism | Increased lipolysis |

Hyperglycemia, glycosuria, osmotic diuresis, electrolyte depletion ← Increased plasma amino acids, nitrogen loss in urine   Increased plasma FFAs, ketogenesis, ketonuria, ketonemia

Dehydration, acidosis

Coma, death

Chronic manifestations   Nonenzymatic glycosylation
1. Small vessel disease (diffuse thickening of BM), retinopathy (hemorrhage, exudates, microaneurysms), nephropathy (nodular sclerosis, progressive proteinuria, chronic renal failure, arteriosclerosis leading to HTN)
2. Large vessel atherosclerosis, coronary artery disease, peripheral vascular occlusive disease and gangrene, cerebrovascular disease
3. Neuropathy (motor, sensory, and autonomic degeneration)
4. Cataracts, glaucoma

Tests   Fasting serum glucose, glucose tolerance test, HbA_{1c} (measures long-term diabetic control)

Type I vs. type II diabetes mellitus

	Type I— juvenile onset (IDDM)	Type II— maturity (adult) onset (NIDDM)
Incidence	15%	85%
Insulin necessary in treatment	Always	Sometimes
Age (exceptions commonly occur)	Under 30	Over 40
Association with obesity	No	Yes
Genetic predisposition	Weak, polygenic	Strong, polygenic
Association with HLA system	Yes (HLA DR 3 & 4)	No
Glucose intolerance	Severe	Mild to moderate
Ketoacidosis	Common	Rare
Beta cell numbers in the islets	Reduced	Variable
Serum insulin level	Reduced	Variable
Classic symptoms of polyuria, polydipsia, thirst, weight loss	Common	Sometimes
Basic cause	?Viral or immune destruction of beta cells	?Increased resistance to insulin

SIADH

Syndrome of inappropriate antidiuretic hormone secretion:
  Excessive water retention
  Hyponatremia
  Serum hypo-osmolarity with urine osmolarity > serum osmolarity
Very low serum sodium levels can lead to seizures.

Causes include:
  Ectopic ADH (small cell lung cancer)
  CNS disorders
  Pulmonary disease
  Drugs

hypo osmolar seizures   vs. hyperosmolar coma

Diabetes insipidus

Characterized by intensive thirst and polyuria together with an inability to concentrate urine with fluid restriction owing to lack of ADH (central DI) or to a lack of renal response to ADH (nephrogenic DI).

Findings — Urine specific gravity < 1.006; serum osmolality > 290 mOsm/L.

Treatment — Adequate fluid intake. For central DI: intranasal desmopressin (ADH analog) once or twice daily. For nephrogenic DI: hydrochlorothiazide, indomethacin, or amiloride.

PATHOLOGY—FINDINGS

Aortic insufficiency

Pistol shot sound heard over femoral vessels (Traube sign).
Water hammer pulse over carotid artery (Corrigan pulse).
Quincke's capillary pulsations (pressure on fingernail results in visible pulsations).

Argyll–Robertson pupil

Argyll–Robertson pupil constricts with accommodation but not reactive to light. Pathognomonic for 3° syphilis.

"life & prostitute"

Argyll–**R**obertson **P**upil
  ARP: Accommodation **R**esponse **P**resent.
  PRA: Pupillary (light) **R**eflex **A**bsent.

Aschoff body

Aschoff bodies (granuloma with giant cells) and Anitschkow's cells (activated histiocytes) are found in rheumatic heart disease.

Think of two **RH**ussians with **RH**eumatic heart disease (Aschoff and Anitschkow).

[handwritten in margin: ...tic of OGENOUS line.]

Auer bodies (rods)

Auer rods are cytoplasmic inclusions in granulocytes and myeloblasts. Primarily seen in acute promyelocytic leukemia.

Casts

Casts of nephron:
RBC casts = glomerular inflammation, ischemia, or malignant hypertension.
WBC casts = inflammation in renal interstitium, tubules, and glomeruli. *[handwritten: pathognomonic of pyelo]*
Hyaline casts often seen in normal urine. *[handwritten: — Tamm-Horsfall protein]*
Waxy casts seen in chronic renal failure.

Presence of casts indicates that hematuria/pyuria is of renal origin.

Erythrocyte sedimentation rate

Very nonspecific test that measures acute-phase reactants. Dramatically increased with infection, *[handwritten: trauma]* malignancy, connective tissue disease. Also increased with pregnancy, inflammatory disease, anemia. Decreased with sickle cell anemia, polycythemia, congestive heart failure.

Simple, cheap, but nonspecific. Should not be used for asymptomatic screening; can be used to diagnose and monitor temporal arteritis and polymyalgia rheumatica.

Ghon complex

TB granulomas with lobar or perihilar lymph node involvement (Ghon focus and lymph node involvement). Reflects primary infection or exposure.

Ghon complex is the lung and the node; Ghon focus is just the focus of lung involvement.

Hyperlipidemia signs

Atheromata = plaques in blood vessel walls.
Xanthelasma = Plaques or nodules composed of lipid-laden histiocytes in the skin, especially the eyelids.
Tendinous xanthoma = lipid deposit in tendon, especially Achilles.
Corneal arcus = lipid deposit in cornea, nonspecific (arcus senilis).

Psammoma bodies

Laminated, concentric, calcific spherules seen in:
1. Papillary adenocarcinoma of thyroid
2. Serous papillary cystadenocarcinoma of ovary

3. Meningioma
4. Malignant mesothelioma

Papillary (thyroid)
Serous (ovary)
a
Meningioma
Mesothel**ioma**

RBC forms

Biconcave = normal.
Spherocytes = hereditary spherocytosis, autoimmune hemolysis.
Elliptocyte = hereditary elliptocytosis.
Macro-ovalocyte = megaloblastic anemia, marrow failure.
Helmet cell, schistocyte = DIC, traumatic hemolysis.
Sickle cell = sickle cell anemia.

Reed–Sternberg cells	Distinctive tumor giant cell seen in Hodgkin's disease; large cell that is binucleate or bilobed with the 2 halves as mirror images ("owl's eyes"). Necessary but not sufficient for a diagnosis of Hodgkin's disease.	There are 4 types of Hodgkin's disease; nodular sclerosis variant is the only one seen in women > men (excellent prognosis).
Roth's spots	White spots of coagulated fibrin in retina seen on funduscopic exam. Associated with bacterial endocarditis.	
Sentinel loop (x-ray)	Represents a distended bowel loop suggestive of a localized ileus secondary to an inflamed abdominal viscus, as in pancreatitis, appendicitis, cholecystitis.	
Virchow's (sentinel) node	A firm supraclavicular lymph node, often on left side, easily palpable (can be detected by medical students), also known as "jugular gland." Presumptive evidence of malignant visceral neoplasm (classically stomach).	

Anemia

Type	Etiology	
Microcytic, hypochromic	Iron deficiency: $\uparrow$ TIBC, $\downarrow$ ferritin, $\downarrow$ serum iron Anemia of chronic disease: $\downarrow$ TIBC, $\uparrow$ ferritin, $\downarrow$ serum iron, $\uparrow$ storage iron in marrow macrophages Thalassemias Lead poisoning	Vit. B_{12} and folate deficiencies are associated with hypersegmented PMNs. Unlike folate deficiency, vit. B_{12} deficiency is associated with neurologic problems.
Macrocytic	Megaloblastic: Vitamin B_{12}/folate deficiency Drugs that block DNA synthesis (e.g., sulfa drugs, AZT) Marked reticulocytosis	Serum haptoglobin and serum LDH are used to determine
Normocytic, normochromic	Hemorrhage Enzyme defects (e.g., G6PD deficiency, PK deficiency) RBC membrane defects (e.g., hereditary spherocytosis) Bone marrow disorders (e.g., aplastic anemia, leukemia) Hemoglobinopathies (e.g., sickle cell disease) Autoimmune hemolytic anemia ⊕ Coomb's	RBC hemolysis. Direct Coombs' test is used to distinguish between immune vs. nonimmune mediated RBC hemolysis.

Aplastic anemia

	Pancytopenia characterized by severe anemia, neutropenia, and thrombocytopenia caused by failure or destruction of multipotent myeloid stem cells, with inadequate production or release of differentiated cell lines.
Causes	Radiation, benzene, chloramphenicol, alkylating agents, antimetabolites, viral agents (HCV, CMV, EBV, herpes zoster-varicella), Fanconi's syndrome, idiopathic (immune-mediated, primary stem-cell defect). Parvovirus r/ SCA
Symptoms All	Fatigue, malaise, pallor, purpura, mucosal bleeding, petechiae, infection.
Pathologic features	Pancytopenia with normal cell morphology; hypocellular bone marrow with fatty infiltration. myelophthisis
Treatment	Withdrawal of offending agent, allogenic bone marrow transplantation, RBC and platelet transfusion, G-CSF or GM-CSF.

Peripheral blood smears

Normal

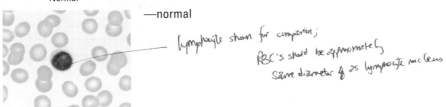

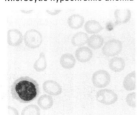

—normal

lymphocyte shown for comparison; RBC's should be approximately same diameter of as lymphocyte nucleus

Microcytic hypochromic anemia

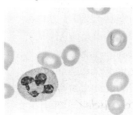

—normally 2° to **iron deficiency**
—low serum ferritin
—elevated serum iron binding capacity

RBC's smaller than lymphocyte nucleus

Megaloblastic anemia

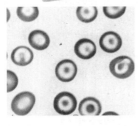

—2° to **folate or B$_{12}$ deficiency**
—hypersegmented (5–7 lobes) PMN's
—large red blood cells (MCV > 100)
—**never** give folate to a patient who is deficient in B$_{12}$
—**pernicious anemia**—autoimmune disease which causes B$_{12}$ deficiency by depleting
  intrinsic factor, which is needed to absorb B$_{12}$ in **terminal ileum**

Target cells

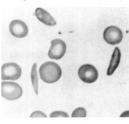

—thalassemia
—hemoglobin C disease
—liver disease

Hemoglobin SS with sickle cells

—**Hb^s**—β-globin GLU → VAL at #6; 8% of US blacks are Hb^s carriers   *sickle cell trait.*
—cells will sickle 2° to hypoxia, dehydration, and ↑ blood viscosity
—anemia
—vaso-occlusive crises +/− chest pain
—aplastic crises (B19 virus)
—splenic sequestration crises
—strokes

Enzyme markers

Serum enzyme	Major diagnostic use
Aminotransferases (AST and ALT)	Myocardial infarction (AST only)
	Viral hepatitis (ALT > AST)
	Alcoholic hepatitis (AST > ALT)
Amylase	Acute pancreatitis, mumps
Ceruloplasmin (decreased)	Wilson's disease
CPK (creatine phosphokinase)	Muscle disorders (e.g., DMD) and myocardial infarction (CPK-MB)
γ-glutamyl transpeptidase *EtOH*	Various liver diseases
LDH-1 (lactate dehydrogenase fraction 1)	Myocardial infarction (LDH1 > LDH2)
Lipase	Acute pancreatitis
Alkaline phosphatase	Bone disease, obstructive liver disease

PATHOLOGY—PHOTOMICROGRAPHS

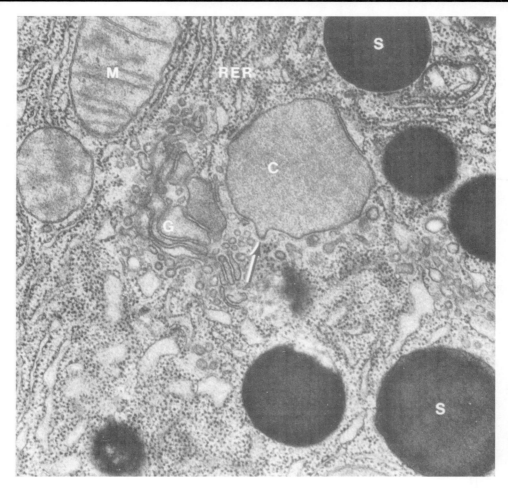

Electron micrograph of a part of a pancreatic acinar cell. A condensing vacuole (C) is receiving secretory product (arrow) from the Golgi complex (G). M, mitochondrion; RER, rough endoplasmic reticulum; S, mature condensed secretory (zymogen) granule.

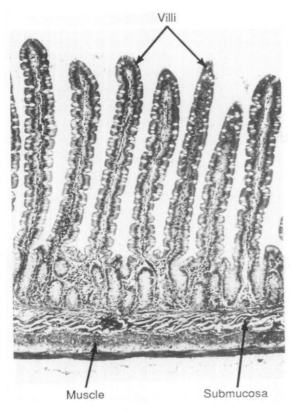

Photomicrograph of the small intestine.

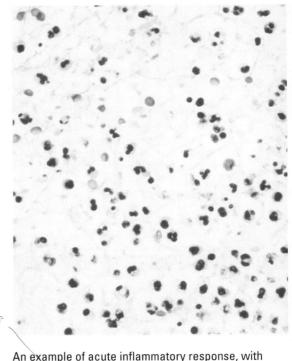

An example of acute inflammatory response, with many polymorphonuclear cells mixed with strands of fibrin. Some macrophages are also present.

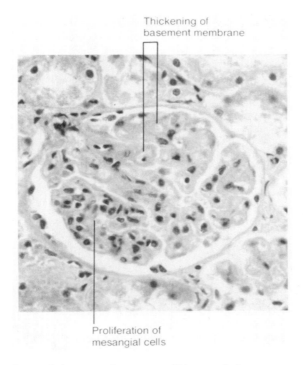

Systemic lupus erythematosus; kidney pathology.

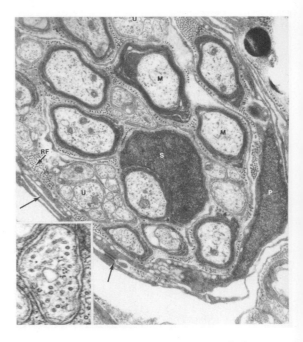

Electron micrograph of a peripheral nerve. (M) myelinated and (U) unmyelinated nerve fibers. (RF) reticular fibers (part of the endoneurium), (S) Schwann cell nucleus, (P, arrows) perineurial cells. Inset shows part of an axon with numerous neurofilaments.

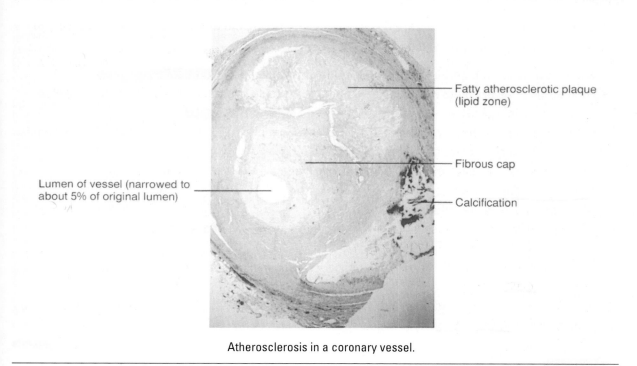

Fatty atherosclerotic plaque
(lipid zone)

Fibrous cap

Calcification

Lumen of vessel (narrowed to
about 5% of original lumen)

Atherosclerosis in a coronary vessel.

These abstracted case vignettes are designed to demonstrate the thought processes necessary to answer multistep clinical reasoning questions.

- Patient presents with aortic regurgitation → describe pulse → water hammer pulse. *Corrigan's*
- 60-year-old male presents with bone pain and anemia, also hypercalcemia and gamma spike on serum electrophoresis → what is the diagnosis? → multiple myeloma.
- Patient has multiple fractures, anemia, cranial nerve deficits → in which of the following cell types is there a defect? → osteoclasts (e.g., osteopetrosis).
- 35-year-old man has high pressure in arms and low pressure in legs → what is the diagnosis? → coarctation of the aorta.
- Man has flank pain, hematuria, and erythrocytosis → cancer of what organ? → kidney. *RCC*
- Woman presents with diffuse goiter and hyperthyroidism → what are the expected values of TSH and thyroid hormones? *↓TSH, ↑T4,T3*
- Patient exhibits an extended expiratory phase → what is the disease process? → obstructive lung disease. *COPD*
- Woman presents with headache, visual disturbance, galactorrhea, and amenorrhea → what is the diagnosis? → prolactinoma.
- Baby has foul-smelling stool and recurrent pulmonary infection → what is the diagnosis? → cystic fibrosis.
- Obese woman presents with hirsutism and increased levels of serum testosterone → what is the diagnosis? → polycystic ovarian syndrome. ~~Kruckel Wilson~~ *Stein-Leventhal*
- 45-year-old female has ruddy complexion and erythrocytosis → increased levels of erythropoietin and hemoglobin are found→ what is the diagnosis? → renal cell carcinoma. *PV: low erythropoietin.*
- Elderly gentleman has large ecchymoses but no problems with coagulation factors or peripheral blood components → what is the diagnosis? *Vasculitis?*
- Pregnant woman in 20th week of gestation develops masklike hyperpigmentation → what is the diagnosis? → systemic lupus erythematosus.
- Chronic smoker develops worsening hoarseness → laryngoscopy shows one vocal cord covered with white material → what is the diagnosis? *Sq cell CA*
- Man presents with extensive destruction of knees, subcutaneous nodules, and exquisite pain in the metatarsophalangeal joint → biopsy shows needle-like crystals → what is the diagnosis? → gouty arthritis.
- 48-year-old female with progressive lethargy and cold intolerance → what is the diagnosis? → hypothyroidism.
- Patient with elevated serum cortisol levels undergoes dexamethasone suppression test. One milligram of dexamethasone does not decrease cortisol levels; 8 mg does → what is the diagnosis? → pituitary tumor.
- During a game, a basketball player collapses and dies immediately → what type of cardiomyopathy? → hypertrophic cardiomyopathy.
- Listless girl has severe iron deficiency → to confirm diagnosis of pica, ask about what? → ingestion of clay.
- Child has been anemic since birth. Splenectomy would result in increased hematocrit in what disease? *hereditary spherocytosis*

- 43-year-old man experiences dizziness and tinnitus → CT shows enlarged internal acoustic meatus → what is the diagnosis? → schwannoma.
- Woman with long history of diabetes has renal insufficiency and pitting edema → what is the fluid change? → hypotonic volume expansion.
- Child exhibits weakness and enlarged calves → Duchenne muscular dystrophy → how is disease inherited? → X-linked recessive.
- Patient shows hemoptysis and signs of malabsorption → cystic fibrosis is diagnosed → by means of what test? → sweat chloride test.
- Person with pancreatic insufficiency demonstrates fat intolerance → what can he not eat? → fat.

- Gross photograph of abdominal aorta with aneurysm → what is the most likely process? → atherosclerosis.
- Gross photograph of hydatidiform mole ("bunch of grapes") → high levels of what substance are present? → hCG.
- Gross photograph of focally hemorrhagic small intestine of weight lifter → what is the process responsible for this? → strangulation of a hernia.
- Chest x-ray shows collapse of middle lobe of right lung; recurrent pneumonia and growth in bronchus → diagnosis? → bronchogenic carcinoma.
- Middle-aged woman with intermittent syncope has a mass removed from the right atrium → H&E shows wispy, mucus-like tissue → what is the diagnosis? → myxoma.
- Chest x-ray shows pneumothorax → what are the clinical findings? → pleuritic chest pain.
- 1-year-old baby present with big red spot on face → what is the likely course of this lesion? → regression vs. Sturge-Weber.
- Gross photograph of lung with caseous necrosis → what is the diagnosis? → TB.
- H&E of lung tissue with multinucleated giant cells → what is the diagnosis?
- H&E of lung biopsy from plumber shows elongated structures in tissue → ferruginous bodies → what is the diagnosis? → malignant mesothelioma.
- H&E of glomerulus → looks like Kimmelstiel-Wilson nodules → lesion is indicative of what disease? diabetes mellitus.
- H&E of granuloma → what is activated? → macrophages.
- Chest x-ray of spine from softball player who developed back pain and lost sensation in a dermatome of the leg → what is the diagnosis? → herniated lumbar disk.
- Karyotype with three 21 chromosomes → Down's → what feature would patient have? → flat facies.
- Gross photograph of polycystic kidneys in adult male → what is the mode of inheritance? → autosomal dominant.
- Patient with hypercalcemia → bone marrow biopsy shows lots of plasma cells → what is the diagnosis? → multiple myeloma.

Congenital
1. Maternal complications of birth (e.g., Sheehan's syndrome, puerperal infection).
2. Failure to thrive: common causes.
3. Causes of kernicterus (hemolytic disease of the newborn).

Neoplasia
1. Bone and cartilage tumors (e.g., osteosarcoma, giant cell tumor, Ewing's sarcoma).
2. Clinical features of lymphomas (Burkitt's and other non-Hodgkin's lymphomas).
3. Risk factors for common carcinomas (e.g., lung, breast).
4. Prostate cancer: epidemiology, presentation (most commonly in peripheral zone/posterior lobe), screening, treatment.
5. Chemical carcinogens (e.g., vinyl chloride, nitrosamines, aflatoxin) and mechanisms of carcinogenesis (e.g., initiator vs. promoter).
6. Malignancies associated with pulmonary pneumoconiosis (e.g., asbestos, silicosis).
7. AIDS-associated neoplasms (Kaposi's sarcoma, B-cell lymphoma).
8. Pituitary tumors (e.g., prolactinomas) and other sellar lesions (e.g., craniopharyngioma).
9. Tumors of the mouth, pharynx, and larynx (e.g., vocal cord tumors in smokers). *squll cA*
10. Modes of spread of certain cancers (e.g., transitional cell carcinoma).
11. Clinical features of leukemias (e.g., demographics, pathology, prognosis).
12. Breast cancer versus benign fibrocystic changes (epidemiology, clinical presentation).

Nervous System
1. Hydrocephalus: types (e.g., communicating, obstructive), sequelae.
2. CNS manifestations of viral infections (e.g., HIV, HSV).
3. Spinal muscular atrophies (e.g., Werdnig–Hoffmann disease, ALS).

Rheumatic/Autoimmune
1. Transplant rejection (hyperacute, acute, graft versus host disease).
2. Differences between rheumatoid arthritis and graft versus host disease.
3. Psoriasis: skin/joint involvement.
4. Autoantibodies (e.g., antimicrosomal) and disease associations.

Vascular/Hematology
1. Hypertension: essential versus secondary hypertension, complications (e.g., cerebral vascular accidents, renal disease).
2. Common hematologic diseases (e.g., thrombocytopenia, clotting factor deficiencies, lymphoma, leukemia).
3. Valvular heart disease (e.g., mitral stenosis, mitral regurgitation, aortic stenosis, aortic regurgitation, tricuspid regurgitation), including clinical presentation, associated murmurs, and cardiac catheterization results.
4. Thoracic and abdominal aortic aneurysms: similarities and differences.
5. Polycythemia: primary (polycythemia) and secondary (e.g., hypoxia) causes, clinical manifestations (e.g., pruritus, fatigue).

General

1. Common clinical features of AIDS (e.g., CNS, pulmonary, GI, dermatologic manifestations).
2. Dermatologic manifestations of systemic disease (e.g., neoplasia, inflammatory bowel disease, meningococcemia, systemic lupus erythematosus).
3. Geriatric pathology: diseases common in the elderly, normal physiologic changes with age.
4. Renal failure: acute versus chronic, features of uremia.
5. Acid–base disturbances, including renal tubular acidosis.
6. Wound repair.
7. Dehydration (e.g., hyponatremic vs. isotonic vs. hypernatremic), including appropriate treatment.
8. Gynecologic pathology (e.g., menstrual disorders).
9. Cell injury and death.
10. Malabsorption (e.g., celiac sprue, bacterial overgrowth, disaccharidase deficiency).
11. EKG tracings of arrhythmias (e.g., atrial fibrillation, torsade de pointes).

Pharmacology

Preparation for questions on pharmacology is straightforward. Memorizing all the key drugs and their characteristics (e.g., mechanisms, clinical use, and important side effects) is high yield. Focus on understanding the prototype drugs in each class. Avoid memorizing obscure derivatives. Learn the "classic" and distinguishing toxicities of the major drugs. Do not bother with drug dosages or trade names. Reviewing associated biochemistry, physiology, and microbiology can be useful while studying pharmacology. There is a strong emphasis on autonomic nervous system, central nervous system, antimicrobial, and cardiovascular agents as well as on NSAIDs. Much of the material is clinically relevant.

Antimicrobial
CNS
Cardiovascular
Cancer Drugs
Toxicology
Miscellaneous
High-Yield Clinical
   Vignettes
High-Yield Topics

Antimicrobial therapy

Mechanism of action	Drugs
Block cell wall synthesis by inhibition of peptidoglycan cross-linking	Penicillin, cephalosporins, imipenem, aztreonam
Block peptidoglycan synthesis	Bacitracin, vancomycin
Block protein synthesis at 50S ribosomal subunit	Chloramphenicol, erythromycin/macrolides, lincomycin, clindamycin
Block protein synthesis at 30S ribosomal subunit	Aminoglycosides, tetracyclines
Block nucleotide synthesis	Sulfonamides, trimethoprim
Block DNA topoisomerases	Quinolones
Block mRNA synthesis	Rifampin
Disrupt bacterial/fungal cell membranes	Polymyxins
Disrupt fungal cell membranes	Amphotericin B, nystatin, fluconazole/azoles
Unknown	Isoniazid, metronidazole, pentamidine

Penicillin

	Penicillin G (IV form), penicillin V (oral):
Mechanism	1. Binds penicillin-binding proteins
	2. Blocks transpeptidase cross-linking of cell wall
	3. Activates autolytic enzymes
Clinical use	Bactericidal for gram-positive cocci, gram-positive rods, gram-negative cocci, and spirochetes. Not penicillinase-resistant.
Toxicity	Hypersensitivity reactions.

Methicillin, nafcillin, dicloxacillin

Mechanism	Same as penicillin. Narrow spectrum, penicillinase resistant because of bulkier R group.
Clinical use	*Staphylococcus aureus.*
Toxicity	Hypersensitivity reactions; methicillin: interstitial nephritis.

Ampicillin, amoxicillin

Mechanism	Same as penicillin. Wider spectrum, penicillinase sensitive. Also, combine with clavulanic acid (penicillinase inhibitor) to enhance spectrum. Amoxicillin has greater oral bioavailability than ampicillin.
Clinical use	Extended-spectrum penicillin: certain gram-positive bacteria and gram-negative rods (*Haemophilus influenzae*, *Escherichia coli*, *Listeria monocytogenes*, *Proteus mirabilis*, *Salmonella*).
Toxicity	Hypersensitivity reactions; ampicillin: rash.

> Coverage: ampicillin/amoxicillin **HELPS**

Carbenicillin, ticarcillin

MEGAPENICILLINS: piperacillin, mezlocillin. (handwritten)

Mechanism	Same as penicillin. Extended spectrum.
Clinical use	*Pseudomonas* species and gram-negative rods.
Toxicity	Hypersensitivity reactions.

Cephalosporins

Mechanism	β-lactam drugs that inhibit cell wall synthesis but are less susceptible to penicillinases. Bactericidal.	
Clinical use	First generation: gram-positive cocci, *Proteus mirabilis*, *E. coli*, *Klebsiella pneumoniae*.	1st generation: **PEcK**
	Second generation: gram-positive cocci, *Haemophilus influenzae*, *Enterobacter aerogenes*, *Neisseria* species, *Proteus mirabilis*, *E. coli*, *K. pneumoniae*, *Serratia marcescens*.	2nd generation: **HEN PEcKS**
	Third generation: serious gram-negative infections. Cefot**ax**ime and ceftri**ax**one can penetrate the CNS (use for meningitis).	*Pseudomonas* (handwritten) Think of an "**ax** to the head" (CNS).
Toxicity	Hypersensitivity reactions, increased nephrotoxicity of aminoglycosides, disulfiram-like reaction with ethanol (in cephalosporins with a methylthiotetrazole group, e.g., cefamandole).	

(handwritten note on left: *better for rods*)

Penicillin

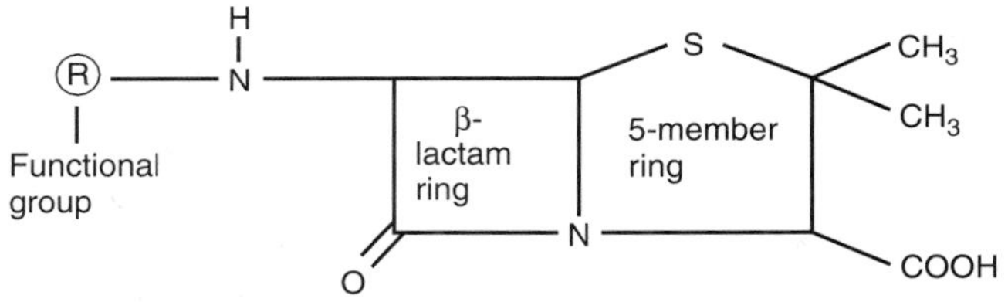

Cephalosporin

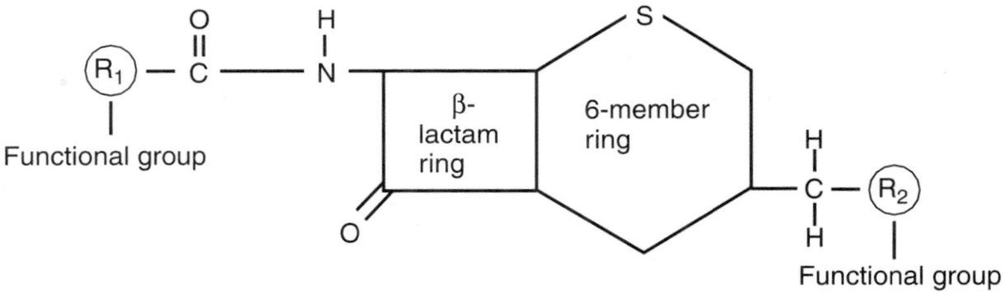

Aztreonam

Mechanism	A monobactam resistant to β-lactamases. Inhibits cell wall synthesis (binds to PBP3). Synergistic with aminoglycosides. No cross-allergenicity with penicillins.
Clinical use	Gram-negative rods: *Klebsiella* species, *Pseudomonas* species, *Serratia* species. No activity against gram-positives or anaerobes.
Toxicity	GI upset with possible superinfections, vertigo, headache.

Imipenem

Mechanism	A carbapenem. Wide spectrum. β-lactamase resistant. Always administered with cilastatin (inhibitor of renal dihydropeptidase I).	With imipenem, "the kill is **lastin** with cil**astatin**."
Clinical use	Gram-positive cocci, gram-negative rods, and anaerobes.	*Primaxin.*
Toxicity	GI distress, skin rash, and CNS toxicity (at high plasma levels).	

Vancomycin

Mechanism	Inhibits cell wall mucopeptide formation. Bactericidal.
Clinical use	Used for serious, gram-positive multidrug-resistant organisms, including *Staphylococcus aureus* and *Clostridium difficile* (pseudomembranous colitis).
Toxicity	**N**ephrotoxicity, **O**totoxicity, **T**hrombophlebitis, diffuse flushing—"red man syndrome" (can largely prevent by pretreatment with antihistamines and slow infusion rate). Well tolerated in general. Does **NOT** have many problems.

Protein synthesis inhibitors

30S inhibitors:

A = Aminoglycosides (streptomycin, gentamicin, tobramycin, amikacin) [bactericidal]

T = Tetracyclines [bacteriostatic]

"Buy **AT 30, CELL** at **50**"

50S inhibitors:

C = Chloramphenicol [bacteriostatic] — *can be 'cidal'*

E = Erythromycin [bacteriostatic] — *all static* — *applies to macrolides*

L = Lincomycin [bacteriostatic]

L = cLindamycin [bacteriostatic]

Aminoglycosides

Gentamicin, streptomycin, tobramycin, amikacin

Mechanism	Bactericidal, inhibits formation of initiation complex and causes misreading of mRNA. Requires O_2 for uptake, therefore ineffective against anaerobes.
Clinical use	Severe gram-negative rod infections.
Toxicity	**N**ephrotoxicity (especially when used with cephalosporins), **O**totoxicity (especially when used with loop diuretics). Ami**NO**glycosides. *reverse relation w/ interactions drgs*

(ADH antagonist.

Tetracyclines
Tetracycline, doxycycline, demeclocycline, minocycline

Mechanism	Bacteriostatic, binds to 30S and prevents attachment of aminoacyl-tRNA, limited CNS penetration. Doxycycline fecally eliminated and can be used in patients with renal failure. Must NOT take with milk or antacids because divalent cations inhibit its absorption in the gut.
Clinical use	***B**orrelia burgdorferi* (Lyme disease), ***C**hlamydia,* ***U**reaplasma,* ***M**ycoplasma pneumoniae,* ***R**ickettsiae,* ***A**cne,* ***T**ularemia,* ***C**holera* (*Vibrio cholerae*)
Toxicity	GI distress, discolors teeth in children, inhibits bone growth in children, Fanconi's syndrome, photosensitivity.

Coverage: **B CUM RATC:** "Become rats."

Erythromycin
Azithromycin a good substitute

Mechanism	Inhibits protein synthesis by blocking translocation, binds to the 23S rRNA of the 50S ribosomal subunit. Bacteriostatic.
Clinical use	Gram-positive cocci, *Mycoplasma, Legionella, Chlamydia, Neisseria.*
Toxicity	Acute cholestatic hepatitis, eosinophilia, skin rashes, GI discomfort.

Chloramphenicol

Mechanism	Inhibits 50S peptidyl transferase. Bacteriostatic.
Clinical use	Meningitis (*H. influenzae, Neisseria meningitidis, Streptococcus pneumoniae*).
Toxicity	Anemia, aplastic anemia, *severe; may be prev.* gray baby syndrome (overdose in premature infants lacking liver UDP-glucuronyl transferase).

Nonsurgical antimicrobial prophylaxis

Meningococcal infection	Rifampin (drug of choice), minocycline
Gonorrhea	Ceftriaxone
Syphilis	Benzathine penicillin G
History of recurrent UTI	Trimethoprim-sulfamethoxazole (TMP-SMX) *Bactrim*
PCP	TMP-SMX (drug of choice), aerosolized pentamidine

Cipro for uncomplicated UTI (and pyelo)

Sulfonamides *Sulfa Rx*

	Sulfamethoxazole (SMX), sulfisoxazole, triple sulfas
Mechanism	PABA antimetabolites inhibit dihydropteroate synthase. Bacteriostatic.
Clinical use	Gram-positive, gram-negative, *Nocardia, Chlamydia.* Triple sulfas or SMX for simple UTI.
Toxicity	Hypersensitivity reactions, hemolysis if G6PD deficient, nephrotoxicity, kernicterus in infants, displace other drugs from albumin.

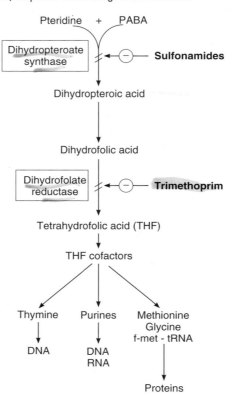

Trimethoprim

Mechanism	Inhibits dihydrofolate reductase. Bacteriostatic.	**T**rimethoprim = **TMP:** "**T**reats **M**arrow **P**oorly."
Clinical use	Used in combination with sulfonamides (trimethoprim–sulfamethoxazole), causing sequential block of folate synthesis. Combination used for recurrent UTI, *Shigella, Salmonella, Pneumocystis carinii* pneumonia.	(folate antagonist.
Toxicity	Megaloblastic anemia, leukopenia, granulocytopenia.	

Fluoroquinolones

	Ciprofloxacin and norfloxacin (fluoroquinolones), nalidixic acid (a quinolone).	Fluoro**quinolones** hurt attachments to your **bones.**
Mechanism	Inhibits DNA gyrase (topoisomerase II). Bactericidal.	
Clinical use	Gram-negative rods (including *Pseudomonas*), *Neisseria,* some gram-positive organisms.	
Toxicity	GI upset, superinfections, skin rashes, headache, dizziness. Contraindicated in pregnant women and in children because animal studies show damage to cartilage. Tendonitis and tendon rupture in adults.	

Metronidazole

Mechanism	Forms toxic metabolites in the bacterial cell. Bactericidal.
Clinical use	Antiprotozoal, trichomoniasis, giardiasis, amebiasis, *Gardnerella vaginalis,* anaerobes (*Bacteroides, Clostridium*). Used with bismuth and amoxicillin or tetracycline for "triple therapy" against *H. pylori*.
Toxicity	Disulfiram-like reaction with alcohol, vestibular dysfunction, headache.

"I took the **metro,** which made me dizzy (vestibular dysfunction) and made me vomit (disulfiram-like reaction with alcohol)."

Polymyxins

Polymyxin B, polymyxin E

Mechanism	Bind to cell membranes of bacteria and disrupt their osmotic properties. Polymyxins are cationic, basic proteins that act like detergents.
Clinical use	Resistant gram-negative cocci, gram-negative rods.
Toxicity	Neurotoxicity, acute renal tubular necrosis.

Use vs. fungi?

Isoniazid (INH)

Mechanism	Decreases synthesis of mycolic acids.
Clinical use	*Mycobacterium tuberculosis.* The only agent used as solo prophylaxis against TB.
Toxicity	Hemolysis if G6PD deficient, neurotoxicity, hepatotoxicity. Pyridoxine (vit. B_6) can prevent neurotoxicity.

INH:

Injures **N**eurons and **H**epatocytes.

Rifampin

Mechanism	Inhibits DNA-dependent RNA polymerase.
Clinical use	*M. tuberculosis,* delays resistance to dapsone when used for leprosy. Always used in combination with other drugs except in the treatment of meningococcal carrier state, and chemoprophylaxis in contacts of children with *H. influenzae* type B.
Toxicity	Increased elimination of HIV protease inhibitors, anticoagulants and methadone, hepatotoxicity, thrombocytopenia, skin rashes, flu response, decreased antibody responses.

Rifampin's **4 R's:**

RNA polymerase inhibitor
Revs up microsomal P450
Red/orange body fluids
Rapid resistance if used alone

Anti-TB drugs:
Rifampin (oral)   *or rifabutin.*
Ethambutol (oral)
Streptomycin (IM)
Pyrazinamide (oral)
Isoniazid (oral)
R
E

Amphotericin B

Mechanism	Binds ergosterol (unique to fungi), forms membrane pores that disrupt homeostasis.
Clinical use	*Cryptococcus, Blastomyces, Coccidioides, Histoplasma, Candida, Mucor* (systemic mycoses). Intrathecally for fungal meningitis; does not cross blood–brain barrier.
Toxicity	Fever/chills ("shake and bake"), hypotension, nephrotoxicity, arrhythmias ("amphoterrible").

Amphotericin "tears" holes in the fungal membrane by forming pores.

Fluconazole, ketoconazole, clotrimazole, miconazole

Mechanism	Inhibit fungal steroid synthesis.
Clinical use	Fluconazole for cryptococcus in AIDS patients and candidal infections of all types. Ketoconazole for *Blastomyces, Coccidioides, Histoplasma, C. albicans.*
Toxicity	Hormone synthesis inhibition (gynecomastia), liver dysfunction (inhibits cyt. P450), fever, chills.

ketoconazole, not fluconazole

Griseofulvin

— much like colchicine, save acts on fungi.

Mechanism	Interferes with microtubule function, disrupts mitosis. Deposits in keratin-containing tissues (e.g., nails).
Clinical use	Oral treatment of superficial infections, inhibits growth of dermatophytes (tinea, ringworm) and *C. albicans.*
Toxicity	Teratogenic, carcinogenic, confusion, headaches, ↑ coumarin metabolism.

Antiviral chemotherapy

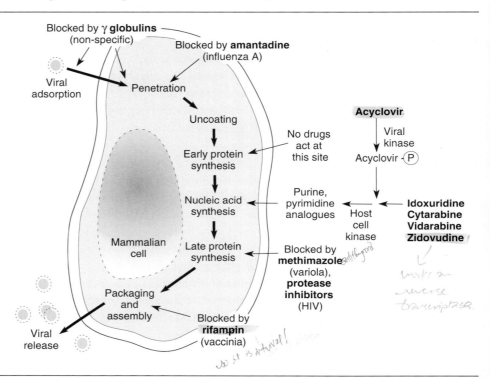

Blocked by γ **globulins** (non-specific)

Blocked by **amantadine** (influenza A)

Viral adsorption

Penetration

Uncoating

No drugs act at this site

Acyclovir

Viral kinase

Acyclovir - Ⓟ

Early protein synthesis

Nucleic acid synthesis

Purine, pyrimidine analogues

Host cell kinase

Idoxuridine Cytarabine Vidarabine Zidovudine

Mammalian cell

Late protein synthesis

Blocked by **methimazole** (variola), **protease inhibitors** (HIV)

works on reverse transcriptase

Packaging and assembly

Blocked by **rifampin** (vaccinia)

Viral release

so it is antiviral!

Amantadine

Mechanism	Blocks viral penetration/uncoating; may buffer pH of endosome. Also causes the release of dopamine from intact nerve terminals.
Clinical use	Prophylaxis for influenza A and rubella. Parkinson's disease.
Toxicity	Ataxia, dizziness, slurred speech.

Amantadine blocks influenza **A** and rubell**A** and causes problems with the cerebell**A**.

Ribavirin

Mechanism	Inhibits synthesis of guanine nucleotides by competitively inhibiting IMP dehydrogenase.
Clinical use	RSV.
Toxicity	Hemolytic anemia.

Acyclovir
Mechanism	Preferentially inhibits viral DNA polymerase when phosphorylated by viral thymidine kinase.
Clinical use	HSV, VZV, EBV. Mucocutaneous and genital herpes lesions. Prophylaxis in immunocompromised patients.
Toxicity	Delirium, tremor, renal crystals.

Ganciclovir
	DHPG (dihydroxy-2-propoxymethyl guanine)
Mechanism	Phosphorylation by viral kinase preferentially inhibits CMV DNA polymerase.
Clinical use	CMV, especially in immunocompromised patients.
Toxicity	Leukopenia, thrombocytopenia, renal toxicity.

Foscarnet
Mechanism	Viral DNA polymerase inhibitor that binds to the pyrophosphate binding site of the enzyme. Does not require activation by viral kinase.
Clinical use	CMV retinitis in immunocompromised patients when ganciclovir fails.
Toxicity	Nephrotoxicity.

Zidovudine (AZT)
Mechanism	Preferentially inhibits reverse transcriptase of HIV. **AZT: A**lways **Z**aps **T**hrombocytes.
Clinical use	HIV-infected patients.
Toxicity	Thrombocytopenia, granulocytopenia, anemia.

Antiparasitic drugs
Ivermectin	Onchocerciasis ("river blindness" ⇒ r**IVER**-mectin).
Mebendazole	Nematode/roundworm (e.g., pinworm, whipworm) infections.
Praziquantel	Trematode/fluke (e.g., schistosomes, *Paragonimus, Clonorchis)* and cysticerci infections.
Niclosamide	Cestode/tapeworm (e.g., *D. latum, Taenia* species) infections.
Pentavalent antimony	Leishmaniasis.　　aka sodium stibogluconate
Chloroquine, quinine, mefloquine	Malaria.
Primaquine	Latent hypnozoite (liver) forms of malaria (*P. vivax, P. ovale*).
Metronidazole	Giardiasis, amoebic dysentery (*E. histolytica*), bacterial vaginitis (*Gardnerella vaginalis*).
Pentamidine	*Pneumocystis carinii* pneumonia.
Nifurtimox	Chagas' disease (*Trypanosoma cruzi*).

Central and peripheral nervous system

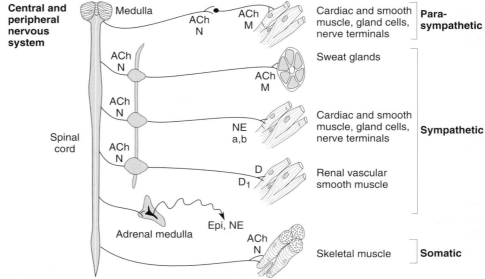

Central and peripheral nervous system

Medulla

ACh N — ACh M — Cardiac and smooth muscle, gland cells, nerve terminals — **Para-sympathetic**

ACh N — ACh M — Sweat glands — **Sympathetic**

Spinal cord

ACh N — NE a,b — Cardiac and smooth muscle, gland cells, nerve terminals

ACh N — D D₁ — Renal vascular smooth muscle

Adrenal medulla — Epi, NE

ACh N — Skeletal muscle — **Somatic**

Autonomic second messengers

Receptor	Major functions
α_1	$\uparrow$ Ca^{2+}, causes contraction, secretion
α_2	$\downarrow$ transmitter release, causes contraction
β_1	$\uparrow$ heart rate, $\uparrow$ contractility; $\uparrow$ renin release
β_2	Relaxes smooth muscle; $\uparrow$ glycogenolysis; $\uparrow$ heart rate, $\uparrow$ contractility
β_3	$\uparrow$ lipolysis
D_1	Relaxes renal vascular smooth muscle

Receptor (M_1, M_3, α_1) $\xrightarrow{G_q}$ Phospholipase C — Lipids ↓ PIP$_2$ → IP$_3$ → $\uparrow$ Ca ; PIP$_2$ → DAG → Protein kinase

Receptor (β, D_1) $\xrightarrow{G_s}$ Adenylcyclase — ATP ↓ $\uparrow$ cAMP → Channels ; cAMP → Enzymes

Receptor (α_2, M_2) $\xrightarrow{G_i}$ Adenylcyclase → $\downarrow$ cAMP

Autonomic drugs

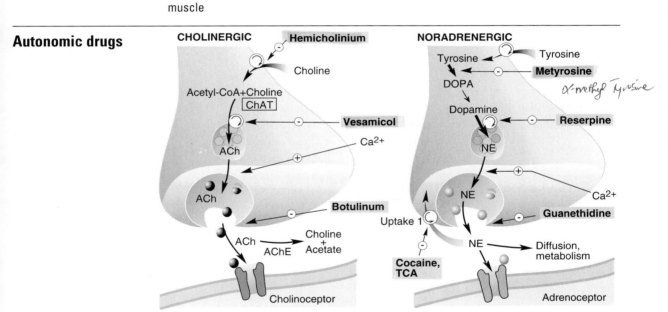

CHOLINERGIC — Hemicholinium · Choline · Acetyl-CoA+Choline [ChAT] · Vesamicol · ACh · Ca^{2+} · ACh · Botulinum · ACh → Choline + Acetate (AChE) · Cholinoceptor

NORADRENERGIC — Tyrosine · Metyrosine · *α-methyl Tyrosine* · DOPA · Dopamine · Reserpine · NE · Ca^{2+} · NE · Guanethidine · Uptake 1 · Cocaine, TCA · NE → Diffusion, metabolism · Adrenoceptor

Circles with rotating arrows represent transporters; ChAT, choline acetyltransferase; ACh, acetylcholine; AChE, acetylcholinesterase; NE, norepinephrine.

Cholinomimetics

	Clinical applications	Action
Direct agonists		
Bethanechol	Postoperative and neurogenic ileus and urinary retention	Activates bowel and bladder smooth muscle
Carbachol, pilocarpine	Glaucoma	Activates ciliary muscle of eye (open angle), pupillary sphincter (narrow angle)
Indirect agonists (anticholinesterases)		
Neostigmine	Postoperative and neurogenic ileus and urinary retention	↑ endogenous ACh
Neostigmine, pyridostigmine, edrophonium	Myasthenia gravis, reversal of NMJ blockade (neostigmine does not cross blood–brain barrier).	↑ endogenous ACh; ↑ strength
Physostigmine	Glaucoma (crosses blood–brain barrier → CNS).	↑ endogenous ACh
Echothiophate	Glaucoma	↑ endogenous ACh

(handwritten in margin: RA OD)

Cholinoreceptor blockers

Muscarinic antagonists	Atropine: used to dilate pupil, reduce acid secretion in acid-peptic disease, reduce urgency in mild cystitis, reduce airway secretions. Causes increased body temperature, rapid pulse, dry mouth, flushed skin, disorientation, mydriasis with cycloplegia.	Atropine parasympathetic block effects: Red as a beet Mad as a hatter Hot as a hare
Nicotinic antagonists	Hexamethonium: ganglionic blocker.	Dry as a bone
Cholinesterase regenerator	Pralidoxime: regenerates active cholinesterase, chemical antagonist, used to treat organophosphate exposure.	Bloated as a bladder Blocks **SLUD: S**alivation, **L**acrimation, **U**rination, **D**efecation. *Emesis*

Antimuscarinic drugs

Organ system	Drugs	Application
CNS	Benztropine	Parkinson's disease
	Scopolamine	Motion sickness
Eye	Atropine, homatropine, tropicamide	Produce mydriasis and cycloplegia
GU	Oxybutynin	Transient cystitis, post-op bladder spasms
Respiratory	Ipratropium	Asthma, COPD

Sympathomimetics

Drug	Mechanism/selectivity	Applications
Catecholamines		
Epinephrine	Direct general agonist (α_1, α_2, β_1, β_2)	Anaphylaxis, glaucoma, asthma, to cause vasoconstriction
Norepinephrine	α_1, α_2, β_1	To cause vasoconstriction in hypotension
Isoproterenol	$\beta_1 = \beta_2$	Asthma, AV block (rare)
Dopamine	$D_1 = D_2 > \beta > \alpha$	Shock, heart failure
Dobutamine	$\beta_1 > \beta_2$	Shock, heart failure
Other		
Amphetamine	Indirect general agonist, releases stored catecholamines	Narcolepsy, obesity, attention deficit disorder — *methylphenidate*
Ephedrine	Indirect general agonist, releases stored catecholamines	Nasal congestion, urinary incontinence, to cause vasoconstriction in hypotension
Phenylephrine	$\alpha_1 > \alpha_2$	To cause mydriasis, vasoconstriction, nasal decongestion
Albuterol, terbutaline	$\beta_2 > \beta_1$	Asthma
Cocaine	Indirect general agonist, uptake inhibitor	To cause vasoconstriction and local anesthesia

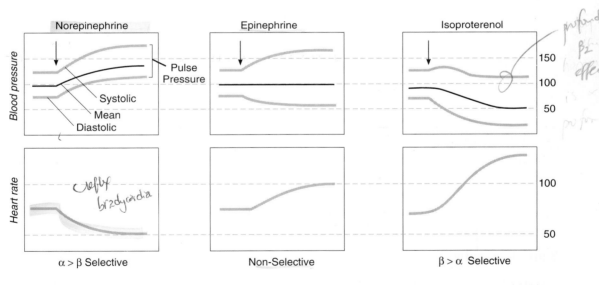

profound β_2 effects. *is x not prior*

reflex bradycardia

249

α Blockers

	Application	Toxicity
Nonselective		
Phenoxybenzamine (irreversible)	Pheochromocytoma	Orthostatic hypotension, reflex tachycardia
Phentolamine (reversible)	Pheochromocytoma	Orthostatic hypotension, reflex tachycardia
α_1-selective		
Prazosin, terazosin, doxazosin	Hypertension, urinary retention in BPH	First-dose orthostatic hypotension, dizziness, headache
α_2-selective		
Yohimbine	Impotence (effectiveness is controversial)	

β Blockers

Propranolol, metoprolol, atenolol, nadolol, timolol, pindolol, esmolol, labetalol *[nonselective. 2: α₁ effects.]*

Application	Effect
Hypertension	↓ cardiac output, ↓ renin secretion *P,N*
Angina pectoris	↓ heart rate and contractility, resulting in decreased oxygen consumption
SVT (propranolol, esmolol)	↓ AV conduction velocity
Glaucoma (timolol)	↓ secretion of aqueous humor
Toxicity	Impotence, exacerbation of asthma, cardiovascular adverse effects (bradycardia, AV block, CHF), CNS adverse effects (sedation, sleep alterations)
Selectivity	Nonselective ($\beta_1 = \beta_2$): propranolol, timolol, pindolol, nadolol, and labetalol (also blocks α_1 receptors)
	β_1 selective ($\beta_1 > \beta_2$): metoprolol, atenolol, esmolol (short-acting) *A-M AME*

Synaptic. rely- (margin note)

Barbiturates

Phenobarbital, pentobarbital, thiopental, secobarbital

BarbiDURATe (↑ DURATion). Contraindicated in porphyria.

Mechanism	Facilitate GABA action by ↑ **duration** of Cl⁻ channel opening.
Clinical use	Anxiety, seizures, insomnia, induction of anesthesia (thiopental).
Toxicity	Dependence, additive CNS depression effects with alcohol, respiratory or cardiovascular depression, drug interactions owing to induction of liver microsomal enzymes (cyt. P450).

Benzodiazepines

Diazepam, lorazepam, triazolam, *short-acting*, temazepam, oxazepam, midazolam, chlordiazepoxide

FREnzodiazepines (↑ FREquency)

Mechanism	Facilitates GABA action by ↑ **frequency** of Cl⁻ channel opening. Most have long half-lives and active metabolites.
Clinical use	Anxiety, spasticity, status epilepticus (diazepam), detoxification (especially alcohol withdrawal–delirium tremens).
Toxicity	Dependence, additive CNS depression effects with alcohol. Less risk of respiratory depression and coma than with barbiturates.
	Treat overdose with flumazenil.

Short acting = **TOM** thumb = **T**riazolam, **O**xazepam, **M**idazolam

Antipsychotics (neuroleptics)

Thioridazine, haloperidol, chlorpromazine.

Evolution of EPS side effects:

Mechanism	Most antipsychotics block dopamine D_2 receptors *extrapyramidal effects.* (excess dopamine effects connected with schizophrenia).

4 h acute dystonia
4 d akinesia

Clinical use — Schizophrenia, psychosis.

4 wk akathisia

Toxicity — Extrapyramidal system side effects, sedation, endocrine side effects, and side effects arising from blocking muscarinic, α, and histamine receptors. Retinal deposits from thioridazine. Neuroleptic malignant syndrome: rigidity, autonomic instability, hyperpyrexia — *may also have poikilothermia!* (treat with dantrolene and dopamine agonists). Tardive dyskinesia: stereotypic oral–facial movements probably due to dopamine receptor sensitization; results of long-term antipsychotic use.

4 mo tardive dyskinesia (irreversible).

Clozapine

Mechanism — Atypical—blocks dopamine D_4 receptors.

Clinical use — 2nd line drug for treatment of schizophrenia, psychosis.

Toxicity — Less sedation, anticholinergic, and extrapyramidal symptoms than typical antipsychotics. Causes agranulocytosis requiring weekly WBC monitoring.

Lithium

Mechanism — Not established; possibly related to inhibition of phosphoinositol cascade.

Clinical use — Mood stabilizer for bipolar affective disorder, blocks relapse and acute manic events.

Toxicity — Tremor, hypothyroidism, polyuria (ADH antagonist causing nephrogenic DI), teratogenesis. Narrow therapeutic window requiring close monitoring of serum levels.

Tricyclic antidepressants

Imipramine, amitriptyline, desipramine, nortriptyline, clomipramine, doxepin

Mechanism — Block reuptake of norepinephrine and serotonin.

Clinical use — Endogenous depression, bedwetting (imipramine), obsessive–compulsive disorder (clomipramine).

Side effects — Sedation, α-blocking effects, atropine-like (anticholinergic) side effects (tachycardia, urinary retention). Tertiary TCAs (amitriptyline) have more anticholinergic effects than secondary TCAs (nortriptyline). Desipramine is the least sedating.

Toxicity — Convulsions, coma, respiratory depression, hyperpyrexia, arrhythmias. Confusion and hallucinations in elderly.

SSRIs

Fluoxetine, sertraline, paroxetine

Mechanism — Serotonin-specific reuptake inhibitors.

Clinical use — Endogenous depression.

Toxicity — Anxiety, insomnia, tremor, anorexia, nausea, and vomiting.

It normally takes 2–3 wk for antidepressants to have an effect.

"Serotonin syndrome" w/ toxicity of other agents.

Monoamine oxidase (MAO) inhibitors

Phenelzine, isocarboxazid, tranylcypromine

Mechanism	Nonselective MAO inhibition.
Clinical use	Atypical depressions (i.e., with psychotic or phobic features), anxiety, hypochondriasis.
Toxicity	Hypertensive crisis with tyramine ingestion (in many foods) and meperidine; CNS stimulation.

Selegiline

Mechanism	Selectively inhibits MAO-B, thereby increasing the availability of dopamine.
Clinical use	Adjunctive agent to L-dopa in treatment of Parkinson's disease.
Toxicity	May enhance adverse effects of L-dopa.

L-dopa

Mechanism	Increases level of dopamine in brain. Parkinsonism thought to be due to loss of dopaminergic neurons and excess cholinergic function. Unlike dopamine, L-dopa can cross blood–brain barrier and is converted by dopa decarboxylase in the CNS to dopamine.
Clinical use	Parkinsonism.
Toxicity	Arrhythmias from peripheral conversion to dopamine. Carbidopa, a peripheral decarboxylase inhibitor, is given with L-dopa in order to reduce the effective dose of L-dopa and to limit peripheral side effects. Dyskinesias also occur.

Opioid analgesics

Morphine, codeine, heroin, methadone, meperidine, dextromethorphan

Mechanism	Act as agonists at opioid receptors (mu - morphine, delta - enkephalin, kappa - dynorphin) to modulate synaptic transmission.
Clinical use	Pain, cough suppression, diarrhea, acute pulmonary edema, maintenance programs for addicts (methadone).
Toxicity	Addiction, respiratory depression, constipation, miosis, additive CNS depression with other drugs. Tolerance does not develop to miosis and constipation. Toxicity treated with naloxone (opioid receptor antagonist).

Sumatriptan

Mechanism	5-HT_{1d} agonist. Half-life < 2 hours. Very expensive.
Clinical use	Acute migraine, cluster headache attacks.
Toxicity	Chest discomfort, mild tingling (contraindicated in patients with CAD or Prinzmetal's angina).

Ondansetron

Mechanism	5-HT_3 antagonist. Powerful central-acting antiemetic.
Clinical use	Control vomiting postoperatively and in patients undergoing cancer chemotherapy.
Toxicity	Headache, diarrhea.

You will not vomit, so you can go **on danc**ing.

Epilepsy drugs

Indications	Drugs of choice
Grand mal (tonic-clonic)	Phenytoin, carbamazepine, phenobarbital
Status epilepticus	Diazepam, lorazepam, phenytoin, phenobarbital
Complex partial (temporal lobe)	Carbamazepine, phenytoin, primidone
Petit mal (absence)	Ethosuximide, valproic acid, clonazepam
Trigeminal neuralgia	Carbamazepine

Epilepsy drug toxicities

Benzodiazepines	Sedation, tolerance, dependence.
Carbamazepine	Diplopia, ataxia, induction of cyt. P450, blood dyscrasias.
Ethosuximide	Gastrointestinal distress, lethargy, headache.
Phenobarbital	Sedation, induction of cyt. P450, tolerance, dependence.
Phenytoin	Nystagmus, diplopia, ataxia, sedation, gingival hyperplasia, hirsutism, anemias, birth defects (teratogenic).
Valproic acid	Gastrointestinal distress, rare but fatal hepatotoxicity, neural tube defects in fetus.

Phenytoin

Mechanism	Use-dependent blockade of Na^+ channels.
Clinical use	Grand mal seizures.
Toxicity	Nystagmus, ataxia, diplopia, lethargy. Chronic use produces gingival hyperplasia in children, peripheral neuropathy, hirsutism, megaloblastic anemia, teratogenic.

Inhaled anesthetics

Halothane, enflurane, isoflurane, sevoflurane, methoxyflurane, nitrous oxide   *in blood*

Principle	The lower the solubility, the quicker the anesthetic induction and the quicker the recovery.
Effects	Myocardial depression, respiratory depression, nausea/emesis, ↑ cerebral blood flow.
Toxicity	Hepatotoxicity (halothane), nephrotoxicity (methoxyflurane), proconvulsant (enflurane).

note differences

Intravenous anesthetics

Barbiturates	Thiopental: high lipid solubility, rapid entry into brain. Used for induction of anesthesia and short surgical procedures. Effect terminated by redistribution from brain. ↓ cerebral blood flow.
Benzodiazepines	Midazolam: used adjunctively with gaseous anesthetics and narcotics. May cause severe postoperative respiratory depression and amnesia.
Arylcyclohexylamines	Ketamine: dissociative anesthetic. Cardiovascular stimulant. Causes disorientation, hallucination, and bad dreams. Increases cerebral blood flow.
Narcotic analgesics	Morphine, fentanyl: used with other CNS depressants during general anesthesia.
Other	Propofol: used for rapid anesthesia induction and short procedures. Less postop nausea than thiopental.

Local anesthetics

Esters: procaine, cocaine, tetracaine

Amides: lidocaine, bupivacaine (amides have 2 **i**'s in name).

Mechanism	Block Na$^+$ channels by binding to specific receptors on inner portion of channel. Tertiary amine local anesthetics penetrate membrane in uncharged form, then bind in charged form.
Principle	1. In infected (acidic) tissue, anesthetics are charged and cannot penetrate membrane effectively. Therefore more anesthetic is needed in these cases.
	2. Small-diameter fibers are blocked more easily than large-diameter ones. Myelinated fibers (nerves) are blocked more easily than unmyelinated fibers of the same diameter. Overall, the size factor predominates such that small, unmyelinated pain fibers (type C) and small, myelinated autonomic fibers (type B) are more easily blocked than very large myelinated motor nerves (type A, alpha).
	3. Given with vasoconstrictors (usually epinephrine) to enhance local action.
Clinical use	Minor surgical procedures, spinal anesthesia.
Toxicity	CNS excitation, severe cardiovascular toxicity (bupivacaine), hypertension and arrhythmias (cocaine).

Parkinson's disease drugs

Dopamine agonists	L-dopa/carbidopa, bromocriptine (an ergot alkaloid and partial dopamine agonist), amantadine (enhance dopamine release)
MAO inhibitors	Selegiline (selective MAO type B inhibitor)
Antimuscarinics	Benztropine (improve tremor and rigidity but have little effect on bradykinesia)

Antihypertensive drugs

Drug	Adverse effects	
Diuretics		
Hydrochlorothiazide	Hypokalemia, slight hyperlipidemia, hyperuricemia, lassitude	
Sympathoplegics		
Clonidine	Dry mouth, sedation, severe rebound hypertension	
Methyldopa	Sedation, positive Coombs' test	
Ganglionic blockers	Severe orthostatic hypotension, blurred vision, constipation, sexual dysfunction	
Reserpine	Sedation, depression, nasal stuffiness, diarrhea	
Guanethidine	Orthostatic and exercise hypotension, sexual dysfunction, diarrhea	
Prazosin	First-dose orthostatic hypotension, dizziness, headache	You'll be sur**praz**ed when you first stand up.
β blockers	Impotence, asthma, CV effects (bradycardia, CHF, AV block), CNS effects (sedation, sleep alterations)	
Vasodilators *zrknze*		
(Hydralazine)	Nausea, headache, lupus-like syndrome, tachycardia, angina, salt retention	
Minoxidil	Hirsutism, pericardial effusion, tachycardia, angina, salt retention	
Nifedipine, verapamil	Dizziness, flushing, constipation (verapamil), nausea	
Nitroprusside	Cyanide toxicity (releases CN) — *do Not take orally.*	
ACE inhibitors		
Captopril	**C**ough, **A**ngioedema, **P**roteinuria, **T**aste changes, hyp**O**tension, **P**regnancy problems (fetal renal damage), **R**ash, **I**ncreased renin, **L**ower AT II	**CAPTOPRIL**

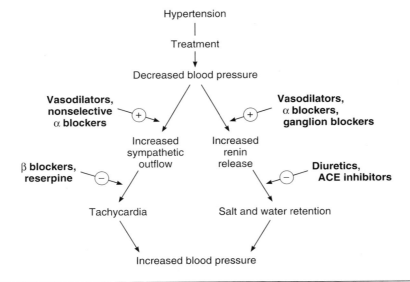

Anti-anginal therapy

Goal: Reduction of myocardial O_2 consumption (MVO_2) by decreasing one or more of the determinants of MVO_2: end diastolic volume, blood pressure, heart rate, contractility, ejection time.

Component	Nitrates	β blockers	Nitrates + β blockers
End diastolic volume	↓	↑	No effect or ↓
Blood pressure	↓	↓ / ↑ varies	↓
Contractility	↑ (reflex response)	↓	Little/no effect
Heart rate	↑ (reflex response)	↓	↓
Ejection time	↓	↑	Little/no effect
MVO_2	↓	↓	↓↓

Calcium channel blockers
—**N**ifedipine is similar to **n**itrates in effect
—Verapamil is similar to β blockers in effect

Calcium channel blockers

Nifedipine, verapamil, diltiazem

Mechanism

Block voltage-dependent calcium channels of cardiac and smooth muscle and thereby reduce muscle contractility.
    Vascular smooth muscle: nifedipine > diltiazem > verapamil.
    Heart: verapamil > diltiazem > nifedipine.

Clinical use

Hypertension, angina, arrhythmias.

Toxicity

Cardiac depression, peripheral edema, flushing, dizziness, and constipation.

ACE inhibitors

Captopril, enalapril, lisinopril

Mechanism

Inhibit angiotensin-converting enzyme, reducing levels of angiotensin II and preventing inactivation of bradykinin, a potent vasodilator. Renin release is ↑ due to loss of feedback inhibition.

Clinical use

Hypertension, congestive heart failure, diabetic renal disease.

Toxicity

Cough, angioedema, proteinuria, taste changes, hypotension, fetal renal damage, rash.

Losartan is a new angiotensin II receptor antagonist. It is **not** an ACE inhibitor and does not cause cough.

Furosemide

Mechanism	Sulfonamide loop diuretic. Inhibits cotransport system (Na^+, K^+, 2 Cl^-) of thick ascending limb of loop of Henle. Abolishes hypertonicity of medulla, preventing concentration of urine. Increases Ca^{2+} excretion.
Clinical use	Edematous states (CHF, cirrhosis, nephrotic syndrome, pulmonary edema), HTN, hypercalcemia.
Toxicity	**O**totoxicity, **H**ypokalemia, **D**ehydration, **A**llergy (sulfa), **N**ephritis (interstitial), **G**out.

Loops **L**ose calcium.

Toxicity: **OH DANG!**

Ethacrynic acid

Mechanism	Phenoxyacetic acid derivative (NOT a sulfonamide). Essentially same action as furosemide.
Clinical use	Diuresis in patients allergic to sulfa drugs.
Toxicity	Similar to furosemide except no hyperuricemia, no sulfa allergies.

Hydrochlorothiazide

Mechanism	Thiazide diuretic. Inhibits NaCl reabsorption in early distal tubule, reducing diluting capacity of the nephron. Decreases Ca^{2+} excretion.
Clinical use	Hypertension, congestive heart failure, calcium stone formation, nephrogenic diabetes insipidus.
Toxicity	Hypokalemic metabolic alkalosis, hyponatremia, hyper**G**lycemia, hyper**L**ipidemia, hyper**U**ricemia, and hyper**C**alcemia. "Hyper**GLUC**." Sulfa allergy.

Acetazolamide

Mechanism	Carbonic anhydrase inhibitor. Causes self-limited $NaHCO_3$ diuresis and reduction in total-body HCO_3^- stores. Acts at the proximal convoluted tubule.
Clinical use	Glaucoma, urinary alkalinization, metabolic alkalosis.
Toxicity	Hyperchloremic metabolic acidosis, neuropathy, NH_3 toxicity, sulfa allergy.

ACIDazolamide causes **acid**osis.

K+-sparing diuretics

Spironolactone, **T**riamterene, **A**miloride

The K+ **STA**ys.

Mechanism	Spironolactone is a competitive aldosterone antagonist in the cortical collecting tubule. Triamterene and amiloride act at same site by blocking Na^+ channels in the CCT.
Clinical use	Hyperaldosteronism, K^+ depletion.
Toxicity	Hyperkalemia, endocrine effects (gynecomastia, anti-androgen effects).

Diuretics: electrolyte changes

Urine NaCl	↑ (all diuretics: carbonic anhydrase inhibitors, loop diuretics, thiazides, K^+-sparing diuretics)
Urine K^+	↑ (all except K^+-sparing diuretics)
Blood pH	↓ (acidosis): carbonic anhydrase inhibitors, K^+-sparing diuretics ↑ (alkalosis): Loop diuretics, thiazides

Diuretics: site of action

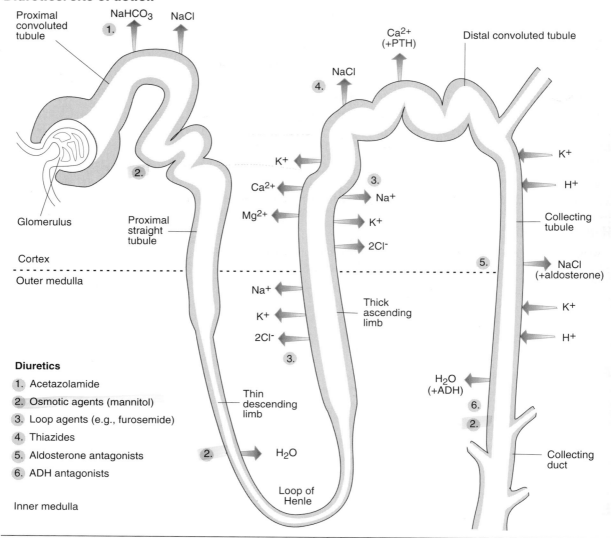

Diuretics

1. Acetazolamide
2. Osmotic agents (mannitol)
3. Loop agents (e.g., furosemide)
4. Thiazides
5. Aldosterone antagonists
6. ADH antagonists

Nitroglycerin, isosorbide dinitrate

Mechanism	Vasodilate by releasing nitric oxide in smooth muscle, causing increase in cGMP and smooth muscle relaxation. Dilate veins >> arteries.
Clinical use	Angina, pulmonary edema. Also used as an aphrodisiac and erection-enhancer.
Toxicity	Tachycardia, hypotension, headache, "Monday disease" in industrial exposure (alternating development of tolerance during the work week and loss of tolerance over the weekend for the vasodilating action, resulting in tachycardia, dizziness, and headache every Monday).

Cardiac glycosides	Digoxin: 75% bioavailability, 20–40% protein bound, $T_{1/2} = 40$ hr, urinary excretion
	Digitoxin: > 95% bioavailability, 70% protein bound, $T_{1/2} = 168$ hrs, biliary excretion (enterohepatic recycling; no need to ↓ dose of digitoxin in renal failure)
Mechanism	Inhibits the Na^+-K^+-ATPase of cell membrane, causing ↑ intracellular Na^+. Na^+-Ca^{2+} antiport does not function as efficiently, causing ↑ intracellular Ca^{2+}; leads to positive inotropy.
Clinical use	CHF, atrial fibrillation.
Toxicity	Nausea, vomiting, diarrhea. Yellow vision. Gynecomastia. Arrhythmia:
	Early ECG changes—↑ PR interval, bradycardia, flattened T wave.
	Later ECG changes—inverted T wave, ST depression, decreased QT.
	Late ECG changes—↑ automaticity, delayed after depolarizations, bigeminy, PVCs, fibrillation.
	Toxicities of digoxin are increased by renal failure (↓ excretion), hydrochlorothiazide (via hypokalemia), and quinidine (↓ digoxin clearance; displaces digoxin from tissue binding sites).
Antidote	Slowly normalize K^+, lidocaine, cardiac pacer, anti-dig Fab fragments.
	Digibind

Antiarrhythmics—Na⁺ channel blockers

Local anesthetics. Slow or block (↓) conduction (especially in depolarized cells) and ↓ abnormal pacemakers that are Na⁺ channel dependent. Are state dependent (i.e., selectively depress tissue that is frequently depolarized, e.g., fast tachycardia).

Class IA

Quinidine, amiodarone, procainamide, disopyramide. *[handwritten: class III]*

↑ AP duration, ↑ effective refractory period (ERP), ↑ QT interval. Affect both atrial and ventricular arrhythmias.

Toxicity: quinidine (cinchonism: headache, tinnitus; thrombocytopenia, torsade de pointes); procainamide (reversible SLE-like syndrome).

Class IB

Lidocaine, mexiletine, tocainide.

↓ AP duration. Affect ischemic or depolarized Purkinje and ventricular tissue. Useful in acute ventricular arrhythmias (especially post-MI) and in digitalis-induced arrhythmias.

Toxicity: local anesthetic toxicity (CNS stimulation/depression, cardiovascular depression).

Class IC

Flecainide, encainide, propafenone.

No effect on AP duration. Useful in V-tachs that progress to VF, and in intractable SVT. Are usually used only as last resort in refractory tachyarrhythmias because of toxicities.

Toxicity: proarrhythmic, CNS stimulation.

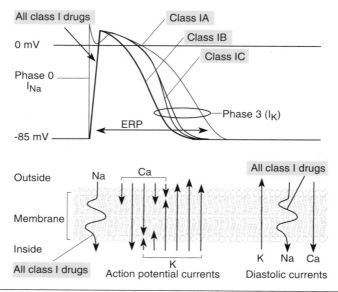

Antiarrhythmics—β blockers

Propranolol, esmolol, metoprolol, timolol.

↓ cAMP, ↓ Ca²⁺ currents. Suppress abnormal pacemakers. AV node particularly sensitive: ↑ PR interval. Esmolol very short-acting. *[handwritten: β₁-selective.]*

Toxicity: impotence, exacerbation of asthma, CV effects (bradycardia, AV block, CHF), CNS effects (sedation, sleep alterations).

Antiarrhythmics—K⁺ channel blockers

Sotalol, ibutilide, bretylium, amiodarone.

↑ AP duration, ↑ ERP. Bretylium is rarely used, and only in post-MI arrhythmias (e.g., recurrent VF).

Toxicity: sotalol (torsade de pointes, excessive β block); ibutilide (torsade) Bretylium (new arrhythmias, hypotension).

Amiodarone (pulmonary fibrosis, corneal deposits, skin deposits resulting in photodermatitis, neurologic effects, constipation, CV effects [bradycardia, heart block, CHF], hypo/hyperthyroidism).

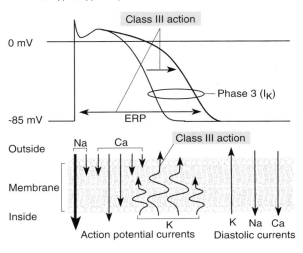

Antiarrhythmics—Ca²⁺ channel blockers

Verapamil, diltiazem, bepridil.

↓ conduction velocity, ↑ ERP, ↑ PR interval. Used in prevention of nodal arrhythmias (e.g., SVT).

Toxicity: constipation, flushing, edema, nausea, CV effects (CHF, AV block, sinus node depression).

Bepridil (torsade de pointes).

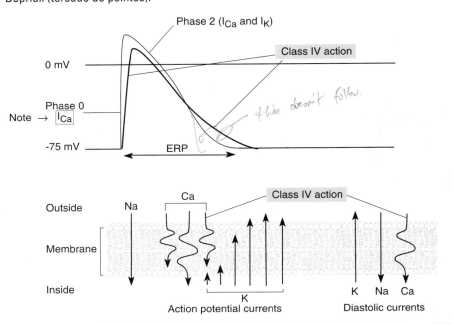

Antiarrhythmics—Miscellaneous

Adenosine	Drug of choice in abolishing AV nodal arrhythmias.
K^+	Depresses ectopic pacemakers, especially in digoxin toxicity.
Mg^+	Effective in torsade de pointes and digoxin toxicity.

Lipid-lowering agents

Drug	Effect on LDL "bad cholesterol"	Effect on HDL "good cholesterol"	Effect on triglycerides	Side effects/problems
Bile acid resins (cholestyramine, colestipol)	↓↓	No effect	Slight ↑	Patients hate it—tastes bad and causes GI discomfort
HMG-CoA reductase inhibitors (lovastatin, provastatin, simvastatin, atorvastatin)	↓↓↓	↑	↓	$, common Reversible ↑ LFTs *(hepatotoxicity)* Muscle damage
Niacin	↓↓	↑↑	↓	Red, flushed face which is ↓ by aspirin or long-term use
Lipoprotein lipase stimulators (gemfibrozil)	↓	↑	↓↓↓	Muscle damage, ↑ LFTs *(hepatotoxicity)*
Probucol	↓	↓	No effect	↓ HDL

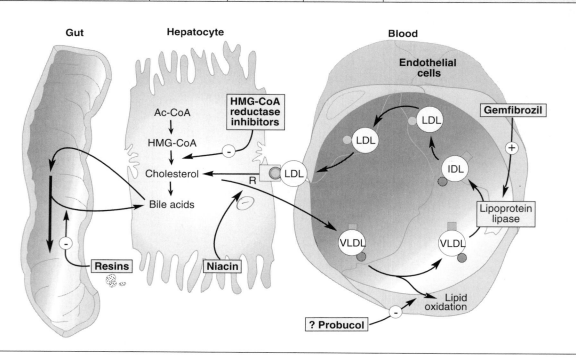

Cyclophosphamide

Mechanism	Alkylating agent; covalently x-links (interstrand) DNA at guanine N-7. Requires bioactivation by liver.
Clinical use	Non-Hodgkin's lymphoma, breast and ovarian carcinomas.
Toxicity	Myelosuppression, hemorrhagic cystitis.

Nitrosureas

	Carmustine, lomustine, semustine, streptozocin
Mechanism	Alkylates DNA. Requires bioactivation. Crosses blood–brain barrier → CNS.
Clinical use	Brain tumors (including glioblastoma multiforme). Streptozocin used for insulinomas.
Toxicity	CNS toxicity (dizziness, ataxia).

Cisplatin

Pt.

Mechanism	Acts like an alkylating agent. X-links via hydrolysis of Cl⁻ groups and reaction with platinum.	Platinum (cisplatin) is a precious metal. Testicles are also precious (testicular cancer).
Clinical use	Testicular and lung carcinomas.	
Toxicity	Nephrotoxicity and acoustic nerve damage.	

Doxorubicin (adriamycin)

Mechanism	Anthracycline antibiotic; noncovalently intercalates in DNA to decrease replication and transcription and generate free radicals.
Clinical use	Part of the **ABVD** combo regimen for myelomas, sarcomas, and lymphomas.
Toxicity	Cardiotoxicity; also myelosuppression and marked alopecia.

Methotrexate

Mechanism	S-phase specific antimetabolite. Folic acid analog that inhibits dihydrofolate reductase, resulting in decreased dTMP and therefore decreased DNA and protein synthesis.
Clinical use	Leukemias, sarcomas, abortion, ectopic pregnancy, rheumatoid arthritis. *osteosarcoma*
Toxicity	Myelosuppression, which is reversible with leucovorin "rescue."

5-fluorouracil (5-FU)

Mechanism	S-phase-specific antimetabolite. Pyrimidine analog bioactivated to 5FdUMP, which covalently complexes folic acid. This complex inhibits thymidylate synthase, resulting in decreased dTMP and same effects as methotrexate.
Clinical use	Colon cancer, basal cell carcinoma (topical).
Toxicity	Myelosuppression, which is NOT reversible with leucovorin; photosensitivity.

Vincristine and vinblastine

Mechanism	M-phase-specific alkaloid from the periwinkle plant (*Vinca rosea*) that binds to tubulin and blocks polymerization of microtubules so that mitotic spindle can't form. *like colchisine, griseof*
Clinical use	Part of **MOPP** (**O**ncovin) combo regimen for lymphoma, Wilms' tumor, choriocarcinoma.
Toxicity	Vincristine—neurotoxicity (areflexia, peripheral neuritis), paralytic ileus. *alopecia* Vin**Blast**ine **Blast**s **B**one marrow (suppression).

Taxol *Paclitaxel*

Mechanism	M-phase-specific agent obtained from yew tree that binds to tubulin and hyperstabilizes polymerized microtubules so that mitotic spindle can't break down (anaphase cannot occur).
Clinical use	Ovarian and breast carcinomas.
Toxicity	Myelosuppression and cardiotoxicity.

Etoposide

Mechanism	G_2-phase-specific podophyllotoxin that inhibits topoisomerase II so that double-strand breaks remain in DNA following replication, with subsequent DNA degradation.
Clinical use	Oat cell carcinoma of the lung and prostate, testicular carcinoma.
Toxicity	Myelosuppression, GI irritation, alopecia.

Prednisone

Mechanism	May trigger apoptosis. May even work on non-dividing cells.
Clinical use	Most commonly used glucocorticoid in cancer chemotherapy. Used in CLL, Hodgkin's lymphomas, rheumatoid arthritis, asthma.
Toxicity	Cushing-like symptoms; immunosuppression.

Tamoxifen

Mechanism	Estrogen receptor mixed agonist/antagonist that blocks the binding of estrogen to ER+ cells.
Clinical use	Breast cancer.
Toxicity	May increase the risk of endometrial carcinoma via partial agonist effects; "hot flashes."

Specific antidotes

Toxin	Antidote/treatment
1. Acetaminophen	1. N-acetylcysteine
2. Anticholinesterases, organophosphates	2. Atropine, pralidoxime
3. Iron salts	3. Deferoxamine, Ca²⁺ EDTA
4. Methanol, ethylene glycol (antifreeze)	4. Ethanol, dialysis
5. Lead	5. CaEDTA, dimercaprol,(BAL) succimer
6. Arsenic, mercury, gold	6. Dimercaprol (BAL), succimer
7. Copper, arsenic, lead, gold	7. Penicillamine
8. Antimuscarinic, anticholinergic agents	8. Physostigmine salicylate
9. Cyanide	9. Nitrite, hydroxocobalamin amyl nitrite / Sodium nitrite
10. Salicylates	10. Alkalinize urine, dialysis
11. Heparin	11. Protamine
12. Methemoglobinemia	12. Methylene blue
13. Opioids	13. Naloxone
14. Benzodiazepines	14. Flumazenil
15. Tricyclic antidepressant arrhythmias	15. NaHCO₃ (nonspecific)
16. Warfarin	16. Vitamin K⁺, FFP
17. Carbon monoxide	17. 100% O₂, hyperbaric O₂
18. Digitalis	18. Stop dig, normalize K⁺, lidocaine, anti-dig Fab fragments Digibind.
19. β blockers	19. Glucagon
20. t-PA, streptokinase	20. Aminocaproic acid
21. PCP	21. Nasogastric suction NH₄Cl

Lead poisoning

Lead **L**ines on gingivae and on epiphyses of long bones on x-ray.

Encephalopathy and **E**rythrocyte basophilic stippling.

Abdominal colic and sideroblastic **A**nemia.

Drops: wrist and foot drop. **D**imercaprol and EDTA as first line of treatment.

LEAD

High risk in houses with chipped paint.

Urine pH and drug elimination

Weak acids (phenobarbital, methotrexate, aspirin) ⇒ alkalinize urine to increase clearance

Weak bases (amphetamines) ⇒ acidify urine to increase clearance.

Drug reactions

Drug reaction	Causal agent
1. Pulmonary fibrosis	1. Bleomycin, amiodarone
2. Hepatitis	2. Isoniazid (INH)
3. Focal to massive hepatic necrosis	3. Halothane, valproic acid
4. Anaphylaxis	4. Penicillin
5. SLE-like syndrome	5. Hydralazine, procainamide, INH
6. Blood dyscrasias	6. Ibuprofen, quinidine, methyldopa, chemotherapy, *clozapine*
7. Hemolysis in G6PD-deficient patients	7. Sulfonamides, INH, aspirin, ibuprofen, primaquine
8. Breast and endometrial cancer	8. Estrogens
9. Thrombotic complications	9. Oral contraceptives (e.g., estrogens and progestins)
10. Adrenocortical insufficiency	10. Glucocorticoids (HPA axis suppression)
11. Photosensitivity reactions	11. Tetracyclines, amiodarone, sulfonamides *Quinolones*
12. Gynecomastia	12. Cimetidine, ketoconazole, spironolactone
13. Induce ($\uparrow$) P450 system	13. Barbiturates, phenytoin, carbamazapine, rifampin
14. Inhibit ($\downarrow$) P450 system	14. Cimetidine, ketoconazole, itraconazole
15. Tubulointerstitial nephritis	15. Sulfonamides
16. Teratogenic effects	16. Ethanol, lithium, warfarin, valproic acid, thalidomide, isotretinoin, androgens
17. Carcinogenic effects	17. Aflatoxin, vinyl chloride, coal tar, polycyclic aromatic hydrocarbons (in tobacco smoke)
18. Mutagenic effects	18. Aflatoxin, cancer chemotherapeutic drugs
19. Hot flashes	19. Tamoxifen
20. Cutaneous flushing	20. Niacin, Ca^{2+} channel blockers, adenosine, vancomycin *red man syndrome*
21. Cardiac toxicity	21. Doxorubicin (Adriamycin)
22. Agranulocytosis	22. Clozapine, carbamazepine
23. Stevens-Johnson syndrome	23. Ethosuximide, sulfonamides
24. Cinchonism	24. Quinidine, quinine
25. Tendonitis, tendon rupture	25. Fluoroquinolones
26. Disulfiram-like reaction	26. Metronidazole, certain cephalosporins, procarbazine

Alcohol toxicity

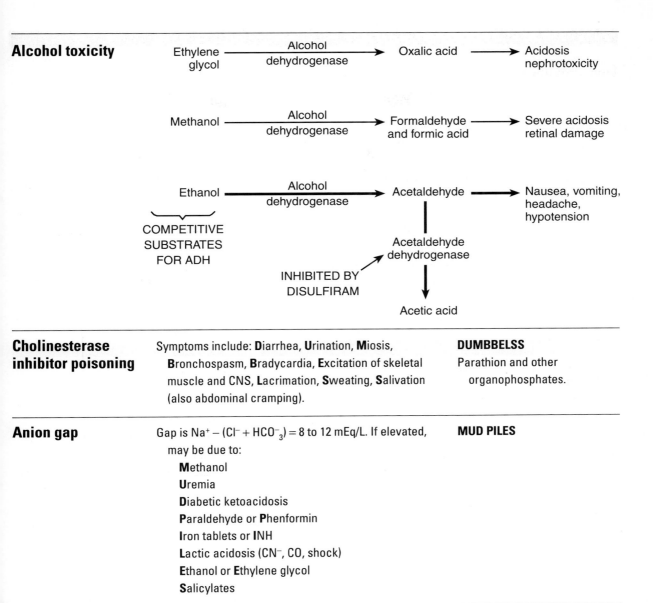

Ethylene glycol →(Alcohol dehydrogenase)→ Oxalic acid → Acidosis nephrotoxicity

Methanol →(Alcohol dehydrogenase)→ Formaldehyde and formic acid → Severe acidosis retinal damage

Ethanol →(Alcohol dehydrogenase)→ Acetaldehyde → Nausea, vomiting, headache, hypotension

COMPETITIVE SUBSTRATES FOR ADH

Acetaldehyde dehydrogenase

INHIBITED BY DISULFIRAM

Acetic acid

Cholinesterase inhibitor poisoning

Symptoms include: **D**iarrhea, **U**rination, **M**iosis, **B**ronchospasm, **B**radycardia, **E**xcitation of skeletal muscle and CNS, **L**acrimation, **S**weating, **S**alivation (also abdominal cramping).

DUMBBELSS
Parathion and other organophosphates.

Anion gap

Gap is $Na^+ - (Cl^- + HCO_3^-) = 8$ to 12 mEq/L. If elevated, may be due to:

Methanol
Uremia
Diabetic ketoacidosis
Paraldehyde or **P**henformin
Iron tablets or **I**NH
Lactic acidosis (CN^-, CO, shock)
Ethanol or **E**thylene glycol
Salicylates

MUD PILES

Coma treatment

ER treatment	Airway (protect)	ABCD (in that order).
	Breathing (assist)	
	Circulation (assist)	
	Dextrose (and thiamine, naloxone IV)	

Rule out	Infections (lumbar puncture)	IT'S COMA
	Trauma (bleeding, consider CT scan)	
	Seizure	
	Carbon monoxide (give O_2)	
	Overdose (pills)/Opioids (give naloxone)	
	Metabolic (hypo/hyperthermia, hypo/hyperglycemia, thiamine deficiency)	
	Alcohol (check serum osmolality)	

H$_2$ blockers
Cimetidine, ranitidine, famotidine, nizatidine

Mechanism	Reversible block of histamine H_2 receptors.
Clinical use	Peptic ulcer, gastritis, esophageal reflux, Zollinger-Ellison syndrome.
Toxicity	Cimetidine is a potent inhibitor of hepatic drug-metabolizing enzymes; it also has an antiandrogenic effect. Other H_2 blockers are relatively free of these effects.

Omeprazole, lansoprazole

Mechanism	Irreversibly inhibits H^+/K^+ ATPase in stomach cells.
Clinical use	Peptic ulcer, gastritis, esophageal reflux, Zollinger-Ellison syndrome.

Sucralfate

Mechanism	Aluminum sucrose sulfate polymerizes in the acid environment of the stomach and selectively binds necrotic peptic ulcer tissue. Acts as a barrier to acid, pepsin, and bile. Sucralfate cannot work in the presence of antacids or H_2 blockers (requires acidic environment to polymerize).
Clinical use	Peptic ulcer disease.
Toxicity	GI upset (minor and rare).

Misoprostol

Mechanism	A PGE_1 analog. Increases production and secretion of gastric mucous barrier.
Clinical use	Prevention of NSAID-induced peptic ulcers.
Toxicity	Diarrhea. Contraindicated in women of childbearing potential (abortifacient).

Heparin

Mechanism	Catalyzes the activation of antithrombin III. Short half-life. Check the aPTT.
Clinical use	Immediate anticoagulation, used in pregnancy (does not cross placenta).
Toxicity	Bleeding, thrombocytopenia, drug-drug interactions. Use protamine sulfate for rapid reversal of heparinization (positively charged molecule that acts by binding negatively charged heparin).

Antacid overuse

Can affect absorption, bioavailability, or urinary excretion of other drugs by altering gastric and urinary pH or by delaying gastric emptying.

Overuse can also cause the following problems:

1. Aluminum hydroxide: constipation and hypophosphatemia
2. Magnesium hydroxide: diarrhea
3. Calcium carbonate: hypercalcemia

All can cause hypokalemia.

AluMINIMUM amount of feces

Mg = Must go to the bathroom

Warfarin (Coumadin)

Mechanism	Interferes with normal synthesis and γ-carboxylation of vit. K-dependent clotting factors II, VII, IX, and X via vitamin K antagonism. Long half-life. Check PT.	**WARFARE** kills babies (teratogenic). **WEPT: W**arfarin affects the **E**xtrinsic pathway and prolongs the **PT**.
Clinical use	Chronic anticoagulation. Not used in pregnant women (because warfarin, unlike heparin, can cross the placenta).	
Toxicity	Bleeding, teratogen, drug–drug interactions.	

Heparin vs. warfarin

	Heparin	Warfarin
Structure	Large anionic polymer, acidic	Small lipid-soluble molecule
Route of administration	Parenteral (IV, SC)	Oral
Site of action	Blood	Liver
Onset of action	Rapid (seconds)	Slow, limited by half-lives of normal clotting factors
Mechanism of action	Activates antithrombin III	Impairs the synthesis of vit. K–dependent clotting factors II, VII, IX, and X (vit. K antagonist)
Duration of action	Acute (hours)	Chronic (weeks or months)
Inhibits coagulation *in vitro*	Yes	No
Treatment of acute overdose	Protamine sulfate	IV vit. K and fresh frozen plasma
Monitoring	aPTT (intrinsic pathway)	PT (extrinsic pathway)

Thrombolytics

	Streptokinase, urokinase, tPA (alteplase), APSAC (anistreplase)	tPA: human protein produced in bacteria.
Mechanism	Directly or indirectly aid conversion of plasminogen to plasmin. Note that tPA specifically converts fibrin-bound plasminogen to plasmin.	Urokinase: from cultured human kidney cells.
Clinical use	Early myocardial infarction.	Streptokinase: from bacteria.
Toxicity	Bleeding.	APSAC: prodrug made of streptokinase plus recombinant human plasminogen.

Neuromuscular blocking drugs

Depolarizing	Succinylcholine
	Reversal of blockade: Phase I—No antidote. Block potentiated by cholinesterase inhibitors. Phase II—Cholinesterase inhibitors (e.g., neostigmine).
Nondepolarizing	Tubocurarine, atracurium, mivacurium, pancuronium, vecuronium.
	Reversal of blockade: Neostigmine, edrophonium, and other cholinesterase inhibitors.

Dantrolene

Used in the treatment of malignant hyperthermia, which is caused by the concomitant use of halothane and succinylcholine. Also used to treat neuroleptic malignant syndrome (a toxicity of antipsychotic drugs).

Mechanism: Prevents the release of Ca^{2+} from the sarcoplasmic reticulum of skeletal muscle.

Ritodrine, terbutaline

β_2 agonists used to delay labor by inhibiting uterine smooth muscle contraction.

Asthma drugs

Nonspecific β agonists	Isoproterenol: relaxes bronchial smooth muscle (β_2). Adverse effect is tachycardia (β_1).
β_2 agonists	Albuterol: relaxes bronchial smooth muscle (β_2). } *status asthmaticus.* Adverse effects are tremor and arrhythmia.
Methylxanthines	Theophylline: mechanism unclear—may cause bronchodilation by inhibiting phosphodiesterase, enzyme involved in degrading cAMP (controversial).
Muscarinic antagonists	Ipratropium: competitive block of muscarinic receptors preventing bronchoconstriction.
Cromolyn	Prevents release of mediators from mast cells. Effective only for the prophylaxis of asthma. Not effective during an active asthmatic attack. Toxicity is very rare.
Corticosteroids	Block synthesis of leukotrienes from arachidonic acid by phospholipase A_2. Are drugs of choice in a patient with status asthmaticus (in combination with albuterol).
Antileukotrienes	Zileuton: blocks synthesis by lipoxygenase; zafirlukast: blocks leukotriene receptors.

— omits new mechanism of A₁

Treatment strategies in asthma

Aspirin

Mechanism	Acetylates and irreversibly inhibits cyclooxygenase (both COX I and COX II) to prevent conversion of arachidonic acid to prostaglandins.
Clinical use	Antipyretic, analgesic, anti-inflammatory, antiplatelet drug.
Toxicity	Gastric ulceration, bleeding, hyperventilation, Reye's syndrome, tinnitus, and dizziness (CN VIII).

Ticlopidine

Mechanism	Inhibits platelet aggregation by irreversibly inhibiting the ADP pathway involved in the binding of fibrinogen.
Clinical use	Decreases the incidence of thrombotic stroke or recurrence.
Toxicity	Neutropenia; reserved for those who cannot tolerate aspirin.

NSAIDs

	Ibuprofen, naproxen, indomethacin
Mechanism	Reversibly inhibit cyclooxygenase (both COX I and COX II). Block prostaglandin synthesis.
Clinical use	Antipyretic, analgesic, anti-inflammatory. Indomethacin is used to close a patent ductus arteriosus. Misoprostol, a PGE$_1$ analog, keeps it open.
Toxicity	Renal damage, aplastic anemia. *dann (phenylbutazone)*

Acetaminophen

Mechanism	Weak prostaglandin inhibitor.
Clinical use	Antipyretic, analgesic, but lacking anti-inflammatory properties.
Toxicity	Overdose produces hepatic necrosis; acetaminophen metabolite depletes glutathione and forms toxic tissue adducts in liver.

Glucocorticoids

	Hydrocortisone, prednisone, triamcinolone, dexamethasone
Mechanism	Decrease the production of leukotrienes and prostaglandins by inhibiting phospholipase A$_2$ and expression of COX II.
Clinical use	Addison's disease, inflammation, and immune suppression.
Toxicity	Iatrogenic Cushing's syndrome: buffalo hump, moon facies, truncal obesity, muscle wasting, thin skin, easy bruisability, osteoporosis, adrenal cortical atrophy, peptic ulcers.

Arachidonic acid products

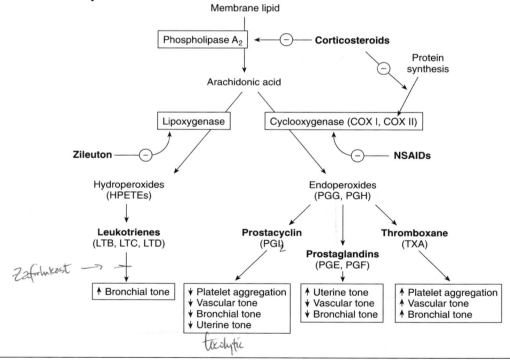

Gout drugs

Colchicine	Acute gout. Depolymerizes microtubules, impairing leukocyte chemotaxis and degranulation. GI side effects, especially if given orally. *N/V/D*
Probenecid	Chronic gout. Inhibits reabsorption of uric acid (also inhibits secretion of penicillin). *Effects many antimetab*
Allopurinol	Chronic gout. Inhibits xanthine oxidase, decreasing conversion of xanthine to uric acid.

Sulfonylureas

Tolbutamide, chlorpropamide, glyburide, glipizide.

Mechanism	Oral hypoglycemic agents used to stimulate release of endogenous insulin. Close K^+ channels in β cell membrane: cell depolarizes, insulin release triggered. Inactive in insulin-dependent diabetics; requires some residual islet cell function.
Clinical use	Non-insulin-dependent (type II) diabetes mellitus.
Toxicity	Hypoglycemia (more common with 2nd generation drugs: glyburide, glipizide). Disulfiram-like effects (not seen with 2nd generation drugs: glyburide, glipizide).

Leuprolide *fertility drug*

Mechanism	GnRH analog with agonist properties when used in pulsatile fashion and antagonist properties when used in continuous fashion.	When used in continuous fashion, it causes a transient initial burst of LH and FSH.
Clinical use	Infertility (pulsatile), prostate cancer (continuous: use with flutamide).	
Toxicity	Antiandrogen, nausea, vomiting. *Multiple for this*	

Propylthiouracil

Mechanism	Inhibits organification and coupling of thyroid hormone synthesis. Also decreases peripheral conversion of T_4 to T_3.
Clinical use	Hyperthyroidism. *Methimazole*
Toxicity	Skin rash, agranulocytosis (rare).

Vasoactive peptides

Angiotensin II (AII)	↑IP_3, DAG. Constricts arterioles, ↑ aldosterone secretion. Also acts at the level of the hypothalamus to increase thirst.
Atrial natriuretic peptide (ANP)	↑ cGMP. Dilates vessels, ↓ aldosterone secretion and effects, ↑ GFR.

Antiandrogens

Finasteride	A 5α-reductase inhibitor (↓ conversion of testosterone to dihydrotestosterone). Useful in BPH. *Extremely teratogenic.*
Flutamide	A nonsteroidal competitive inhibitor of androgens at the testosterone receptor. Used in prostate carcinoma.
Leuprolide	A GnRH analog. Used in prostate cancer, infertility, and uterine fibroids.
Ketoconazole, spironolactone	Inhibit steroid synthesis, used in the treatment of polycystic ovarian syndrome to prevent hirsutism.

Open-angle glaucoma drugs

	Mechanism	Side effects
α agonists		
Epinephrine	↑ outflow of aqueous humor	Mydriasis, stinging. Do not use in closed-angle glaucoma.
β blockers		
Timolol, betaxolol, carteolol	↓ aqueous humor secretion	No pupillary or vision changes.
Cholinomimetics		
Pilocarpine, carbachol, physostigmine, echothiophate	Ciliary muscle contraction, opening of trabecular meshwork; ↑ outflow of aqueous humor	Miosis, cyclospasm.
Diuretics		
Acetazolamide, dorzolamide	↓ aqueous humor secretion due to ↓ HCO_3^- (via inhibition of carbonic anhydrase)	No pupillary or vision changes.

Immunosuppressive agents: sites of action

Agent	Site
Prednisone	2, 6
Cyclosporine	2, 3
Azathioprine	2
Methotrexate	2
Dactinomycin	2, 3
Cyclophosphamide	2
Antilymphocytic globulin and monoclonal anti-T-cell antibodies	1, 2, 3
Rh₃(D) immune globulin	1

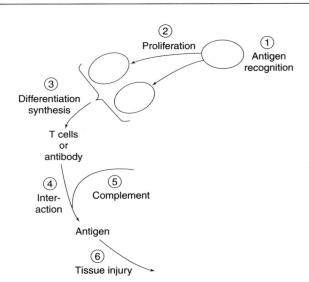

Cyclosporine

Mechanism	Binds to cyclophilins (peptidyl proline *cis-trans* isomerase), blocking the differentiation and activation of T cells mainly by inhibiting the production of IL-2 and its receptor.
Clinical use	Suppresses organ rejection after transplantation; selected autoimmune disorders.
Toxicity	Predisposes patients to viral infections and lymphoma; nephrotoxic (preventable with mannitol diuresis).

Azathioprine

Mechanism	Antimetabolite derivative of 6-mercaptopurine that interferes with the metabolism and synthesis of nucleic acid. Toxic to proliferating lymphocytes after Ag exposure.
Clinical use	Kidney transplantation, autoimmune disorders (including glomerulonephritis and hemolytic anemia).

Drug development and testing

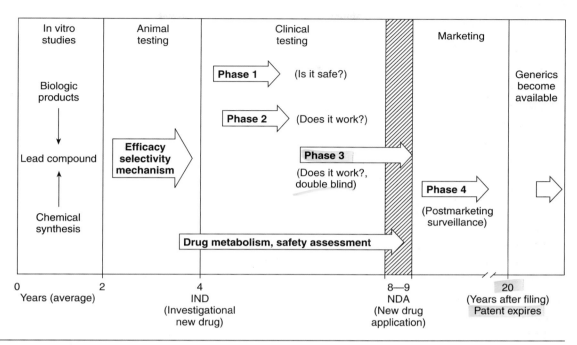

	In vitro studies	Animal testing	Clinical testing	Marketing	

Biologic products

Phase 1 → (Is it safe?)

Phase 2 (Does it work?)

Phase 3 (Does it work?, double blind)

Phase 4 (Postmarketing surveillance)

Generics become available

Lead compound

Efficacy selectivity mechanism

Chemical synthesis

Drug metabolism, safety assessment

0	2	4	8—9	20
Years (average)		IND (Investigational new drug)	NDA (New drug application)	(Years after filing) Patent expires

Pharmacokinetics

Volume of distribution (V_d)	Relates the amount of drug in the body to the plasma concentration. V_d of plasma protein-bound drugs can be altered by liver and kidney disease.

$$V_d = \frac{\text{amount of drug in the body}}{\text{plasma drug concentration}}$$

Clearance (CL)	Relates the rate of elimination to the plasma concentration.

$$CL = \frac{\text{rate of elimination of drug}}{\text{plasma drug concentration}}$$

Half-life ($t_{1/2}$)	The time required to change the amount of drug in the body by one-half during elimination (or during a constant infusion). A drug infused at a constant rate reaches 94% of steady state after four $t_{1/2}$.

$$t_{1/2} = \frac{0.7 \times V_d}{CL}$$

# of half-lives	1	2	3	3.3
Concentration	50%	75%	87.5%	90%

Dosage calculations

Loading dose = $C_p \times V_d/F$

Maintenance dose = $C_p \times CL/F$

where C_p = target plasma concentration and F = bioavailability

In patients with impaired renal or hepatic function, the loading dose remains unchanged, although the maintenance dose is decreased.

Elimination of drugs

Zero-order elimination	Rate of elimination is constant regardless of C_p. C_p decreases linearly with time. Examples of drugs: ethanol, phenytoin and aspirin (at high or toxic concentrations).
First-order elimination	Rate of elimination is proportional to the drug concentration. Drug's concentration in plasma (C_p) decreases exponentially with time.

Phase I versus phase II metabolism

Phase I (reduction, oxidation, hydrolysis) yields slightly polar, water-soluble metabolites (often still active).

Phase II (acetylation, glucuronidation, sulfation) yields very polar inactive metabolites (renally excreted).

Phase I: P450

Phase II: conjugation. Geriatric patients lose phase I first.

Drug name

Ending	Category	Example
-ane	Inhalational general anesthetic	Halothane
-azepam	Benzodiazepine	Diazepam
-azine	Phenothiazine (neuroleptic, antiemetic)	Chlorpromazine
-azole	Antifungal	Ketoconazole
-barbital	Barbiturate	Phenobarbital
-caine	Local anesthetic	Lidocaine
-cainide	Class IC antiarrhythmic	Flecainide
-cillin	Penicillin	Methicillin
-cycline	Antibiotic, protein synthesis inhibitor	Tetracycline
-ipramine	Tricyclic antidepressant	Imipramine
-ol	Beta agonist	Isoproterenol
-olol	Beta antagonist	Propranolol
-operidol	Butyrophenone (neuroleptic)	Haloperidol
-oxin	Cardiac glycoside (inotropic agent)	Digoxin
-phylline	Methylxanthine	Theophylline
-pril	ACE inhibitor	Captopril
-relin	GnRH	Buserelin
-rinone	Antiarrhythmic (inotropic agent)	Amrinone
-terol	β_2 agonist	Albuterol
-tidine	H2 antagonist	Cimetidine
-triptyline	Tricyclic antidepressant	Amitriptyline
-tropin	Pituitary hormone	Somatotropin
-zosin	Alpha antagonist	Prazosin

These abstracted case vignettes are designed to demonstrate the thought processes necessary to answer multistep clinical reasoning questions.

- 28-year-old chemist presents with MPTP overdose → what neurotransmitter is depleted? → dopamine.
- Woman taking tetracycline exhibits photosensitivity → what are the clinical manifestations? → rash on sun-exposed regions of the body.
- Young girl with congenital valve disease is given penicillin prophylactically → develops bacterial endocarditis → what do you give now? → beta-lactamase-resistant penicillin.
- Patient presents with hyperthyroidism but low levels of C peptide → what is the diagnosis? → surreptitious insulin. *C?*
- African-American man who goes to Africa develops anemia after taking prophylactic medicine → what is the enzyme deficiency? → glucose-6-phosphate dehydrogenase.
- 27-year-old female with a history of psychiatric illness now has urinary retention → due to neuroleptic → what do you treat it with? → bethanechol. *(urecholl)*
- Farmer presents with dyspnea, salivation, miosis, diarrhea, cramping, and blurry vision → what caused this? → insecticide poisoning → what is the mechanism of action? → inhibition of acetylcholinesterase.
- 55-year-old man undergoing treatment for BPH has decreased levels of testosterone and DHT as well as gynecomastia and edema → what is the drug? → estrogen (DES).
- Prevention of recurrence of transient ischemic attacks in a 70-year-old man can best be achieved with what drug? *antiplatelet agents   sulfinpyrazon, dypyridamole*
- Patient with recent kidney transplant is on cyclosporine for immunosuppression. Requires antifungal agent for candidiasis → what drug would result in cyclosporine toxicity? → ketoconazole.
- Young man with history of schizophrenia on neuroleptics presents with tremor and rigidity → what is the reason for side effects? *anti-DA → tardive dyskinesia (EPS)*
- Man on several medications, including antidepressants and antihypertensives, has mydriasis and becomes constipated → what is the cause of his symptoms? → tricyclic antidepressant.
- Patient presents with renal insufficiency → what alterations in doses of digoxin and digitoxin, respectively? → decreased, same.
- 55-year-old postmenopausal woman is on tamoxifen therapy → what is she at increased risk of acquiring? → endometrial carcinoma.
- Woman on MAO inhibitor has hypertensive crisis after a meal → what did she ingest? → tyramine (wine or cheese).
- 17-year-old overdoses on acetaminophen → massive hepatic necrosis → what is the appearance of the liver years later?
- After taking clindamycin, patient develops toxic megacolon and diarrhea → gross photograph of large intestine → what is the mechanism of diarrhea? *pseudomembranous*

Mechanism, clinical use, and toxicity of:

1. Motion sickness drugs (e.g., scopolamine).
2. Antipsychotics (neuroleptics), low and high potency.
3. Opiates (e.g., analgesic, antidiarrheal, antitussive), receptor types, agonists, mixed agonist-antagonists.
4. New pharmacologic agents (erythropoietin, RU486, acarbose, losartan).
5. Myasthenia gravis drugs.
6. Hormonal treatments of cancer (e.g., leuprolide, flumetanide, aminoglutethimide).
7. New oral hypoglycemic agents (acarbose, metformin).
8. Stool softeners (e.g., psyllium, methylcellulose).
9. Angiotensin II receptor blockers (e.g., losartan).
10. Dermatologic agents (e.g., corticosteroids, retinoids, antifungal agents).

Know about:

1. Complications of empiric antibiotic use (e.g., resistance, fungal infection, psuedomembranous colitis).
2. Secondary effects of common drugs (e.g., heparin and osteoporosis, thiazides and hyperlipidemia).
3. Common drugs that block/increase hepatic drug metabolism (e.g., cimetidine, ethanol, phenobarbital, phenytoin, rifampin).
4. Fundamental pharmacodynamics (e.g., partial agonists, physiologic antagonists, efficacy).
5. Drug efficacy and potency as demonstrated on dose-response curves.
6. Pharmacogenetics: drugs whose metabolism is affected by inheritance (e.g., procainamide).
7. Anesthesia: physical properties of gaseous agents (MAC, blood:gas partition coefficient, rate of induction), different IV agents, toxicities (e.g., malignant hyperthermia).
8. Drugs that cause lupus-like syndromes (e.g., procainamide, hydralazine).
9. Treatment of anemia (e.g., erythropoietin, B_{12}, folate, testosterone, iron supplements).
10. Prevention/treatment of cerebrovascular disease (e.g., aspirin, thrombolytics).
11. Treatment of rheumatoid arthritis.
12. Bacteriostatic versus bactericidal antibiotics.
13. Vaccines: indications, potential side effects.
14. Chemotherapeutic agents: risk of possible secondary cancer.

Physiology

The portion of the examination dealing with physiology is broad and concept oriented and does not lend itself as well to fact-based review. Diagrams are often the best study aids from which to learn, especially given the increasing number of questions requiring the interpretation of diagrams. It may be useful to get help (tutor or group study) if you are weak with basic concepts, as they may be hard to learn from books. Learn to work with basic physiologic relationships in a variety of ways (e.g., Fick equation, clearance equations). You are seldom asked to perform complex calculations. Hormones are the focus of many questions. Learn their sites of production and action as well as their regulatory mechanisms.

A large portion of the physiology tested on the USMLE Step 1 is now clinically relevant and involves understanding physiologic changes associated with pathologic processes (e.g., changes in pulmonary function testing with chronic obstructive pulmonary disease). Thus, it is worthwhile to review the physiologic changes that are found with common pathologies of the major organ systems (e.g., heart, lungs, kidneys, and gastrointestinal tract).

Cardiovascular
Respiratory
Gastrointestinal
Renal
Endocrine
High-Yield Topics

Myocardial action potential

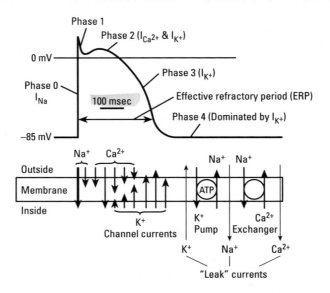

[handwritten note: Notes: no fast acting Na⁺ channels.]

Occurs in atrial and ventricular myocytes and Purkinje fibers.

Phase 0 = Rapid upstroke—voltage-gated Na⁺ channels open.

Phase 1 = Partial repolarization—inactivation of voltage-gated Na⁺ channels. Voltage-gated K⁺ channels begin to open.

Phase 2 = Plateau—Ca²⁺ influx from voltage-gated Ca²⁺ channels balances K⁺ efflux. Ca²⁺ influx triggers myocyte contraction.

Phase 3 = Rapid repolarization—massive K⁺ efflux due to opening of voltage-gated slow K⁺ channels and closure of voltage-gated Ca²⁺ channels.

Phase 4 = Resting potential—high K⁺ permeability through K1 channels.

Cardiac output

Cardiac output = (stroke volume) (heart rate)

Fick principle:

$$CO = \frac{\text{rate of O}_2 \text{ consumption}}{\text{arterial O}_2 \text{ content} - \text{venous O}_2 \text{ content}}$$

$$\begin{pmatrix}\text{Mean arterial} \\ \text{pressure}\end{pmatrix} = \begin{pmatrix}\text{cardiac} \\ \text{output}\end{pmatrix} \times \begin{pmatrix}\text{total peripheral} \\ \text{resistance}\end{pmatrix}$$

During exercise, CO increases primarily as a result of increased HR. If HR is too high, CO drops (e.g., ventricular tachycardia).

[handwritten note: MAP = diastolic + ⅓ PP = C.O × TPR]

Cardiac output variables	Stroke volume affected by **C**ontractility, **A**fterload, and **P**reload.	SV **CAP**

Contractility (and SV) increased with:

Stroke volume increases in anxiety, exercise, and pregnancy.

1. Catecholamines ($\uparrow$ activity of Ca^{2+} pump in sarcoplasmic reticulum).
2. $\uparrow$ extracellular calcium
3. $\downarrow$ extracellular sodium
4. Digitalis ($\uparrow$ intracellular Na^+, resulting in $\uparrow Ca^{2+}$)

Pulse pressure is proportional to stroke volume.

Contractility (and SV) decreased with:

A failing heart has decreased stroke volume.

1. β_1 blockade
2. Heart failure
3. Acidosis
4. Hypoxia/hypercapnea

Myocardial O_2 demand is $\uparrow$ by:
$\uparrow$ afterload ($\propto$ diastolic BP)
$\uparrow$ contractility
$\uparrow$ heart rate
$\uparrow$ heart size ($\uparrow$ wall tension)

Pacemaker action potential

Occurs in the SA and AV nodes. Key differences from the myocardial action potential include:

Phase 0 = slow upstroke—opening of voltage-gated Ca^{2+} channels. These cells lack fast voltage-gated Na^+ channels. Results in a slow conduction velocity that is utilized by the AV node to prolong transmission from the atria to ventricles.

Phase 4 = diastolic depolarization—membrane potential spontaneously depolarizes as K^+ conductance decreases and as Na^+ conductance increases. Accounts for automaticity of SA and AV nodes. Rate of diastolic depolarization in the SA node determines heart rate. Acetylcholine decreases and catecholamines increase the slope of this phase, thus decreasing or increasing heart rate, respectively.

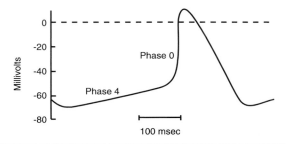

Preload and afterload

Preload = ventricular end-diastolic volume.
Afterload = peripheral resistance.
Venous dilators (e.g., nitroglycerin) decrease preload.
Vasodilators (e.g., hydralazine) decrease afterload.
$\uparrow$ SV when $\uparrow$ preload or $\downarrow$ afterload.

Preload increases with exercise (slightly), extra blood (overtransfusion), and excitement (sympathetics). Preload pumps up the heart.

Starling curve

Energy of contraction is proportional to initial length of cardiac muscle fiber (preload).

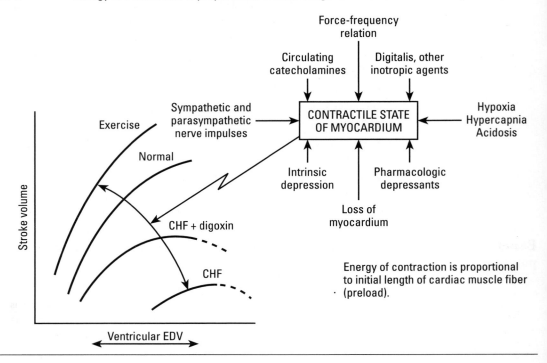

Energy of contraction is proportional to initial length of cardiac muscle fiber (preload).

Ejection fraction

$$\text{Ejection fraction} = \frac{\text{end-diastolic volume} - \text{end-systolic volume}}{\text{end-diastolic volume}}$$

Ejection fraction is an index of ventricular function.

Ejection fraction is normally 60–80%.

Resistance, pressure, flow

$$\text{Resistance} = \frac{\text{driving pressure } (\Delta P)}{\text{flow}} \propto \frac{\text{viscosity } (\eta) \times \text{length}}{(\text{radius})^4}$$

$$\frac{8\eta l}{r^4}$$

Viscosity increases in:

1. Polycythemia
2. Hyperproteinemic states (e.g., multiple myeloma)
3. Hereditary spherocytosis

Viscosity depends mostly on hematocrit.

Capillary fluid exchange

Four forces known as Starling forces determine fluid movement through capillary membranes:

P_c = capillary pressure—tends to move fluid out of capillary

P_i = interstitial fluid pressure—tends to move fluid into capillary

π_c = plasma colloid osmotic pressure—tends to cause osmosis of fluid into capillary

π_i = interstitial fluid colloid osmotic pressure—tends to cause osmosis of fluid out of capillary

K_f = filtration constant   ←permeability.

Thus net filtration pressure = $P_{net} = [(P_c - P_i) - (\pi_c - \pi_i)]$

Net fluid flow = $(P_{net})(K_f)$

Edema: excess fluid outflow into interstitium that is commonly caused by:

1. ↑ capillary pressure (↑ P_c; heart failure)
2. ↓ plasma proteins (↓ π_c; nephrotic syndrome)
3. ↑ capillary permeability (↑ K_f; toxins, infections, burns)
4. ↑ interstitial fluid colloid osmotic pressure (↑ π_i; lymphatic blockage)

Blood

Normal adult blood composition. Note that serum = plasma – clotting factors (e.g., fibrinogen).

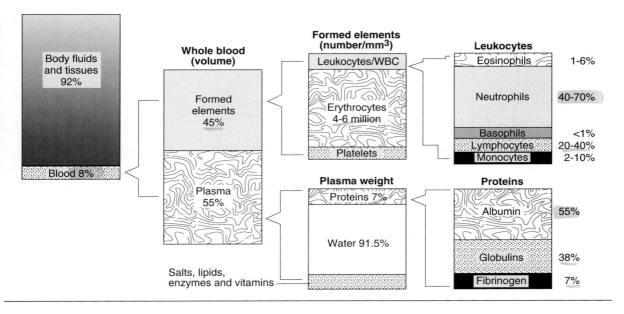

Cardiac cycle

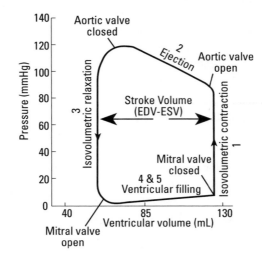

Phases:

1. Isovolumetric contraction—period between mitral valve closure and aortic valve opening; period of highest oxygen consumption
2. Systolic ejection—period between aortic valve opening and closing
3. Isovolumetric relaxation—period between aortic valve closing and mitral valve opening
4. Rapid filling—period just after mitral valve opening
5. Slow filling—period just before mitral valve closure

S1—mitral and tricuspid valve closure.
S2—aortic and pulmonary valve closure.
S3—end of rapid ventricular filling.
S4—high atrial pressure/stiff ventricle.

S3 is associated with dilated CHF.
S4 is associated with hypertrophic CHF ("atrial kick").

a wave: atrial contraction.
c wave: RV contraction (tricuspid valve bulging into atrium).
v wave: ↑ atrial pressure due to filling against closed tricuspid valve.

A: **A**trial contraction.
C: RV **C**ontraction/**C**arotid pulse.
V: **V**enous return against closed **V**alve.
Jugular venous distention is seen in right-heart failure.

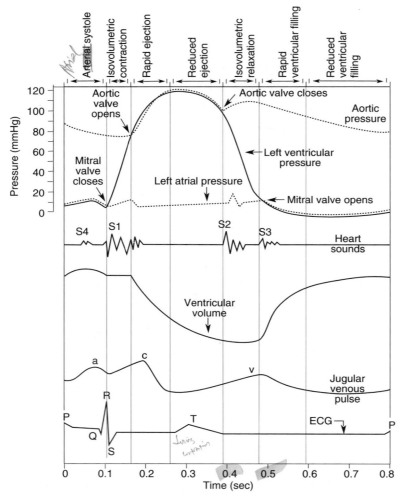

Electrocardiogram

P wave—atrial depolarization.

P-R interval—conduction delay through AV node.

QRS complex—ventricular depolarization.

Q-T interval—mechanical contraction of the ventricles.

T wave—ventricular repolarization.

Atrial repolarization is masked by QRS complex.

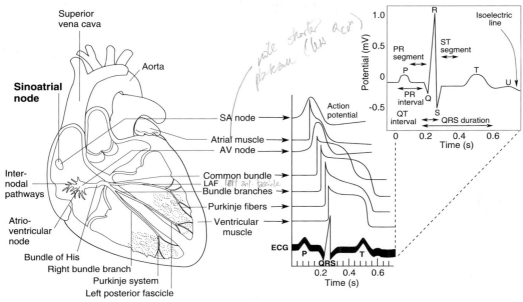

SA node "pacemaker" inherent dominance with slow phase of upstroke
AV node - 100-msec delay-atrial ventricular delay

AV block (heart block)

First degree	Prolonged P-R interval.
Second degree	Type I (Wenckebach) shows a gradual prolongation of P-R interval until a P wave is not conducted ("dropped").
	Type II (Mobitz) shows sporadic/episodic "dropped" P wave.
Third degree	Complete AV block with P waves completely dissociated from QRS complexes.

Arterial baroreceptors

Receptors:

1. Aortic arch transmits via vagus nerve to medulla (responds only to ↑ blood pressure).
2. Carotid sinus transmits via glossopharyngeal nerve to medulla.

Hypotension: ↓ arterial pressure → ↓ stretch → ↓ afferent baroreceptor firing → ↑ sympathetic firing and ↓ efferent parasympathetic stimulation → vasoconstriction, ↑ HR, ↑ contractility, ↑ BP. Important in the response to severe hemorrhage.

Carotid massage: increased pressure on carotid artery → ↑ stretch . . . ↓ HR.

Chemoreceptors

Peripheral

1. Aortic bodies: respond to decreased P_{O_2}, increased P_{CO_2} of blood
2. Carotid bodies: respond to decreased P_{O_2}, increased P_{CO_2}, and decreased pH of blood

Central

Respond to changes in pH and P_{CO_2} of brain interstitial fluid, which in turn are influenced by arterial CO_2. Do not directly respond to P_{O_2}. Responsible for Cushing reaction to increased intracranial pressure: hypertension and bradycardia.

Electrophysiologic differences between skeletal and cardiac muscle

In contrast to skeletal muscle:

1. Cardiac muscle action potential has a plateau, which is due to Ca^{2+} influx
2. Cardiac nodal cells spontaneously depolarize, resulting in automaticity
3. Cardiac myocytes are electrically coupled to each other by gap junctions
4. Cardiac muscle contraction is dependent on extracellular calcium, which stimulates calcium release from the cardiac muscle sarcoplasmic reticulum (calcium-induced calcium release)

Fetal circulation

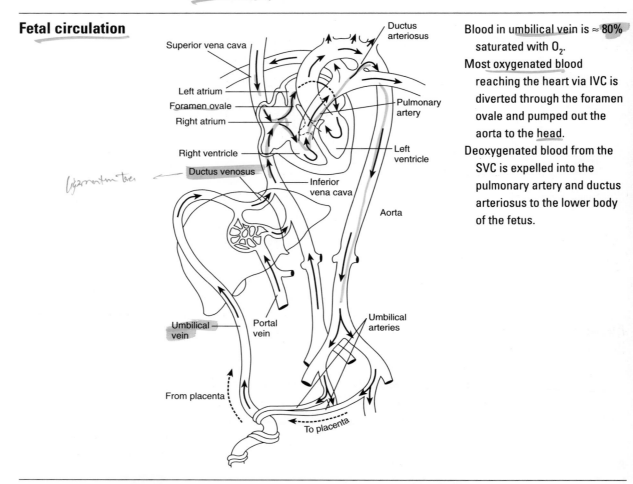

Superior vena cava
Left atrium
Foramen ovale
Right atrium
Right ventricle
Ductus venosus
Inferior vena cava
Umbilical vein
Portal vein
From placenta
Ductus arteriosus
Pulmonary artery
Left ventricle
Aorta
Umbilical arteries
To placenta

Blood in umbilical vein is ≈ 80% saturated with O_2.

Most oxygenated blood reaching the heart via IVC is diverted through the foramen ovale and pumped out the aorta to the head.

Deoxygenated blood from the SVC is expelled into the pulmonary artery and ductus arteriosus to the lower body of the fetus.

Control of mean arterial pressure

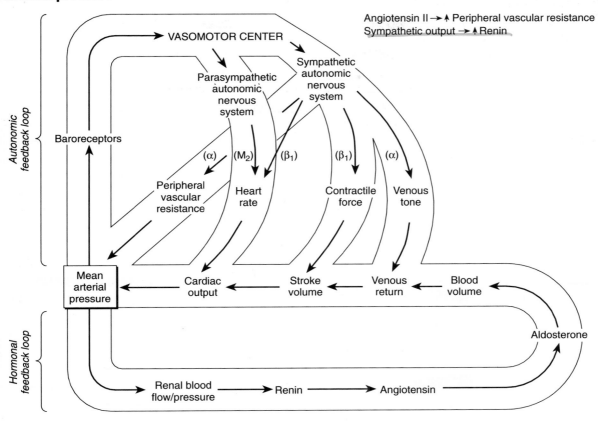

Angiotensin II → ↑ Peripheral vascular resistance
Sympathetic output → ↑ Renin

Circulation through organs

Liver: largest share of systemic cardiac output.
Kidney: highest blood flow per gram of tissue.
Heart: large arteriovenous O_2 difference. Increased O_2 demand is met by increased coronary blood flow, not by increased extraction of O_2.

Normal pressures

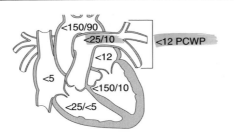

PCWP = pulmonary capillary wedge pressure (in mmHg).

Autoregulation

Sites: brain, kidney, heart
Mechanism: in the brain and heart, blood flow is altered to meet demands of tissue via local metabolites (e.g., nitric oxide, adenosine). In the kidney, local metabolites maintain renal artery pressure constant.

The pulmonary vasculature is unique in that hypoxia causes vasoconstriction (in other organs hypoxia causes vasodilation).

Response to high altitude

1. Acute increase in ventilation by 65%
2. Chronic increase in ventilation
3. ↑ erythropoietin → ↑ hematocrit and hemoglobin (chronic hypoxia)
4. Increased 2,3-DPG (binds to Hb so that Hb releases more O_2)
5. Cellular changes (increased mitochondria)
6. Increased renal excretion of bicarbonate to compensate for the respiratory alkalosis
7. Chronic hypoxic pulmonary vasoconstriction results in right ventricular hypertrophy

Important lung products

1. Surfactant: ↓ alveolar surface tension, ↑ compliance
2. Prostaglandins
3. Histamine
4. Angiotensin converting enzyme (ACE): AI → AII; inactivates bradykinin (ACE inhibitors ↑ bradykinin and cause cough, angioedema)
5. Kallikrein: activates bradykinin

Surfactant: dipalmitoyl phosphatidylcholine (lecithin) deficient in neonatal RDS.

Particle size and lung entrapment

Diameter of:
> 10 μm: Trapped by nostril hairs or settle on mucous membranes in nose and pharynx.
2–10 μm: Fall on bronchial walls → reflex bronchial constriction and coughing. Also removed by cilia.
0.5–2 μm: Reach alveoli → ingested by macrophages.
< 0.5 μm: Remain suspended in air.

Kartagener's syndrome = immotile cilia due to a dynein arm defect. Bacteria and particles not pushed out (also sperm cilia inactive). Results in bronchiectasis, situs inversus, sterility, and recurrent sinusitis.

Lung volumes

1. Residual volume (RV) = air in lung at maximal expiration
2. Expiratory reserve volume (ERV) = air that can still be breathed out after normal expiration
3. Tidal volume (TV) = air that moves into lung with each inspiration
4. Inspiratory reserve volume (IRV) = air in excess of tidal volume that moves into lung on maximum inspiration
5. Vital capacity (VC) = TV + IRV + ERV
6. Functional reserve capacity (FRC) = RV + ERV
7. Inspiratory capacity (IC) = IRV + TV
8. Total lung capacity = TLC = IRV + TV + ERV + RV

Vital capacity is everything but the residual volume.

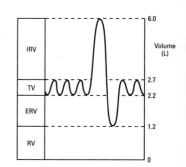

Pulmonary flow volume loops

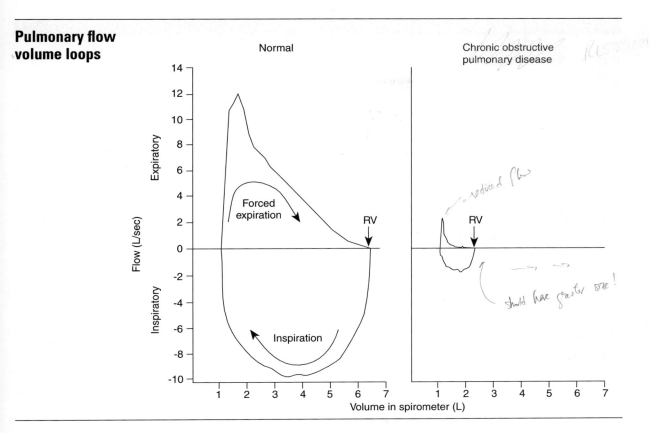

Normal

Chronic obstructive pulmonary disease

RESTRICTIVE

Flow (L/sec)

Expiratory

Inspiratory

Forced expiration

RV

Inspiration

reduced flow

RV

should have greater size!

Volume in spirometer (L)

Oxygen dissociation curve

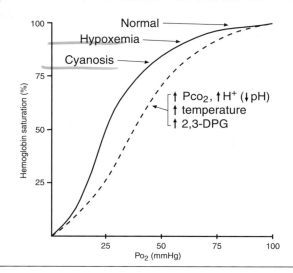

When curve shifts to the right, ↓ affinity of hemoglobin for O_2 (facilitates unloading of O_2 to tissue).

An ↑ in all factors (except pH) causes a shift of the curve to the right.

Acid-base physiology

	pH	Pco_2	$[HCO_3^-]$	Cause	Compensatory response
Metabolic acidosis	↓	↓	↓	Diabetic ketoacidosis; diarrhea	Hyperventilation
Respiratory acidosis	↓	↑	↑	COPD; airway obstruction	Renal $[HCO_3^-]$ reabsorption
Respiratory alkalosis	↑	↓	↓	High altitude; hyperventilation	Renal $[HCO_3^-]$ secretion
Metabolic alkalosis	↑	↑	↑	Vomiting	Hypoventilation

Pulmonary circulation

Normally a low-resistance, high-compliance system keeps pulmonary blood pressure low. With increased Pco_2 (e.g., exercise), a low pulmonary blood pressure is maintained by vasodilating normally closed apical capillaries, thereby lowering pulmonary resistance.

A consequence of pulmonary hypertension is cor pulmonale and subsequent right ventricular failure (jugular venous distension, edema, hepatomegaly).

V/Q mismatch

Ideally, ventilation is matched to perfusion (i.e., V/Q = 1) in order for adequate oxygenation to occur efficiently.

Lung zones:
Apex of the lung: V/Q = 3 (wasted ventilation)
Base of the lung: V/Q = 0.6 (wasted perfusion)
Both ventilation and perfusion are greater at the base of the lung than at the apex of the lung.

With exercise (increased cardiac output), there is vasodilation of apical capillaries, resulting in a V/Q ratio that approaches unity.
Certain organisms that thrive in high O_2 (e.g., TB) flourish in the apex.
V/Q → ∞ = dead space
V/Q → 0 = shunt

CO₂ transport

Carbon dioxide is transported from tissues to the lungs in 3 forms:

1. Bicarbonate (65%)

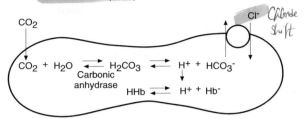

2. Bound to hemoglobin as carbaminohemoglobin (25%)   *carboxy Hb: CO₂ binding*
3. Dissolved CO_2 (10%)

In lungs, oxygenation of Hb promotes dissociation of CO_2 from Hb.

In peripheral tissue, $\uparrow H^+$ shifts curve to right, unloading O_2 (Bohr effect).

Obstructive lung disease

Obstruction of air flow, resulting in air trapping in the lungs. Pulmonary function tests: decreased FEV_1/FVC ratio (hallmark).

Types:

1. Chronic bronchitis ("blue bloater")—productive cough for greater than 3 consecutive months in two or more years. Hypertrophy of mucus-secreting glands in the bronchioles (Reid index > 50%). Leading cause is smoking. Findings: wheezing, crackles, cyanosis.
2. Emphysema ("pink puffer")—enlargement of air spaces and decreased recoil resulting from destruction of alveolar walls. Caused by smoking (centroacinar emphysema) and α_1-antitrypsin deficiency (panacinar emphysema and liver cirrhosis) $\rightarrow \uparrow$ elastase activity. Findings: dyspnea, $\downarrow$ breath sounds, tachycardia, $\downarrow$ I/E ratio.
3. Asthma—Bronchial hyperresponsiveness causes reversible bronchoconstriction. Can be triggered by viral URIs, allergens, and stress. Findings: cough, wheezing, dyspnea, tachypnea, hypoxemia, $\downarrow$ I/E ratio, pulsus paradoxus.
4. Bronchiectasis—chronic necrotizing infection of bronchi $\rightarrow$ dilated airways, purulent sputum, recurrent infections, hemoptysis. Associated with bronchial obstruction, cystic fibrosis, poor ciliary motility.

Restrictive lung disease	Decreased lung volumes (decreased VC and TLC).

Types:
1. Poor breathing mechanics (extrapulmonary):
   a. Poor muscular effort: polio, myasthenia gravis.
   b. Poor apparatus: scoliosis, *obesity.*
2. Poor lung expansion (pulmonary):
   a. Defective alveolar filling: pneumonia, ARDS, pulmonary edema.
   b. Interstitial fibrosis: causes increased recoil, thereby limiting alveolar expansion. PFTs reveal an FEV_1/FVC ratio > 90%. Complications include cor pulmonale. Can be seen in diffuse interstitial pulmonary fibrosis and bleomycin toxicity. Symptoms include gradual progressive dyspnea and cough. *Amiodarone*

PHYSIOLOGY—GASTROINTESTINAL

Pancreatic exocrine secretion	Secretory acini synthesize and secrete zymogens, stimulated by acetylcholine and CCK. Pancreatic ducts secrete mucus and alkaline fluid when stimulated by secretin.

Pancreatic enzymes	Alpha-amylase: starch digestion, secreted in active form.

Lipase, phospholipase A, colipase: fat digestion.

Proteases (trypsin, chymotrypsin, elastase, carboxypeptidases): protein digestion, secreted as proenzymes. *aminopeptidases*

self-activate?

Trypsinogen is converted to active enzyme trypsin by enteropeptidase, a duodenal brush-border enzyme. Trypsin then activates the other proenzymes and can also activate trypsinogen (positive-feedback loop).

Pancreatic insufficiency is seen in CF and other conditions. Patients present with malabsorption, steatorrhea (greasy, malodorous stool). Limit fat intake, monitor for signs of fat-soluble vitamin (A, D, E, K) deficiency.

Stimulation of pancreatic functions

Secretin	Stimulates flow of bicarbonate-containing fluid.
Cholecystokinin	Major stimulus for zymogen release, weak stimulus for alkaline fluid flow.
Acetylcholine	Major stimulus for zymogen release, poor stimulus for bicarbonate secretion.
Somatostatin	Inhibits the release of gastrin and secretin.

Bilirubin

Product of heme metabolism, actively taken up by hepatocytes. Conjugated version is water soluble. Jaundice (yellow skin, scleral icterus) results from elevated bilirubin levels.

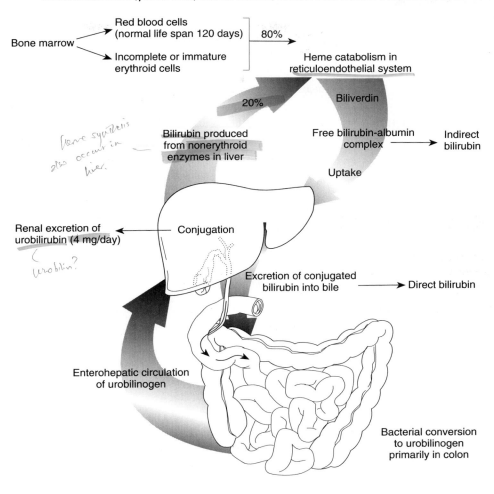

Bone marrow → Red blood cells (normal life span 120 days)
Bone marrow → Incomplete or immature erythroid cells

80% → Heme catabolism in reticuloendothelial system

20%

Biliverdin

Bilirubin produced from nonerythroid enzymes in liver

heme synthesis also occurs in liver.

Free bilirubin-albumin complex → Indirect bilirubin

Uptake

Renal excretion of urobilirubin (4 mg/day)

urobilin?

Conjugation

Excretion of conjugated bilirubin into bile → Direct bilirubin

Enterohepatic circulation of urobilinogen

Bacterial conversion to urobilinogen primarily in colon

Bile

Secreted by hepatocytes. Composed of bile salts, phospholipids, cholesterol, bilirubin, water (97%). Bile salts are amphipathic (hydrophilic and hydrophobic domains) and solubilize lipids in micelles for absorption.

Carbohydrate digestion

Only monosaccharides are absorbed.

Salivary amylase

Starts digestion, hydrolyzes alpha-1,4 linkages to give maltose, maltotriose, and α-limit dextrins.

Pancreatic amylase

Highest concentration in duodenal lumen, hydrolyzes starch to oligosaccharides, maltose, and maltotriose.

Oligosaccharide hydrolases

At brush border of intestine, is the rate-limiting step in carbohydrate digestion, produces monosaccharides (glucose, galactose, fructose).

Salivary secretion

Source	Parotid, submandibular, and sublingual glands.
Function	1. Alpha-amylase (ptyalin) begins starch digestion
	2. Neutralizes oral bacterial acids, maintains dental health
	3. Mucins (glycoproteins) lubricate food

Salivary secretion is stimulated by both sympathetic and parasympathetic activity.

[handwritten: mucous]
[handwritten: serous]

Glucose absorption

Occurs at duodenum and proximal jejunum.

Absorbed across cell membrane by sodium-glucose-coupled transporter.

Stomach secretions

	Purpose	Source
Mucus	Lubricant, protects surface from H^+	Mucous cell — *[handwritten: goblet cell]*
Intrinsic factor	Vitamin B_{12} absorption (in small intestine)	Parietal cell
H^+	Kills bacteria, breaks down food, converts pepsinogen	Parietal cell
Pepsinogen	Broken down to pepsin (a protease)	Chief cell
Gastrin	Stimulates acid secretion	G cell — *[handwritten: []'d in antrum]*

GI secretory products

Product	Source	Function	Regulation	Notes
Intrinsic factor	Parietal cells (stomach)	Vitamin B_{12} binding protein required for vitamin's uptake in terminal ileum		Autoimmune destruction of parietal cells → chronic gastritis → pernicious anemia [*handwritten:* type A]
Gastric acid	Parietal cells	Lowers pH to optimal range for pepsin function. Sterilizes chyme	Stimulated by histamine, ACh, gastrin. Inhibited by prostaglandin	Not essential for digestion. Inadequate acid → ↑ risk of *Salmonella* infections
Pepsin	Chief cells (stomach)	Begins protein digestion; optimal function at pH 1.0–3.0	Stimulated by vagal input, local acid	Inactive pepsinogen converted to pepsin by H^+
Gastrin	G cells of antrum and duodenum	1. Stimulates secretion of HCl, IF and pepsinogen 2. Stimulates gastric motility	Stimulated by stomach distention, amino acids, peptides, vagus (via GRP); inhibited by secretin and stomach acid pH < 1.5	Hypersecreted in Zollinger–Ellison syndrome → peptic ulcers. Phenylalanine and tryptophan are potent stimulators.
Bicarbonate	Surface submucosal cells of stomach and duodenum [*handwritten:* ?]	Neutralizes acid; present in unstirred layer with mucus on luminal surface, preventing autodigestion	Stimulated by secretin (potentiated by vagal input, CCK)	
Cholecystokinin (CCK)	I cells of duodenum and jejunum	1. Stimulates gallbladder contraction 2. Stimulates pancreatic enzyme secretion 3. Inhibits gastric emptying	Stimulated by fatty acids, amino acids	In cholelithiasis, pain worsens after eating fatty foods due to CCK release
Secretin	S cells of duodenum	Nature's antacid: 1. Stimulates pancreatic HCO_3^- secretion 2. Inhibits gastric acid secretion	Stimulated by acid and fatty acids in lumen of duodenum [*handwritten:* high potein contbut hypertonicity]	Alkaline pancreatic juice in duodenum neutralizes gastric acid, allowing pancreatic enzymes to function
Somatostatin	D cells in pancreatic islets, gastrointestinal mucosa	Inhibits: 1. Gastric acid and pepsinogen secretion 2. Pancreatic and small intestine fluid secretion 3. Gallbladder contraction 4. Release of both insulin and glucagon	Stimulated by acid; inhibited by vagus	Very inhibitory hormone; anti-growth hormone effects (↓ digestion and ↓ absorption of substances needed for growth)

Regulation of gastric acid secretion

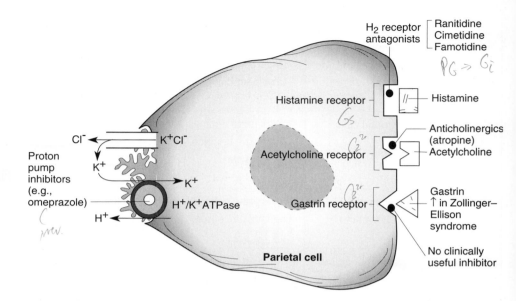

H₂ receptor antagonists
[Ranitidine
  Cimetidine
  Famotidine]

$PG > Gi$

Histamine receptor — Histamine

Gs

Cl⁻
K⁺Cl⁻
K⁺

Anticholinergics (atropine) / Acetylcholine

Acetylcholine receptor

C^{2+}

Proton pump inhibitors (e.g., omeprazole)

K⁺
H⁺/K⁺ATPase
H⁺

Gastrin receptor

C^{2+}

Gastrin ↑ in Zollinger–Ellison syndrome

No clinically useful inhibitor

Parietal cell

PHYSIOLOGY—RENAL

Filtration fraction

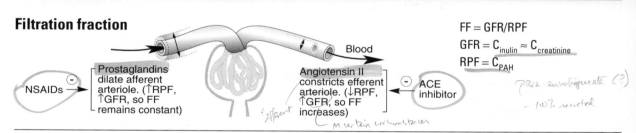

NSAIDs ⊖

Prostaglandins dilate afferent arteriole. (↑RPF, ↑GFR, so FF remains constant)

Blood

Angiotensin II constricts efferent arteriole. (↓RPF, ↑GFR, so FF increases)

⊖ ACE inhibitor

$FF = GFR/RPF$
$GFR = C_{inulin} \approx C_{creatinine}$
$RPF = C_{PAH}$

para-aminohippurate (?)
— 10% secreted

Renal clearance	$C_x = U_x V / P_x$ = volume of plasma from which the substance is cleared completely per unit time. If $C_x <$ GFR, then there is net tubular reabsorption of X. If $C_x >$ GFR, then there is net tubular secretion of X. If $C_x =$ GFR, then there is no net secretion or reabsorption.	
Glomerular filtration rate	$GFR = U_{Inulin} \times V / P_{Inulin} = C_{Inulin}$ $= K_f [(P_{GC} - P_{BS}) - (\pi_{GC} - \pi_{BS})]$ (GC = glomerular capillary; BS = Bowman's space)	Inulin is freely filtered and is neither reabsorbed nor secreted.
Effective renal plasma flow	$ERPF = U_{PAH} \times V / P_{PAH} = C_{PAH} = RBF (1 - Hct)$	PAH is filtered and secreted.
PAH	Secreted in proximal tubule. Active transport process, requires ATP, inhibited by cyanide. Mediated by a carrier system for organic acids, competitively inhibited by probenecid.	
Glucose clearance	Glucose at a normal level is completely reabsorbed (99% in proximal tubule, 1% in collecting ducts). At plasma glucose of 200 mg/dL, glucosuria begins. At 300 mg/dL, transport mechanism is completely saturated.	Glucosuria is an important clinical clue to diabetes mellitus.

Amino acid clearance	Reabsorption by at least 3 distinct carrier systems, with competitive inhibition within each group. Active transport occurs in proximal tubule and is saturable.

Electrolyte clearance

[handwritten: No, This describes Na⁺ activity. ~1% excreted; ~99% reabs.]

Sodium — >99% of filtered load is absorbed. Reabsorption is active throughout most of nephron.

Chloride — Reabsorption is passive, driven by electrochemical gradients maintained by sodium reabsorption (except at thick ascending loop of Henle). *[handwritten: 2Cl⁻/K⁺/Na⁺ cotransporter]*

[handwritten: 2°ily active actually]

Measuring fluid compartments

Compartment	Direct measurement
Total body water (TBW)	Antipyrine, tritium
Extracellular fluid (ECF) (⅓ TBW)	Inulin, mannitol
Plasma (¼ ECF, ½ TBW)	Evans blue, I^{131}-albumin
	Indirect measurement
Interstitial fluid (¾ ECF, ¼ TBW).	ECF – plasma
Intracellular fluid (⅔ TBW)	TBW – extracellular fluid

Kidney endocrine functions	Endocrine functions of the kidney: 1. Endothelial cells of peritubular capillaries secrete erythropoietin in response to hypoxia 2. Conversion of 25-OH vit. D to 1,25-$(OH)_2$ vit. D by 1α-hydroxylase, which is activated by PTH 3. JG cells secrete renin in response to ↓ renal arterial pressure and ↑ renal nerve discharge 4. Secretion of prostaglandins that vasodilate the afferent arterioles to increase GFR	NSAIDs can cause renal failure by inhibiting the renal production of prostaglandins, which normally keep the afferent arterioles vasodilated to maintain GFR.

[handwritten: not an endocrine fxn; is paracrine]

Glomerular filtration barrier	Composed of: 1. Fenestrated capillary endothelium (size barrier) 2. Fused basement membrane with heparan sulfate (negative charge barrier) 3. Epithelial layer consisting of podocyte foot processes *[handwritten: size barrier]*	The charge barrier is lost in nephrotic syndrome, resulting in albuminuria, hypoproteine-mia, generalized edema, and hyperlipidemia.

Renal failure	Failure to make urine and excrete nitrogenous wastes. Consequences: 1. Anemia (failure of erythropoietin production) 2. Renal osteodystrophy (failure of active vit. D production) 3. Hyperkalemia, which can lead to cardiac arrhythmias 4. Metabolic acidosis due to ↓ acid excretion and ↓ generation of buffers 5. Uremia (increased BUN, creatinine) 6. Sodium and H_2O excess → CHF and pulmonary edema	Two forms of renal failure: acute renal failure (often due to hypoxia) and chronic renal failure.

Hormones acting on kidney

	Stimulus for secretion	Action on kidneys
Vasopressin (ADH)	↑ plasma osmolarity	↑ H_2O permeability of principal cells in collecting ducts
	↓↓ blood volume	
Aldosterone	↓ blood volume (via AII)	↑ Na^+ reabsorption, ↑ K^+ secretion, ↑ H^+ secretion in distal tubule
	↑ plasma $[K^+]$	
Angiotensin II	↓ blood volume (via renin)	Contraction of mesangial cells → ↓ GFR
		↑ Na^+ and HCO_3^- reabsorption in proximal tubule
Atrial natriuretic peptide (ANP)	↑ atrial pressure	↓ Na^+ reabsorption, ↑ GFR
PTH	↓ plasma $[Ca^{2+}]$	↑ Ca^{2+} reabsorption, ↓ PO_4^{3-} reabsorption, ↑ $1,25 (OH)_2$ vitamin D production

(handwritten annotations: also action on principal cells (75%), intact 25%; says TGFR (p. 296); $\downarrow$ GFR = in sae are.)

Renin–angiotensin system

Mechanism   Renin is released by the kidneys upon sensing ↓ BP and serves to cleave angiotensinogen to angiotensin I (AI) (a decapeptide). AI is then cleaved by angiotensin-converting enzyme (ACE), primarily in the lung capillaries, to angiotensin II (AII, an octapeptide).

Actions
1. Potent vasoconstriction
2. Release of aldosterone from the adrenal cortex
3. Release of ADH from posterior pituitary
4. Stimulates hypothalamus → ↑ thirst

Overall, AII serves to ↑ intravascular volume and ↑ BP.

ANP may act as a "check" on the renin-angiotensin system (e.g., in heart failure).

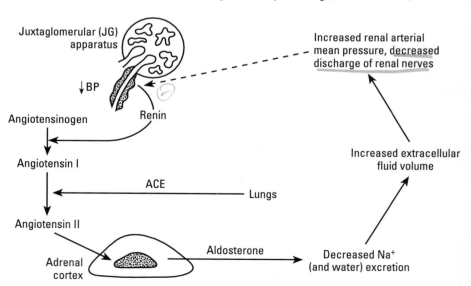

Hyperaldosteronism

Primary hyperaldosteronism (Conn's syndrome). Caused by an aldosterone-secreting tumor, resulting in hypertension, hypokalemia, hypernatremia, metabolic alkalosis, and **low** plasma renin.

Secondary hyperaldosteronism. Due to renal artery stenosis, chronic renal failure, CHF, cirrhosis, or nephrotic syndrome. Kidney misperception of low intravascular volume, resulting in an overactive renin-angiotensin system. Therefore, it is associated with **high** plasma renin.

Treatment includes spironolactone, a diuretic that works by acting as an aldosterone antagonist.

Nephron physiology

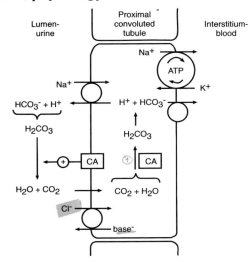

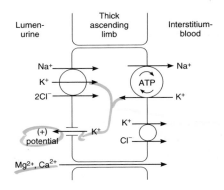

Thin descending loop of Henle—passively reabsorbs water via medullar hypertonicity (impermeable to sodium).

Thick ascending loop of Henle—actively reabsorbs Na^+, K^+, Cl^- and indirectly induces the reabsorption of Mg^{2+} and Ca^{2+}.

Proximal convoluted tubule—"workhorse of the nephron." Reabsorbs all of the glucose and amino acids and most of the bicarbonate, sodium, and water. Secretes ammonia, which acts as a buffer for secreted H^+.

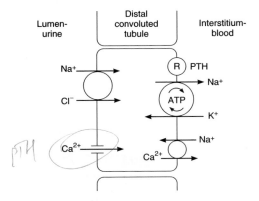

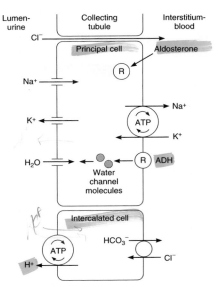

Distal convoluted tubule—actively reabsorbs Na^+, Cl^-. Reabsorption of Ca^{2+} is under the control of PTH.

Collecting tubules—reabsorb Na^+ in exchange for secreting K^+ or H^+ (regulated by aldosterone). Reabsorption of water is regulated by ADH. Osmolarity of medulla can reach 1200–1400 mOsm.

Steroid/thyroid hormone mechanism

The need for gene transcription and protein synthesis delays the onset of action of these hormones.

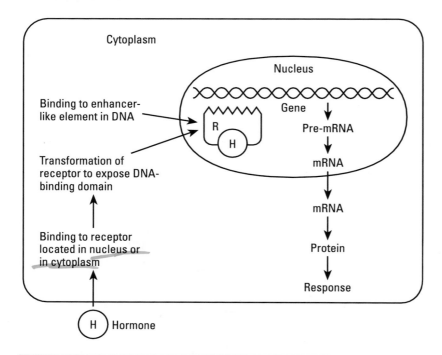

Cytoplasm

Nucleus

Binding to enhancer-like element in DNA

Gene

R

H

Pre-mRNA

Transformation of receptor to expose DNA-binding domain

mRNA

mRNA

Binding to receptor located in nucleus or in cytoplasm

Protein

Response

H Hormone

Insulin-independent organs

Muscle and adipose tissue depend on insulin for increased glucose uptake. Brain and RBCs take up glucose independent of insulin levels.

Brain and RBCs depend on glucose for metabolism under normal circumstances. Brain uses ketone bodies in starvation.

Pituitary glycoprotein hormones

Anterior pituitary glycoprotein hormones are TSH, LH, FSH. GH? ACTH? PRL? – not glycoprotein, tho

α subunit – common subunit to TSH, LH, FSH and hCG.

β subunit – determines hormone specificity.

T.S.H. and TSH = The Sex Hormones and TSH

PTH

Source
: Chief cells of parathyroid.

Function
: 1. Increase bone resorption of calcium
2. Increase kidney reabsorption of calcium
3. Decrease kidney reabsorption of phosphate
4. Increase 1,25 $(OH)_2$ vit. D production (cholecalciferol) by stimulating kidney 1α-hydroxylase.

Regulation
: Increases in serum Ca^{2+} decrease secretion.

PTH: increases serum Ca^{2+}, decreases serum PO_4^{3-}, increases urine PO_4^{3-}.

PTH stimulates both osteoclasts and osteoblasts.

PTH = Phosphate Trashing Hormone

Calcitonin

Source	Parafollicular cells (C cells) of thyroid.	Calcitonin rhymes with **"bone in."**
Function	1. Decrease bone resorption of calcium 2. Increase urinary excretion of calcium	Calcitonin opposes actions of PTH and acts faster than PTH. It is probably not important in normal calcium homeostasis.
Regulation	Increases in serum Ca^{2+} increase secretion.	

Vitamin D

Source	Vitamin D_3 from sun exposure in skin. D_2 from plants. Both converted to 25-OH vit. D in liver and to 1,25-$(OH)_2$ vit. D (active form) in kidney.	If you do not get vit. D, you get rickets (kids) or osteomalacia (adults).
Function	1. Increase absorption of dietary calcium 2. Increase absorption of dietary phosphate 3. Increase bone resorption of Ca^{2+} and PO_4^{3-}	24,25-$(OH)_2$ vit. D is the inactive form of vit. D.
Regulation	Increased PTH causes increased 1,25-(OH_2) vit. D formation. Decreased phosphate causes increased 1,25-$(OH)_2$ vit. D conversion. 1,25-$(OH)_2$ vit. D feedback inhibits its own production.	

Estrogen

Source	Ovary (estradiol), placenta (estriol), blood (aromatization), testes.	Potency: estradiol > estrone > estriol
Function	1. Growth of follicle 2. Endometrial proliferation, myometrial excitability 3. Genitalia development 4. Stromal development of breast 5. Fat deposition 6. Libido 7. Hepatic synthesis of transport proteins 8. Feedback inhibition of FSH 9. LH surge (estrogen feedback on LH secretion switches to positive from negative just before LH surge).	Estrogen hormone replacement therapy after menopause: ↓ risk of heart disease, ↓ hot flashes, and ↓ postmenopausal bone loss. Unopposed estrogen therapy: ↑ risk of endometrial cancer and possibly ↑ risk of breast cancer; use of progesterone with estrogen ↓ those risks.

Menstrual cycle

Follicular growth is fastest during second week of proliferative phase.

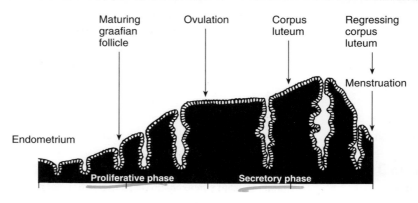

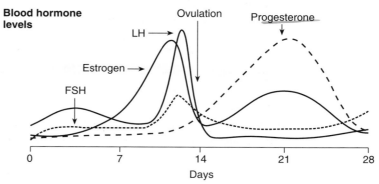

Menopause

Cessation of estrogen production with age-linked decline in number of ovarian follicles. Sx: vasomotor instability (hot flashes), vaginal atrophy (pain, infection), osteoporosis, ↑ CAD.

Average age of onset is 51 y (earlier in smokers). Hormonal changes: ↓ estrogen, ↑↑ FSH, ↑ LH (no surge).

Progesterone

Source Corpus luteum, placenta, adrenal cortex, testes.

Function
1. Stimulation of endometrial glandular secretions and spiral artery development
2. Maintenance of pregnancy
3. Decreased myometrial excitability
4. Production of thick cervical mucus, which inhibits sperm entry into the uterus
5. Increased temperature (0.5 degree)
6. Inhibition of gonadotropins (LH, FSH)
7. Uterine smooth muscle relaxation

Elevation of progesterone is indicative of ovulation.

hCG

Source Trophoblast, placenta

Function
1. Maintains the corpus luteum for the 1st trimester because it acts like LH but is not susceptible to feedback regulation from estrogen and progesterone.
   In the 2nd and 3rd trimester, the placenta synthesizes its own estrogen and progesterone. As a result, the corpus luteum degenerates.
2. Used to detect pregnancy because it appears in the urine 8 days after successful fertilization (blood and urine tests available).
3. Elevated hCG in women with hydatidiform moles or choriocarcinoma.

Norepinephrine vs. epinephrine

	Epinephrine	Norepinephrine	
Predominant receptor effect	$\beta > \alpha$	$\alpha \gg \beta$	Adrenal medullary cells and some neurons contain the enzyme PNMT, which converts norepinephrine to epinephrine.
Total peripheral resistance	↓	↑	
Cardiac output	↑	↓	
Heart rate	↑	↓ (reflex)	
Blood pressure	↑ pulse pressure	↑	

Male spermatogenesis

Pituitary	Testes	Products	Functions of products

FSH ———→ Sertoli cell ———→ Androgen binding protein   Ensures that testosterone in seminiferous tubule is high

Inhibin   Inhibits FSH

LH ———→ Leydig cell ———→ Testosterone   Differentiates male genitalia, has anabolic effects on protein metabolism, maintains gametogenesis, maintains libido, inhibits LH, and fuses epiphyseal plates in bone

DHT

↑EPO

FSH → **S**ertoli cells → **S**perm production
LH → **L**eydig cells

Cardiovascular
1. Basic electrocardiographic changes (e.g., Q waves, ST segment elevation).
2. Effects of electrolyte abnormalities on all major organ systems (e.g., potassium or calcium imbalances).
3. Physiologic effects of the Valsalva maneuver.
4. Cardiopulmonary changes with pregnancy.

Endocrine/Reproductive
1. Physiologic features of hypoparathyroidism, associated laboratory findings.
2. Clinical tests for endocrine abnormalities (e.g., dexamethasone suppression tests, glucose tolerance tests, TSH).
3. Diseases associated with endocrine abnormalities (e.g., Cushing's, Addison's, Conn's).
4. Sites of hormone production during pregnancy (e.g., corpus luteum, placenta).
5. Regulation of prolactin secretion.
6. All aspects of diabetes.

Gastrointestinal
1. Sites of absorption of major nutrients (e.g., ileum: vit. B_{12}).
2. Bile production and enterohepatic circulation.
3. Glucose cotransport into cells of gut and peripheral tissues.
4. Fat digestion and absorption.

Pulmonary
1. Alveolar-arterial oxygen gradient and changes seen in lung disease.
2. Mechanical differences between inspiration and expiration.
3. Characteristic pulmonary function curves for common lung diseases (e.g., bronchitis, emphysema, asthma, interstitial lung disease).
4. Gas diffusion across alveolocapillary membrane.

Renal/Acid-Base
1. Differences among active transport, facilitated diffusion, and diffusion.
2. Differences between central and nephrogenic diabetes insipidus.

General
1. Role of calmodulin and troponin C, and tropomyosin in muscle contraction.
2. Role of ions (e.g., calcium, sodium, magnesium, potassium) in skeletal muscle, cardiac muscle, and nerve cells (e.g., muscle contraction, membrane and action potentials, neurotransmitter release).
3. The clotting cascade, including those factors which require vitamin K for synthesis (II, VII, IX, X).
4. Regulation of core body temperature.

Database of Basic Science Review Resources

Comprehensive
Anatomy
Behavioral Science
Biochemistry
Microbiology
Pathology
Pharmacology
Physiology

Commercial Review Courses
Publisher Contacts

This section is a database of current basic science review books, sample examination books, and commercial review courses marketed to medical students studying for the USMLE Step 1. At the end of this section is a list of publishers and independent bookstores with addresses and phone numbers. For each book, we list the **Title** of the book, the **First Author** (or editor), the **Series Name** (where applicable), the **Current Publisher**, the **Copyright Year**, the **Number of Pages**, the **ISBN Code**, the **Approximate List Price**, the **Format** of the book, and the **Number of Test Questions**. The entries for most books also include **Summary Comments** that describe their style and overall utility for studying. Finally, each book receives a **Rating**. The books are sorted into a comprehensive section as well as into sections corresponding to the seven traditional basic medical science disciplines (anatomy, behavioral science, biochemistry, microbiology, pathology, pharmacology, and physiology). Within each section, books are arranged first by Rating, then by Title, and finally by Author.

For the 1998 edition of *First Aid for the USMLE Step 1,* the database of review books has been expanded and updated, with more than 30 new books and software and more in-depth summary comments. A letter rating scale with ten different grades reflects the detailed student evaluations. Each book receives a rating as follows:

A+	Excellent for boards review.
A A–	Very good for boards review; choose among the group.
B+ B B–	Good, but use only after exhausting better sources.
C+ C C–	Fair, but many better books in the discipline, or low-yield subject material.
D	Not appropriate.
N	Not rated.

The **Rating** is meant to reflect the overall usefulness of the book in preparing for the USMLE Step 1 examination. This is based on a number of factors, including:

■ The cost of the book.
■ The readability of the text.
■ The appropriateness and accuracy of the book.
■ The quality and number of sample questions.
■ The quality of written answers to sample questions.
■ The quality and appropriateness of the illustrations (e.g., graphs, diagrams, photographs).
■ The length of the text (longer is not necessarily better).

- The quality and number of other books available in the same discipline.
- The importance of the discipline on the USMLE Step 1 examination.

Please note that the rating does **not** reflect the quality of the book for purposes other than reviewing for the USMLE Step 1 examination. Many books with low ratings are well written and informative but are not ideal for boards preparation. We have also avoided listing or commenting on the wide variety of general textbooks available in the basic sciences.

Evaluations are based on the cumulative results of formal and informal surveys of thousands of medical students at many medical schools across the country. The summary comments and overall ratings represent a consensus opinion, but there may have been a large range of opinion or limited student feedback on one particular book.

Please note that the data listed are subject to change in that:

- Publishers' prices change frequently.
- Individual bookstores often charge an additional markup.
- New editions come out frequently, and the quality of updating varies.
- The same book may be reissued through another publisher.

We actively encourage medical students and faculty to submit their opinions and ratings of these basic science review books so that we may update our database. (*See* How to Contribute, p. xv.) In addition, we ask that publishers and authors submit review copies of basic science review books, including new editions and books not included in our database for evaluation. We also solicit reviews of new books or suggestions for alternate modes of study that may be useful in preparing for the examination, such as flashcards, computer-based tutorials, and commercial review courses.

Disclaimer/Conflict of Interest Statement

No material in this book, including the ratings, reflects the opinion or influence of the publisher. All errors and omissions will gladly be corrected if brought to the attention of the authors through the publisher. Please note that the book *Underground Step 1 Answers to the NBME Retired and Self-Test Questions* (p. 313) is an independent publication by the authors of this book; its rating is based solely on data from the student survey and feedback forms.

Body Systems Reviews I, II, and III

$24.95 ea   Test/770 q

Board Simulator Series, Gruber

Book I: Williams & Wilkins, 1997, 338 pages, ISBN 0683302981

Book II: Williams & Wilkins, 1997, 350 pages, ISBN 068330299X

Book III: Williams & Wilkins, 1997, 298 pages, ISBN 0683303007

Four exams with approximately 160 questions each. Follows new USMLE content outline (Book I covers hematopoietic/lymphoreticular, respiratory, and cardiovascular systems; Book II tests GI, renal, reproductive, and endocrine systems; and Book III tests nervous, skin/connective tissue, and musculoskeletal systems). Numerous vignettes reflect clinical slant of the exam. Good black-and-white photographs. Comprehensive systems-based approach. Most effective if all three books are used. For the motivated student. Explanations discuss important concepts. New editions not yet reviewed.

Retired NBME Basic Medical Sciences Test Items

—   Test/993 q

NBME

NBME, 1991, 136 pages, out of print

Contains "retired" questions in all seven areas of basic science. Good topics. Letter answers only with no explanations. Content is still relevant, but the format is outdated. Contains old K-type questions. No clinical vignettes. Limited utility for test simulation. Out of print, so try to find an old copy. Not available in bookstores. Explanatory study guide is available as a separate publication (*Underground Step 1 Answers;* see later in this section).

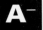

Review for USMLE Step 1 Examination

$33.00   Test/1000+ q

NMS, Lazo

Williams & Wilkins, 1996, 348 pages, ISBN 068306276X

Very good source of practice questions and answers. Features updated clinical questions with a limited number of vignettes. Some questions are too picky or difficult. Good explanations, but occasionally offers unnecessary detail. Good buy for the number of questions. Organized as four 200-question booklets; good for simulating the exam. Helpful color plates.

Ace Basic Sciences: USMLE Step 1

$31.95   Test/800 q

Ace, Mosby

Mosby-Yearbook, 1996, 206 pages, ISBN 081569043 (Windows),

ISBN 081518669X (Mac)

Some clinically focused vignettes interspersed with basic science questions. Answers explain why each choice is right or wrong rather than focusing on didactic teaching of main concepts. Four comprehensive exams with 200 questions each. Money-back guarantee if you fail. Small type may be hard to read. Questions can be done in book or on diskette. Compare with Lazo (*Review for USMLE Step 1 Examination*) and Barton (*Appleton & Lange's Review for the USMLE Step 1*). Very limited student feedback. No photomicrographs. Software not yet examined.

Appleton & Lange's Review for the USMLE Step 1 $36.95   Test/1200 q
Barton

Appleton & Lange, 1996, 331 pages, ISBN 0838502652

Good questions with good answers. Many questions are very picky. Features seven subject-based tests and one 300-plus-question comprehensive exam. Good buy for the number of questions. Few clinical vignettes. A good, straightforward, question-based review to assess your strengths and weaknesses. Revised anatomy section and some mixed-quality color plates. Compare closely with NMS/Lazo.

 General Principles in the Basic Sciences $24.95   Test/770 q
Board Simulator Series, Gruber

Williams & Wilkins, 1997, 306 pages, ISBN 0683302965

Four exams with approximately 160 questions each. Systems-based approach. Follows USMLE content outline. Includes some clinical vignettes. Thorough explanations highlight basic concept tested by each question. Very detailed. Some very difficult questions. For the motivated student. Good black-and-white photographs. New edition not yet reviewed.

 Normal and Abnormal Processes in the Basic Sciences $24.95   Test/770 q
Board Simulator Series, Gruber

Williams & Wilkins, 1997, 304 pages, ISBN 0683302973

Four exams with approximately 160 questions each. This is probably the one book in the series (see above) that students can do without using the other books in the series. Questions cover all seven major subject areas. Many questions are written as clinical vignettes. Limited student feedback. New edition not yet reviewed.

 Rapid Preparation for the USMLE Step 1 $36.00   Test/926 q
Johnson

J&S Publishing, 1997, 406 pages, ISBN 1888308028

A "best of J&S" compendium. Questions are organized by subject and are drawn as exact duplicates from other books in the series. Great explanations with key concepts in boldface. High-quality black-and-white MRIs, CTs, line drawings, histology, and gross photo illustrations. Clinical vignette-based questions. Used by The Princeton Review in its Step 1 review course.

B+ **Self-Test in the Part I Basic Medical Sciences** — Test/630 q

NBME

NBME, 1989, 91 pages, out of print

A very good source of questions, level of difficulty, and detail, although the format is outdated. Ninety items are given per discipline. Letter answers are given with no explanations. No clinical vignettes. Limited utility for test simulation. Some repeated questions from "Retired Items." Out of print; try to find an old copy. Not available in bookstores. Explanatory study guide is available as a separate publication (*Underground Step 1 Answers,* see below).

B+ **Underground Step 1 Answers to the NBME Retired and Self-Test Questions** $22.95 Review/1600 a

Amin

S2S Medical, 1996, 387 pages, ISBN 1890061018

Concise explanatory study guide to 1600+ *NBME Retired* and *Self-Test* questions. Easy read, although some superficial answers. Useful with or without NBME questions (not included). Referenced to current textbooks. Second edition features expanded and updated explanations. Available in some bookstores or can be ordered at (800) 247-6553 or by fax at (419) 281-6883; fully refundable. Note that this book is by the authors of *First Aid for the USMLE Step 1.*

B **Crashing the Boards: USMLE Step 1** $16.00 Review only

Yeh

Lippincott-Raven, 1997, 151 pages, ISBN 0397584091

Brief coverage of high-yield topics. Great diagrams. No photographs. Excellent organization (bulleted facts and highlighted boxing). Appropriate for supplementary review. Mixed student feedback. Incomplete review of books in the back. Compare with Carl's *Medical Boards—Step 1 Made Ridiculously Simple.*

B **Medical Boards—Step 1 Made Ridiculously Simple** $21.95 Review

Carl

MedMaster, 1996, 260 pages, ISBN 0940780259

Quick reading. Table and chart format is organized by subject. Excellent pathology section. Very mixed reviews. Some charts are poorly labeled. Consider as an adjunct. Compare with Yeh's *Crashing the Boards.*

B **MEPC USMLE Step 1 Review** $32.95 Test/1200 q

Fayemi

Appleton & Lange, 1996, 455 pages, ISBN 0838562698

Features questions with explanatory answers. Offers mixed-quality questions with some incomplete or inaccurate explanations. Includes clinical vignettes.

B | Step 1 Success

$40.00   Test/720 q

Zaslau

FMSG, 1996, 240 pages, ISBN 1886468079

Full-length practice examination with four 180-question booklets with explanations (same as actual exam). Features many clinically focused questions similar to USMLE format. Offers small number of black-and-white photographs of moderate quality, but no color pictures. Some typographic and grammatical errors. Limited student feedback. Expensive for the number of questions. Also available on CD-Rom.

B | USMLE Success

$40.00   How-to/540 q

Zaslau

FMSG, 1996, 280 pages, ISBN 1886468095

Broad overview of preparation necessary for all three steps. Has a very useful "what to study" section with a list of classic slides, x-rays, and gross specimens that have appeared on previous USMLE exams. Mnemonic section is helpful. Includes a 180-question mock Step 1 exam with explanations. This exam represents the format and clinical focus of the USMLE exam but contains grammatical errors. Especially appropriate for the IMG student preparing for all three Step exams in a short time period. Expensive.

B⁻ | Preparation for USMLE Step 1 Basic Medical Sciences, Volumes A, B, C

$14.00 ea   Test/315 q

Luder

Maval Medical Education, 1995, 70 pages, ISBN 1884083099 (Vol. A), 1884083102 (Vol. B), 1884083110 (Vol. C)

Appropriate-format questions with explanatory answers. Good color photographs. Poorly edited. Some wrong answers in the key. Many typographic and grammatical errors; expensive for the number of questions.

B⁻ | Preparation for the USMLE Step 1 Basic Medical Sciences, Volumes D, E

$14.00 ea   Test/210 q

Luder

Maval Medical Education, 1995, 54 pages, ISBN 1884083129

Same format and comments as for Volumes A, B, and C, but even more expensive for the number of questions. Numerous errors; poor editing.

B⁻ | Rypin's Questions and Answers for Basic Science Review

$29.95   Test/1640 q

Frohlich

Lippincott, 1993, 211 pages, ISBN 0397512473

Questions with detailed answers to supplement *Rypin's Basic Sciences Review*. Decent overall question-based review of all subjects. Not referenced to a text. Requires time commitment. New edition not yet reviewed.

Step 1 Update—Book A

$16.00   Test/180 q

Zaslau

FMSG, 1996, 66 pages, ISBN 1886468133

Questions and answers with brief explanations. Based on recent examinations. Contains some repeated questions from other books in the series. Many clinical vignettes, but no photographs. Expensive for the number of questions. Limited student feedback.

Basic Science Bank—"NBME"

$88.00   Test/3500 q

FMSG

FMSG, 1991, 301 pages

Advertised as questions "remembered" from past NBME exams. Variable-quality questions with letter answers only. Poor photo quality. Contains outdated K-type and C-type (A/B/both/neither) items. Not available in bookstores. Can be ordered at (800) 443-4194; nonrefundable.

Clinical Anatomy and Pathophysiology for the Health Professional

$18.95   Review only

Stewart

MedMaster, 1997, 260 pages, ISBN 0940780062

Written for non-MD professionals. Not boards oriented. Simplistic, but may be a good place to start for some students. Good diagrams.

Future Test: USMLE Step 1

$59.95   Software

National Learning Corp.

Future Technologies, 1994, ISBN 0837394538

PC software features multiple ways to review and self-test from database of questions with explanations. Question styles are not representative of the current exam. Few clinical vignettes.

Medical Student's Guide to Top Board Scores: USMLE Steps 1 and 2

$15.95   Review

Rogers

Little, Brown, 1996, 146 pages, ISBN 0316754366

Easy to read, but information is low yield and coverage of topics is spotty. Contains some good mnemonics in basic and clinical sciences, but not necessarily boards-relevant. Incomplete and outdated list of recommended books for board review.

The Most Common Manual for Medical Students

$14.95   Review only

Grosso

Stephen Grosso, 1991, 487 pages, ISBN 1883205298

A compilation of more than 3500 "most common questions" of medicine. Well organized, compact. Useful for the wards, with some high-yield basic science material mixed in with the clinical material.

PASS USMLE Step 1: Practice by Assessing Study Skills

$19.95   How-to/500 q

Schwenker

Little, Brown, 1995, 140 pages, ISBN 0316776009

Detailed review of study and testing strategies for standardized exams and medical school. Worth considering if you have study or testing difficulties. Includes diagnostic test.

PreTest Step 1 Simulated Exam

$32.00   Test/420 q

Thornborough

McGraw-Hill, 1996, 178 pages, ISBN 0070520208

Typical PreTest questions, some of which are repeated from PreTest book series. Letter answers with explanations. Free computerized evaluation. Picky topics. Some questions are poorly written, but features some good photomicrographs. Also, beware of similar PreTest "Customized Examinations" offered at some individual medical schools.

Rypin's Basic Sciences Review, Vol. I

$34.95   Review/1000+ q

Frohlich

Lippincott, 1993, 856 pages, ISBN 0397512457

Multitopic textbook with very few figures and tables. A good general reference, but should be used with other subject-specific sources. Well priced for the number of pages and questions. Requires extensive time commitment.

Study Skills and Test-Taking Strategies for Medical Students

$17.95   How-to only

Oklahoma Notes, Shain

Springer-Verlag, 1995, 204 pages, ISBN 038794396X

Very detailed discussion of study skills for medical school. May be useful for some students seeking a structured approach, but probably not necessary for most medical students.

How to Prepare for the USMLE Step 1

$15.95   How-to/575 q

Thornborough

McGraw-Hill, 1996, 261 pages, ISBN 0070645248

A detailed but not very useful "how-to-prepare" book written for the new examination. Uses questions from other PreTest books. Twenty 25-question practice tests divided by topic plus a 75-question pretest. Contains an alphabetical list of 2000 medical terms of dubious value.

C | **New Rudman's Questions and Answers on the USMLE** | $49.95 | Test/280 q

Rudman

National Learning Corporation, 1991, 200 pages, ISBN 0837358043

Combines Step 1 and Step 2 questions but with no explanations. Lacks clinical vignettes and references. Some errors. Very expensive. Limited review of anatomy and physiology at the end of the book.

C | **USMLE Step 1 Review: The Study Guide** | $32.95 | Review

Goldberg

Sage, 1996, 473 pages, ISBN 0803972849

A new comprehensive review that often reads like a textbook. Does not organize ideas in a way that is useful for review purposes. No mnemonics, no questions, very few diagrams or pictures. Requires a large time commitment, but low yield.

NEW BOOKS—COMPREHENSIVE

N | **A&LERT USMLE Step 1** | $59.95 | Test/2400 q

Appleton & Lange

Appleton & Lange, 1998, ISBN 0838584462

Available. Windows/Mac-based testing software. Includes six simulated USMLE-type tests featuring over 2,000 questions with explanations. Also provides timing, scoring, searching, note taking, and bookmarking functions.

N | **A&LERT USMLE Step 1 Deluxe** | $89.95 | Test/3600 q

Appleton & Lange

Appleton & Lange, 1998, ISBN 0838503497

Available. Windows/Mac-based testing software. Includes all the same features of the Standard Edition plus an additional question bank of 1200 questions and answers for each of the basic science topics.

N | **Basic Science Bank—"USMLE"** | $36.00 | Test/500 q

Zaslau

FMSG, 1997, 176 pages, ISBN 1886468176

New edition has three sections designed to simulate the three-hour time periods of the exam. Includes letter answers with explanations and many clinical vignettes. Poor photo quality. Repeated questions from other books in the series. Limited student feedback.

N | **Basic Science Review Success** | $28.00 | Review

Zaslau

FMSG, 1997, 137 pages, ISBN 1886468184

Not yet reviewed.

N **Gold Standard Prep Set**
for USMLE Step 1   **$99.00**   Audio tape

Knouse

Gold Standard, 1997

Not yet reviewed. Set of 15 approximately 90-minute audio tapes covering
USMLE Step 1 material. Available by calling (614) 592-4124 or faxing (614)
592-4045.

N **Passing the USMLE Step 1, Vols. I–IV**   **$30.00 ea** Test/500 q

Gold

Vol. I: Southland Tutorial, 1996, 165 pages, ISBN 1888628006
Vol. II: Southland Tutorial, 1996, 150 pages, ISBN 1888628014
Vol. III: Southland Tutorial, 1996, 166 pages, ISBN 1888628022
Vol. IV: Southland Tutorial, 1996, 150 pages, ISBN 1888628030
Each book contains 500 multiple-choice questions with lengthy explana-
tions. Includes many clinical vignettes. Poor-quality photo illustrations. Lim-
ited student feedback. Compare with *Board Simulator Series*.

N **Passing the USMLE Steps 1, 2, & 3 Photo Diagnosis,** **$30.00 ea** Test/100 q
Vols. I and II

Vol. I: Southland Tutorial, 1996, 75 pages, ISBN 1888628235
Vol. II: Southland Tutorial, 1996, 75 pages, ISBN 1888628243
One hundred picture-based questions with thorough explanations. Pictures
include good CTs, x-rays, MRIs, angiograms, EKGs, etc. May be helpful if
used in conjunction with other Southland Tutorial review books. Limited
student feedback. Expensive for the number of questions.

N **USMLE Step 1 Starter Kit**   **$29.95**   Test/360 q

Kaplan Educational

Appleton & Lange, 1998, 208 pages, ISBN 0838586651

Expected early 1998.

Not yet reviewed. Two 180-question sample exams. Answers can be ana-
lyzed over the Internet, at a Kaplan Center, or by mail. Analysis includes a
diagnostic profile and study-plan summary.

A⁻ High-Yield Embryology

$14.95   Review only

Dudek

Williams & Wilkins, 1996, ISBN 068302714X

Excellent, concise review of embryology. Thorough coverage of subject. Excellent organization with clinical correlations. Crammable list of embryologic origins of tissues. Consider *BRS Embryology* for more complete diagrams.

A⁻ High-Yield Gross Anatomy

$14.95   Review only

Dudek

Williams & Wilkins, 1997, 170 pages, ISBN 0683182153

Excellent, concise review with clinical correlations. Contains well-labeled, high-yield radiologic images. Limited but very positive student feedback.

A⁻ High-Yield Neuroanatomy

$14.95   Review only

Fix

Williams & Wilkins, 1994, 111 pages, ISBN 0683032488

Clean, easy-to-read outline format. Straightforward text with excellent diagrams and illustrations. Just enough detail without anything extra. Very high yield review, especially if the emphasis on neuroanatomy seen on the '97 exam continues. More comprehensive than *Clinical Neuroanatomy Made Ridiculously Simple.* Lacks index.

B⁺ Ace Neuroscience

$29.95   Review/235 q

Ace, Castro

Mosby-Year Book, 1996, 464 pages, ISBN 0815114796 (Windows), ISBN 081511480X (Mac)

Outline format with some good photomicrographs. Covers neuroanatomy, neurophysiology, and neuropathology. Separate chapters on clinical correlations are very high yield. For the motivated student. Would have been very useful for the '97 exam. Limited student feedback. Test software included with text. Money-back guarantee if you fail.

B⁺ Anatomy: Review for New National Boards

$25.00   Test/506 q

Johnson

J & S, 1992, 217 pages, ISBN 0963287303

Easy reading. Clinical case-based questions with detailed explanations. Good, superficial overview of cell biology, histology, gross anatomy, embryology, and neuroanatomy. Discusses clinically relevant anatomic science with adequate explanations, illustrations, and pictures; also covers many clinically relevant genetic diseases. Spotty coverage; many key topics are not covered. Includes good photomicrographs and cross-sectional imaging-based questions.

B+ **Cell Biology: Review for New National Boards**   **$25.00**   Review/524 q
Adelman
J&S, 1995, 203 pages, ISBN 0963287389
Question-based review format like other J&S books. Covers classic topics
in cell biology. Very detailed, but some topics showed up in the '97 exam.
Contains some high-quality micrographs. Recycles some questions and il-
lustrations from J&S *Anatomy.*

B+ **Clinical Anatomy Made Ridiculously Simple**   **$18.95**   Review only
Goldberg
MedMaster, 1991, 187 pages, ISBN 094078002X
Easy reading, simple diagrams, lots of mnemonics and "ridiculous" associations. Incomplete. This style has variable appeal to students, so browse before buying. Some students really love this book. Good review for the relatively low-yield subject of gross anatomy. Best if used during the first year.

B+ **Clinical Neuroanatomy Made Ridiculously Simple**   **$12.95**   Review/Few q
Goldberg
MedMaster, 1995, 89 pages, ISBN 0940780003
Easy to read, memorable, and simplified, with clever hand-drawn diagrams.
Very quick, high-yield review of clinical neuroanatomy. Good emphasis on
clinically relevant pathways, cranial nerves, and neurologic diseases.
Spotty coverage of some key boards topics. No USMLE-style questions.
Good complement to Fix's *High-Yield Neuroanatomy.*

B+ **High-Yield Histology**   **$14.95**   Review only
Dudek
Williams & Wilkins, 1997, 95 pages, ISBN 0683027204
Quick and easy review of relatively low-yield subject. Tables with some
high-yield information. Appendix contains classic EMs. Limited student
feedback.

B+ **Liebman's Neuroanatomy Made Easy**   **$30.00**   Review/Few q
& Understandable
Gertz
Aspen, 1996, 176 pages, ISBN 0834207303
Easy to read. Contains excellent diagrams. A fast, straightforward, high-
yield review. Some humor and interesting facts to help the student remem-
ber pathways. Expensive. Incomplete, but more thorough than Goldberg's
Clinical Neuroanatomy Made Ridiculously Simple.

B⁺ **MEPC Anatomy** $19.95 Test/700 q

Wilson

Appleton & Lange, 1995, 251 pages, ISBN 0838562183

Many clinical vignettes followed by questions. Includes gross anatomy, neuroanatomy, cell biology, and embryology. Worth considering as an alternative to J&S *Anatomy*. Good value. Mixed-quality questions with concise answers. Overly detailed.

B **Ace Anatomy** $29.95 Review/300+ q

Ace, Moore

Mosby-Year Book, 1996, 400 pages, ISBN 0815169051 (Windows), ISBN 0815186711 (Mac)

Thorough coverage of gross anatomy only. Good, but non-boards-style questions with explanations. Helpful summary tables. Detailed coverage of a low-yield topic. More appropriate for coursework. No radiographs. Test software included with text. Money-back guarantee with proof of failure.

B **Ace Histology and Cell Biology** $29.95 Review/286 q

Ace, Burns

Mosby-Year Book, 1996, 250 pages, ISBN 0815113382 (Windows), ISBN 0815113358 (Mac)

Good diagrams of tissues, but no actual photomicrographs. Outline format with dense text. Icons are more distracting than helpful. Non-boards-style review questions are given at the end of each chapter with detailed explanations. Too much detail in some areas. Limited feedback on software. Money-back guarantee if you fail.

B **Embryology** $19.95 Review/500 q

BRS, Fix

Williams & Wilkins, 1995, 266 pages, ISBN 0683032437

Outline-based review of embryology that is typical for books in this series. Good review of important embryology, but too detailed. Good discussion of congenital malformations at the end of each chapter. The comprehensive exam at the end of the book is the most high-yield part of the book.

B⁻ **Anatomy** $17.95 Review/70 q

Oklahoma Notes, Papka

Springer-Verlag, 1995, 231 pages, ISBN 0387943951

Covers embryology, gross anatomy, neuroanatomy, and histology. Broad coverage, but dense text is somewhat difficult to read. Very few illustrations. The student is "encouraged to thoughtfully engage the narrative . . . and incorporate mental images of structures. . . ."

Clinical Anatomy: An Illustrated Review with Questions and Explanations   **$27.95**   Review/500+ q

Snell

Little, Brown, 1996, 308 pages, ISBN 0316803073

Text is a well-organized summary of Snell's major book. Great diagrams and tables. Questions incorporate radiographs, CT scans, and MRIs. Does not cover neuroanatomy or embryology. Neither text nor questions are as clinical as the title implies. Only some of the answers have explanations, most of which are too short.

 Neuropathology and Basic Neuroscience   **$17.95**   Review/101 q

Oklahoma Notes, Brumback

Springer-Verlag, 1996, 289 pages, ISBN 0387946357

Utilizes organ system approach by integrating CNS anatomy, pathology, physiology, and some pharmacology. Easy to read. Good-quality line drawings. Use either with organ system review or as a supplement to a subject review. Limited student feedback.

 Neuroscience   **$17.95**   Test/509 q

Pretest, Siegel

McGraw-Hill, 1996, 209 pages, ISBN 0070520828

Detailed questions and answers. Includes photographs of CT/MRIs and drawings of brain sections. Useful after studying from other sources. For the motivated student.

 Cell Biology & Histology   **$22.95**   Review/500 q

BRS, Gartner

Williams & Wilkins, 1997, 377 pages, ISBN 0683361039

Nice format with mixed-quality reproductions, but too detailed. Nineteen chapters with detailed answers. For the motivated student. New edition not yet reviewed.

 Clinical Anatomy   **$26.00**   Review/500 q

NMS, April

Williams & Wilkins, 1996, 650 pages, ISBN 0683061992

Organized in outline form. Questions with detailed answers. Text is too in-depth and low yield. Limited student feedback. However, contains some very good clinical correlations and boards-style questions.

 Histology QuizBank Vols. 1 & 2   **$69.00**   Software/800+ q

Downing

Keyboard Publishing, 1995, ISBN 1573493171 (Mac), ISBN 1573493198 (Windows)

Database of boards-style questions arranged by subject area. Explanations on demand. Questions cross-referenced to Junqueira's *Histology Text Stack* (sold separately). Expensive for limited-yield topic.

C+ | **Langman's Medical Embryology** | $35.00 | Review only

Sadler

Williams & Wilkins, 1995, 460 pages, ISBN 068307489X

Lengthy text. Good for reference, but too detailed for boards review. Concise summary pages. Good pictures with useful clinical correlations.

C+ | **Molecular Biology QuizBank** | $59.00 | Software/500+ q

Case Western Reserve

Keyboard Publishing, 1995, ISBN 1573493422 (Mac), ISBN 1573493430 (Windows)

Software database of boards-style questions. Expensive for limited-yield topic.

C+ | **Wheater's Functional Histology** | $54.95 | Review only

Burkitt

Churchill-Livingstone, 1993, 407 pages, ISBN 0443046913

Color atlas with pictures of normal histology and accompanying text. Not directed to boards-type review. May be more useful to skim through for photomicrograph-based questions in the glossy booklets.

C | **Anatomy** | $17.95 | Test/500 q

PreTest, April

McGraw-Hill, 1996, 220 pages, ISBN 0070520909

Difficult questions with detailed answers. Some illustrations. Requires time commitment. Limited student feedback.

C | **Basic Histology: Examination and Board Review** | $31.95 | Review/1000+ q

Paulsen

Appleton & Lange, 1996, 379 pages, ISBN 0838522823

Dense, thorough review, but low yield for boards. Good format with many questions. Designed to complement Junqueira's *Basic Histology* textbook. Requires time commitment.

C | **Blond's Anatomy** | $17.99 | Review only

Tesoriero

Sulzburger & Graham, 1994, 282 pages, ISBN 094581920X

Concise review of gross anatomy—a low-yield topic. Easy read. Good tables and illustrations. More appropriate for coursework than for boards review.

C | **Cell Biology and Histology** | $27.00 | Review/500 q

NMS, Johnson

Williams & Wilkins, 1991, 409 pages, ISBN 0683062107

Outline form. Questions with detailed answers. Best if used with course.

C Gross Anatomy

$21.95   Review/500 q

BRS, Chung

Williams & Wilkins, 1995, 388 pages, ISBN 068301563X

Detailed, lengthy text in outline format with illustrations and tables. Better for course review; too detailed for boards review. Good clinical correlation section.

C Guide to Human Anatomy

$34.50   Review/350 q

Philo

Saunders, 1985, 335 pages, ISBN 0721612032

Contains excellent pictorial summaries of body regions, clinical comments, and a section of CTs of key body levels. Covers only gross anatomy. High volume, but low-yield topic. Very expensive. For the dedicated student.

C Histology & Cell Biology

$17.95   Test/500 q

PreTest, Klein

McGraw-Hill, 1996, 307 pages, ISBN 007052081X

Similar to others in the PreTest series. Some difficult questions with explanations that are often too detailed. Requires time commitment.

C Medcharts: Anatomy

$17.95   Review only

Gest

ILOC, 1994, 309 pages, ISBN 1882531019

Tabular summaries of gross anatomy for course and boards review. Chart overkill. Low yield.

C Neuroanatomy

$22.95   Review/500 q

BRS, Fix

Williams & Wilkins, 1995, 416 pages, ISBN 0683032496

Updated text. Covers anatomy and embryology of the nervous system. Compare with *High-Yield Neuroanatomy* by the same author.

C Neuroanatomy

$27.00   Review/300 q

NMS, DeMyer

Williams & Wilkins, 1997, 380 pages, ISBN 068330075X

Outline form. Nice diagrams, but low yield. Good for coursework but too detailed for boards review. Limited student feedback on new edition.

C Review of Gross Anatomy

$39.95   Review/500+ q

Pansky

McGraw-Hill, 1996, 688 pages, ISBN 0071054464

Outline format with pictures on opposite page. New color illustrations and imaging correlations. Very detailed review of only gross anatomy, so low overall yield. Contains good illustrations and a few tables. For the dedicated student.

C

Review Questions: Gross Anatomy and Embryology

$21.95   Test/2500+ q

Gest

Parthenon, 1993, 399 pages, ISBN 1850705038

Contains outdated K-type questions and has no matching questions or clinical vignettes. Huge collection of questions covers only gross anatomy and embryology.

C⁻

Appleton & Lange's Review of Anatomy

$32.95   Test/1400+ q

Montgomery

Appleton & Lange, 1995, 340 pages, ISBN 0838502466

High volume of questions with brief explanations, no text, and few diagrams. Limited student feedback.

C⁻

Essentials of Human Histology

$29.95   Review/100 q

Krause

Little, Brown, 1996, 452 pages, ISBN 0316503363

Review text with some boards-style questions and letter answers. May be more appropriate as a course text than as a review book. Limited student feedback.

C⁻

Gross Anatomy: A Review with Questions and Explanations

$28.95   Review/430+ q

Snell

Little, Brown, 1990, 345 pages, ISBN 0316801976

A preeminent author. Dense but thorough; requires time commitment. Good diagrams. Some questions are outdated. Very little clinical correlation. Still low yield.

C⁻

Keyboard Histology Series Personal Edition

$149.00   Software/800+ q

Keyboard Publishing, 1995, ISBN 1573492973 (Mac), ISBN 1573492981 (Windows)

Includes *Histology QuizBank Vols. 1 & 2* (reviewed previously) and Junqueira's *Histology Text Stack*. QuizBank questions are linked to passages in Text Stack. Text can be exported to a word processor. Very expensive for a limited-yield subject. Better if purchased by the library. Text Stack is more appropriate for reference than for review.

C- **Neuroanatomy: A Review with Questions and Explanations** $29.95   Review/400+ q

Snell

Little, Brown, 1992, 298 pages, ISBN 0316802468

Reasonably easy to read; contains some clinical correlations. Book is too long in relation to the small portion of the exam devoted to neuroanatomy. New edition entitled *Clinical Neuroanatomy: An Illustrated Review with Questions and Explanations* expected in December 1997.

NEW BOOKS—ANATOMY

N **Concepts in Gross Anatomy** $26.95   Review/160 q

Mosenthal

Parthenon, 1997, 250 pages, ISBN 1850709289

Long, detailed narrative format with review questions may be more appropriate for coursework. In-depth coverage of a relatively low-yield subject. Clinical correlations hidden in dense text. Some line drawings and fill-in-the-blank drawings are of questionable value for review. Limited student feedback.

N **Correlative Neuroanatomy** $31.95   Review only

Waxman

Appleton & Lange, 1997, ISBN 0838514774

Not yet reviewed.

N **Embryology: Review for New National Boards** $25.00   Test/500+ q

Gasser

J&S, 1997, 221 pages, ISBN 188830801X

Typical format for this series. Not yet reviewed.

N **Histology** $26.00   Review/q

NMS, Henrickson

Williams & Wilkins, 1997, 350 pages, ISBN 0683062255

Not yet reviewed.

N **PreTest Anatomy Study Disk** $28.00   Software/500 q

April

McGraw-Hill, 1995, ISBN 0078641632 (Mac), ISBN 0078641624 (Windows)

Incomplete copy of exactly the same questions found in PreTest book. Picky, difficult questions with detailed answers. Program can vary length of time allotted per question. Score report of questionable value gives breakdown of questions by type answered correctly (matching versus positive and negatively phrased questions). More expensive than the book. Limited student feedback.

Review Questions for Human Anatomy

$21.95 Test/1000 q

Tank

Parthenon, 1996, 150 pages, ISBN 1850707952

Very detailed questions may be more appropriate for coursework. Extensive coverage of very low yield subject with two comprehensive exams at the end. Some clinical correlations are scattered throughout. May be too time-consuming for boards exam. Limited student feedback.

Review Questions for Human Embryology

$17.95 Test/482 q

Gest

Parthenon, 1995, 104 pages, ISBN 1850705917

Designed for the USMLE Steps 1 and 2; may be too detailed for low-yield embryology section on Step 1. Non-boards-style questions with outdated K-type questions. Letter answers with explanations. Most helpful if the student has already reviewed the subject. Limited student feedback.

Review Questions for Human Histology

$19.95 Test/1042 q

Burns

Parthenon, 1995, 216 pages, ISBN 1850705941

Extensive question bank covering cell biology and histology. No pictures. Many questions for a relatively low-yield subject. Detailed questions with letter answers and explanations. Most helpful if the student has already reviewed the subject. Limited student feedback.

Review Questions for Neuroanatomy

$19.95 Test/965 q

Mosenthal

Parthenon, 1996, 200 pages, ISBN 1850706530

Good, non-boards-style questions with explanations. Some diagrams with quesions on lesions scattered throughout. Includes embryology of nervous system. Limited student feedback.

Basic Concepts in Embryology

$24.95 Review

Sweeney

McGraw-Hill, 1998, 456 pages

Expected in December 1997.

A **High-Yield Behavioral Science** $14.95 Review only

High Yield, Fadem

Williams & Wilkins, 1997, 102 pages, ISBN 0683029401

Clear, concise, very quick review of behavioral science. Logical presentation with charts, graphs, and tables. More compact than Fadem's other review text (*Behavioral Science Review*). Short but adequate statistics chapter. Lacks index.

A⁻ **Behavioral Science Review** $22.95 Review/500 q

BRS, Fadem

Williams & Wilkins, 1994, 237 pages, ISBN 0683029533

Easy reading, outline format, boldfacing of key terms. Good, detailed coverage of high-yield topics. Gives more information than may be needed for the USMLE. Great tables and charts. Short but complete statistics chapter. Contains review questions.

B⁺ **Ace Behavioral Science** $29.95 Review/217+ q

Ace, Cody

Mosby-Year Book, 1996, 200 pages, ISBN 0815118449 (Windows), ISBN 0815114877 (Mac)

Concise content review with boards-style questions and explanations. Thorough, easy-to-read format with numerous tables. Icons may be more distracting than helpful. No biostatistics. Test software is included with text. Money-back guarantee if you fail.

B⁺ **USMLE Behavioral Science Made Ridiculously Simple** $14.95 Review only

Sierles

MedMaster, 1997, 146 pages, ISBN 0940780348

Short, easy reading; reasonable yield. An updated version of *Behavioral Science for the Boreds*. Includes medical sociology and psychopathology. Not enough to achieve a high score. Must supplement with another text. Incomplete biostatistics. Casual style does not appeal to all students. Consider if you have very limited time. Limited student feedback on this revised book.

B **Behavioral Sciences in Psychiatry** $27.00 Review/300 q

NMS, Wiener

Williams & Wilkins, 1995, 375 pages, ISBN 0683062034

Detailed multidisciplinary outline. Neatly organized. Incorporates DSM-IV. Probably more detailed than necessary. For the motivated student starting early, or to be used as a reference. Biostatistics chapter is inadequate. Spotty coverage of some boards topics.

B High-Yield Biostatistics

$15.00   Review only

Glaser

Williams & Wilkins, 1995, 83 pages, ISBN 0683035665

Well-written, illustrated book with extensive coverage of biostatistics.
Good review exercises and tables. Still, limited-yield topic. For the motivated student; not for last-minute cramming. Suitable for a course.

B A & L's Review of Epidemiology and Biostatistics

$24.95   Review/100q

Hanrahan

Appleton & Lange, 1994, 109 pages, ISBN 083850244X

Excellent, concise overview of epidemiology with complete explanations
and diagrams. Does not include other behavioral science subtopics. Expensive and limited yield. Good for the motivated student.

B⁻ Behavioral Sciences

$17.95   Review/169 q

Oklahoma Notes, Krug

Springer-Verlag, 1995, 311 pages, ISBN 0387943935

Typewritten, easy reading. Outline format. Questions of mixed quality. Good
tables. For the motivated student.

B⁻ Digging Up the Bones: Behavioral Sciences

$17.95   Review/Cards

Linardakis

McGraw-Hill/Michaelis, 1996, 85 pages, ISBN 1884084192

Concise narrative review of behavioral sciences; disorganized format covers some high-yield topics. Choppy style with misspellings. New edition
contains flash cards.

C⁺ Behavioral Sciences

$17.95   Test/500 q

PreTest, Pattishall

McGraw-Hill, 1996, 275 pages, ISBN 0070520844

Easy reading. Questions with detailed answers. Requires some time invest-
ment.

C⁺ Medical Biostatistics and Epidemiology: Examination and Board Review

$32.95   Review/100+ q

Essex-Sorlie

Appleton & Lange, 1995, 359 pages, ISBN 0838562191

Too in-depth for USMLE biostatistics. Requires time commitment. Consider
using with a course. Sample questions may not be representative of the
USMLE Step 1.

C Clinical Epidemiology and Biostatistics

$27.00 Review/300 q

NMS, Knapp

Williams & Wilkins, 1992, 435 pages, ISBN 0683062069

Overkill for a limited-yield topic.

C Epidemiology, Biostatistics and Preventive Medicine Review

$19.95 Review/385 q

STARS, Katz

Saunders, 1997, 241 pages, ISBN 0721640842

Detailed and dense text that is excessive for USMLE Step 1 review. May be useful for an in-depth biostatistics course. Limited student feedback.

C A Review of Biostatistics

$22.95 Review only

Leaverton

Little, Brown, 1995, 117 pages, ISBN 0316518832

Review of biostatistics that does not focus on high-yield topics for the USMLE. Last two chapters cover material relevant to USMLE review. More appropriate for coursework than for USMLE review.

C− Psychiatry Made Ridiculously Simple

$12.95 Review only

Good

MedMaster, 1997, 90 pages, ISBN 0940780224

Easy reading. Includes epidemiology. Low basic science yield, but very good clinical material. New edition not yet reviewed.

NEW BOOKS—BEHAVIORAL SCIENCE

N Behavioral Science: Review for New National Boards

$25.00 Test/500+ q

Frank

J&S, 1998, ISBN 1888308001

Expected in 1998.

N Medical BioStats

— Cards

Orlando

Medfiles, 1998, ISBN 0965537323

Not yet reviewed. High-yield biostatistics and medical equations in flash-card format.

Lippincott's Illustrated Reviews: Biochemistry

$29.95 Review/250+ q

Champe

Lippincott, 1994, 443 pages, ISBN 0397510918

Excellent book, but requires time commitment, so an early start is necessary. Best used while taking the course. Excellent diagrams. Emphasizes
concepts. Good clinical correlations. Comprehensive review of biochemistry, including low-yield topics. Not for cramming unless you skim high-
yield diagrams.

Biochemistry

$22.95 Review/500 q

BRS, Marks

Williams & Wilkins, 1994, 337 pages, ISBN 0683055976

Easy-to-read outline with very good boldfaced chapter summaries. More
concise alternative to Lippincott. Outline format is not ideal for some sections. Mixed-quality diagrams. High-yield clinical correlations are given at
the end of each chapter. Questions with short answers. Some questions
are too picky.

Ace Biochemistry

$29.95 Review/326 q

Ace, Pelley

Mosby-Year Book, 1996, 400 pages, ISBN 0815186525 (Windows),
ISBN 0815186681 (Mac)

Concise content review with good clinical correlations. Easy-to-read format. Test software is included with text. Money-back guarantee if you fail.
Limited student feedback.

Biochemistry Review

$19.95 Review/600 q

STARS, Roskoski

Saunders, 1996, 242 pages, ISBN 0721651755

Content review in dense outline format with small type. Chapters are short
and include only relevant pathways. Good for students who prefer outline-
based review. Parallels a core text by the same authors. Comprehensive
exam at the end of the book has some questions with a clinical slant.

Biochemistry: Review for New National Boards

$25.00 Test/505 q

Kumar

J & S, 1993, 211 pages, ISBN 0963287311

Quick question-based review of biochemistry. Includes clinical vignettes
and extended matching questions; few diagrams. Use in conjunction with
other resources.

B⁺ Digging Up the Bones: Biochemistry

$17.95   Review only

Wilson

McGraw-Hill/Michaelis, 1997, 89 pages, ISBN 0070382174

Collection of high-yield biochemistry facts. Use for last-minute review or in conjunction with another review book. Some lists are helpful. New edition features improved formatting. Limited student feedback.

B Biochemistry

$17.95   Review/549+ q

Oklahoma Notes, Briggs

Springer-Verlag, 1995, 287 pages, ISBN 0387943986

Dense text with many hand-drawn diagrams. Good chapter on medical genetics. Non-clinically oriented questions with brief explanations in the margin. Multiple authors; inconsistent style. Easy reading, but not thorough.

B Biochemistry

$17.95   Test/500 q

PreTest, Chlapowski

McGraw-Hill, 1996, 231 pages, ISBN 0070520895

Difficult questions with detailed, referenced explanations. Better than average for this series; best for the motivated student who uses this and a review book. Contains some questions on biochemical disorders but no clinical vignettes.

B Biochemistry: An Illustrated Review with Questions and Explanations

$29.95   Review/220+ q

Friedman

Little, Brown, 1995, 220 pages, ISBN 0316294284

Good-quality, concise text review. Metabolism section is well illustrated. Molecular biochemistry section fails to emphasize important concepts and has few illustrations. Good coverage of vitamin deficiencies and genetic disorders. Too few pathways; too many structures. Questions favor basic biochemistry over clinical correlation. Gives letter answers with occasional short explanations.

B Biochemistry: Examination and Board Review

$32.95   Review/500+ q

Balcavage

Appleton & Lange, 1995, 433 pages, ISBN 0838506615

Comprehensive review of biochemistry. Requires time commitment. Appropriate as a course text. Has some clinical correlations.

B Biochemistry Illustrated

$34.95   Review only

Campbell

Churchill-Livingstone, 1994, 304 pages, ISBN 0443045739

Excellent diagrams with explanations but no questions. Good for students who prefer learning by diagrams. Readable. Very expensive. Requires time commitment.

| **B** | **Blond's Biochemistry** | $17.99 | Review only |

Guttenplan

Sulzburger & Graham, 1994, 269 pages, ISBN 0945819498

Easy reading. Requires moderate time commitment. Some topics are covered only superficially. Not boards oriented; may be more appropriate with coursework.

| **B** | **Clinical Biochemistry Made Ridiculously Simple** | $22.95 | Review only |

Goldberg

MedMaster, 1997, 93 pages, ISBN 0940780305

Conceptual approach to clinical biochemistry, with humor. The casual style does not appeal to all students. Mnemonics tend to be somewhat complicated. A good overview and integration for all metabolic pathways. Includes a 23-page clinical review that is very high yield and crammable. Also contains a unique foldout "road map" of metabolism. Not adequate as sole study source. For students with firm biochemistry background.

| **B** | **Metabolism at a Glance** | $26.95 | Review only |

Salway

Blackwell Science, 1994, 95 pages, ISBN 0632032588

Highly visual. Features diagrams with associated text. Illustrations are attractive but complicated. Use as a supplement to traditional review books. Large-page format.

| **B⁻** | **Biochemistry** | $27.00 | Review/500 q |

NMS, Davidson

Williams & Wilkins, 1994, 584 pages, ISBN 0683062050

Very long, detailed outline. Questions with detailed answers. Good pathway illustrations, but too much chemical-structure detail. Concise review of genetics. Overall, too detailed to use as a review text unless previously used during coursework. For the motivated student.

| **B⁻** | **Essentials of Biochemistry** | $32.95 | Review/100 q |

EBS, Schumm

Little, Brown, 1995, 382 pages, ISBN 0316775312

Review text with some boards-style questions and letter answers. May be more appropriate as a course text than as a review book.

| **B⁻** | **MEPC Biochemistry** | $19.95 | Test/700 q |

Glick

Appleton & Lange, 1995, 228 pages ISBN 0838557791

Picky questions with brief explanations. Few clinical vignettes.

B⁻   **PreTest Biochemistry Study Disk**   **$28.00**   Software/500 q

Chlapowski

McGraw-Hill, 1995, ISBN 0078641659 (Mac), ISBN 0078641640 (Windows)
A subset of exactly the same questions found in *PreTest Biochemistry*.
Picky, difficult questions with detailed answers. Program can vary the
length of time allocated per question. Score report of questionable value
gives breakdown of questions by type answered correctly (matching versus positive and negatively phrased questions). More expensive than the
book. Limited student feedback.

C⁺   **Genetics**   **$27.00**   Review/300 q

NMS, Friedman

Williams & Wilkins, 1995, ISBN 0683062174
Detailed outline format supplemented by numerous charts and diagrams.
Low yield. Some chapters are not relevant for boards review. For the highly
motivated student.

C   **Basic Concepts in Biochemistry:**   **$25.95**   Review only
A Student's Survival Guide

Gilbert

McGraw-Hill, 1992, 298 pages, ISBN 0070234493
Presents concise summaries of difficult biochemical concepts and principles. Because it ignores much of the high-yield material, it is not very useful for boards review. Oriented toward undergraduate courses.

C   **Genetics**   **$17.95**   Test/500 q

PreTest, Finkelstein

McGraw-Hill, 1996, 206 pages, ISBN 0070520836
Detailed questions and answers. Questions of mixed quality. Limited student feedback.

NEW BOOKS—BIOCHEMISTRY

N   **Color Atlas of Biochemistry**   **$29.95**   Review

Koolman

Thieme, 1996, 435 pages, ISBN 0865775842
Well-illustrated four-color diagrams. Not designed for boards review.

N   **Medical Biochemistry at a Glance**   **$21.95**   Review only

Greenstein

Blackwell Science, 1996, 117 pages, ISBN 0865429804
Highly visual. Diagrams with associated text. Not yet reviewed.

N **Molecular Biology QuizBank Personal Edition** $59.00 Software/500 q

Keyboard Publishing, 1995, ISBN 1573493422 (Mac), ISBN 1573493430 (Windows)

Many good questions with clear explanations. Expensive for student purchase. Limited student feedback.

A | **Medical Microbiology & Immunology: Examination and Board Review** | **$31.95** | Review/692 q

Levinson

Appleton & Lange, 1996, 523 pages, ISBN 0838562256

Clear, concise writing, with excellent diagrams and tables. Excellent immunology section. Forty-two-page "Summary of Medically Important Organisms" very crammable. Requires time commitment. Sometimes too detailed and dense. Best if started early with the course. Covers all topics, including low-yield ones. Good practice questions and comprehensive exam, but questions have letter answers only.

A⁻ | **Clinical Microbiology Made Ridiculously Simple** | **$22.95** | Review

Gladwin

MedMaster, 1997, 268 pages, ISBN 0940780321

Very good chart-based review of microbiology. Clever and humorous mnemonics. Best of this series. Text easy to read. Excellent antibiotic review helps for pharmacology as well. "Ridiculous" style does not appeal to everyone. Does not cover immunology. Excellent if you have limited time or are "burning out."

A⁻ | **Microbiology & Immunology** | **$22.95** | Review/500 q

BRS, Johnson

Williams & Wilkins, 1996, 297 pages, ISBN 0683180053

Outline-format, well-organized, organ-based approach. Good questions at the ends of chapters. Too few diagrams. Includes chapters on bacterial genetics and laboratory methods. Immunology section is concise. Compare with Levinson *(Medical Microbiology & Immunology: Examination and Board Review).*

B⁺ | **Ace Microbiology & Immunology** | **$29.95** | Review/262+ q

Ace, Rosenthal

Mosby-Year Book, 1996, 320 pages, ISBN 0815173490 (Windows), ISBN 0815186703 (Mac)

Concise but comprehensive review of microbiology and immunology in outline format. Good diagrams and tables. Icons are designed to help classify information, but overabundance may confuse some students. Additional questions are given on test software included with text. Money-back guarantee if you fail. Limited student feedback.

Appleton & Lange's Review of Microbiology and Immunology $32.95   Test/995 q

Yotis

Appleton & Lange, 1997, 288 pages, ISBN 0838502733

Large number of questions with detailed answers. Updated for USMLE-style questions. Well referenced. Inadequate as a primary source, but a very good supplement. For the motivated student.

 Medical MicroCards $16.95   150 cards

Orlando

Medfiles, 1996, 150 pages, ISBN 0965537307

Concise flash cards cover bacteriology, virology, mycology, and parasitology. Designed for fast review. No extraneous information. Covers disease characteristics, treatment, prevention, and clinical findings. Compare with Topf's *Microbiology Companion.*

B⁺ Microbiology Companion $27.95   Review/Cards

Topf

Alert and Oriented, 1997, 253 pages, ISBN 0964012413

Chart format is well organized; spiral binding makes it easy to read and carry. Most relevant to microbiology topics. Ties in relevant drugs. Has a short immunology review. High-yield flash cards (180) are a plus.

B⁺ Microbiology: Review for New National Boards $25.00   Test/507 q

Stokes

J & S, 1993, 194 pages, ISBN 096328732X

Easy reading. Covers many high-yield topics and includes case-based questions and extended matching questions. Very good question-and-answer–based review of clinically relevant microbiology and immunology, but lacking somewhat in detailed information. Helpful as a supplement to a review book.

B Buzzwords in Microbiology $19.95   Review only

Hurst

Bryan Edwards, 1994, 155 pages, ISBN 1878576089

Spiral-bound flash cards contain important facts about the most medically relevant bacteria and fungi. Directed to boards review. Bullet presentation of information affords easy and quick review. Excellent pictures and buzzwords. Useful as a speedy pocket-sized review after you have studied from a more complete text. Does not cover virology, parasitology, or immunology. Out of print.

B **Digging Up the Bones: Microbiology and Immunology**   **$17.95**   Review/Cards

Linardakis

McGraw-Hill/Michaelis, 1996, 99 pages and flash cards, ISBN 1884084192
Easy to read. Brief collection of phrases and associations. A few tables and
simple diagrams. Expensive for the amount of material given. New edition
features improved organization and promising detachable flash cards. Limited student feedback.

B **Immunology at a Glance**   **$21.95**   Review only

Playfair

Blackwell Science, 1996, 95 pages, ISBN 0865426775
Sophisticated, well-thought-out, diagram-based synopsis of immunology.
Text and figures are on the left, with legends on the right. Expensive given
the length of the book, but worth considering for students who like a
graphic approach. Not designed for the USMLE. Limited student feedback.

B **Microbiology and Immunology**   **$17.95**   Review/312+ q

Oklahoma Notes, Hyde

Springer-Verlag, 1995, 229 pages, ISBN 0387943927
Easy to read, but not adequate as sole study source. Good summary state-
ments are given at the end of each chapter. Extended matching questions.
Poor typeface and diagrams. Unequal coverage.

B **Microbiology & Immunology: An Illustrated Review**   **$29.95**   Review/450+ q
with Questions and Explanations

Hentges

Little, Brown, 1995, 304 pages, ISBN 0316357847
Comprehensive review takes time commitment. Revised edition has updated tables and charts. Improved format and organization. Summation
chapter at the end of the book is of limited value. Limited student feedback.

B⁻ **Blond's Microbiology**   **$15.99**   Review only

Alcamo

Sulzberger & Graham, 1994, 181 pages, ISBN 0945819412
Text review. Spotty coverage of some key topics. Below average for this
series.

B⁻ **Essential Immunology Review**   **$19.95**   Test/422 q

Roitt

Blackwell Science, 1995, 319 pages, ISBN 0865424586
Boards-style questions with explanations that also discuss the incorrect
answers. Required text at some medical schools. Very mixed reviews.

MEPC Microbiology

$19.95   Test/770 q

Kim

Appleton & Lange, 1995, 257 pages, ISBN 0838563082

Includes clinical vignettes. Good infectious-disease questions. Variable-quality questions. Easy read. Explanations are brief and direct.

Microbiology

$17.95   Test/500 q

PreTest, Tilton

McGraw-Hill, 1996, 191 pages, ISBN 0070520887

Mixed-quality questions with detailed, often verbose explanations. Useful for additional question-based review in bacteriology and virology, but not high yield.

Microbiology and Infectious Disease

$26.00   Review/500 q

NMS, Virella

Williams & Wilkins, 1996, 575 pages, ISBN 0683062352

Outline form. Too detailed in some areas. Insufficient immunology; NMS has a separate immunology book. Lacks good explanation of bacterial genetics. Updated material on AIDS. Useful only if previously used as a textbook. Limited student feedback.

Microbiology QuizBanks Vol. 2 & 3

$69.00   Software/800+ q

Gotts

Keyboard Publishing, 1995, ISBN 1573493252 (Mac), 1573493279 (Windows)

Computer-based questions with explanations. Helpful to gauge strengths and weaknesses. Questions are electronically referenced to Sherris Microbiology Text Stack (sold separately). Expensive for a student; consider for library acquisition.

Immunology

$27.00   Review/300 q

NMS, Hyde

Williams & Wilkins, 1995, 316 pages, ISBN 068306231X

Outline form. Very detailed. Good figures and explanations of laboratory methods. Lengthy for immunology alone. Requires time commitment.

The Keyboard Immunology Series Personal Edition

$149.00   Software/400 q

Roitt

Keyboard Publishing, 1995, ISBN 1573492035 (Mac), ISBN 1573492043 (Windows).

Includes *Immunology QuizBank Vol. 1*. More appropriate for use with course work. Includes *Essential Immunology* Text Stack by Roitt. Questions are conveniently cross-linked to Text Stack. Text can be exported to a word processor. Available for PC and Macintosh. Good learning tool, but beyond the student budget. More appropriate as a library purchase.

The Keyboard Microbiology Series Personal Edition $149.00 Software/900+ q

Ryan

Keyboard Publishing, 1995, ISBN 1573492701 (Mac), ISBN 157349271X
(Windows)

Includes two Microbiology QuizBanks and the electronic edition of *Sherris
Medical Microbiology*. Questions cross-linked to Text Stack. Includes immunology and a comprehensive exam. High-quality pictures. Text can be
exported to a word processor. More appropriate for use with course work
and as a reference. Good learning tool but beyond the student budget.
More appropriate as a library purchase.

 Microbiology & Immunology Casebook $17.95 Review/185 q

Barrett

Little, Brown, 1995, 262 pages, ISBN 0316081329

Uses case examples to cover major concepts. Cases do not resemble typical boards vignettes. Useful only as a supplement to a review book.

 PreTest Microbiology Study Disk $28.00 Software/500 q

Tilton

McGraw-Hill, 1995, ISBN 0078641551 (Mac), ISBN 0078641543 (Windows)

Subset of exactly the same questions found in *PreTest Microbiology*. Picky,
difficult questions with detailed answers. Program can vary the length of
time allotted per question. Score report of questionable value gives breakdown of questions by type answered correctly (matching versus positive
and negatively phrased questions). More expensive than the book. Limited
student feedback.

 Immunology Illustrated Outline $19.95 Review only

Male

Raven Press, 1991, ISBN 0397448252

Pocket-sized booklet, well organized, concise. Quick to read and review.
Not targeted for boards review.

NEW BOOKS—MICROBIOLOGY

 Clinical Microbiology Review $31.25 Review

Warinner

Wysteria Ltd., 1995, 140 pages, ISBN 0965116204

Concise but comprehensive review in chart form with some clinical correlations. No immunology. Spatial organization, color coding, and bulleting of
facts facilitate review of subject. Great cross-reference section groups organisms by general characteristics. Limited but quite positive student feedback.

N ## Concepts in Microbiology, Immunology, and Infectious Disease $17.95 Review/100+ q

Gupta

Parthenon, 1997, 150 pages, ISBN 1850707979

Brief paragraphs in outline form on each disease cover most of the important points. Good clinical questions at the end of each section. Good section on immunologic disorders. Format may not appeal to all students. No illustrations. Best for the well-prepared student. Limited student feedback.

N ## Flash Micro — Cards

Ting

Stanford Ink, 1997, 131 pages

Concise flash cards designed for boards review. Includes 190 pathogens. No immunology. Color coded. Compare with Orlando's *Medical Micro Cards*.

N ## The Integrator Series in Microbiology — Chart

Sanford

Integrator, 1996, 26 pages, ISBN 8801612982

Oversize chart-format review of microbiology for boards review.

N ## Lippincott's Illustrated Reviews: Microbiology $27.95 Review

Strohl

Lippincott, 1997, ISBN 0397515685

Expected in late 1997. Features a comprehensive, highly illustrated review of microbiology similar in style to Champe's *Lippincott's Illustrated Reviews: Biochemistry*.

N ## Microbiology Review $19.95 Review/600 q

STARS, Walker

Saunders, 1997, 504 pages, ISBN 0721646425

Will parallel core text by the same authors. Expected in late 1997.

N ## Basic Concepts in Immunology $24.95 Review

Clancy

McGraw-Hill, 1998, 328 pages

Pathology

$22.95   Review/500 q

BRS, Schneider

Williams & Wilkins, 1993, 412 pages, ISBN 0683076086

Excellent, concise review with appropriate emphasis. Outline-format chapters with boldfacing of key facts. Excellent questions with explanations at the end of each chapter and a comprehensive exam at the end of the book. Well-organized tables and diagrams. Some good black-and-white photographs representative of classic pathology. Short on clinical details for vignette questions. Consistently high student recommendations. Must start early, but very worthwhile to master this book. Correlate with color photographs from an atlas.

Pathology: Review for New National Boards

$25.00   Test/509 q

Miller

J & S, 1993, 222 pages, ISBN 0963287338

Question-and-answer–based review of pathology. Includes many case-based questions. Focuses on high-yield topics. Good black-and-white photographs. Some picky questions with incomplete answers. Inadequate as sole source of review. Expensive for number of questions.

Pathophysiology of Disease: An Introduction to Clinical Medicine

$32.95   Review/Few q

McPhee

Appleton & Lange, 1997, 521 pages, ISBN 0838576788

Interdisciplinary course text useful for understanding the pathophysiology of clinical symptoms. Excellent integration of basic sciences with mechanisms of disease. Great graphs, diagrams, and tables. Most helpful if used during coursework due to length. Few non-boards-style questions. Clinical emphasis nicely complements *BRS Pathology*. New edition not yet reviewed.

Ace Pathology

$29.95   Text/414 q

Ace, Wurzel

Mosby-Year Book, 1996, 400 pages, ISBN 0815192762 (Windows), ISBN 0815194285 (Mac)

Features a detailed content review with good photomicrographs. Test software with additional questions is included with text. Money-back guarantee if you fail. Limited student feedback.

Appleton & Lange's Review of General Pathology

$32.95 Test/896 q

Lewis

Appleton & Lange, 1993, 197 pages, ISBN 0838501613

Short text sections followed by lots of questions with answers. Some very useful high-yield tables at the beginning of each section. Good photomicrographs. Covers only general pathology (i.e., no organ-based pathology). Can be used as a supplement to more detailed texts. Reviewable in a short period.

Digging Up the Bones: Pathology

$17.95 Review only

Linardakis

McGraw-Hill/Michaelis, 1997, 130 pages, ISBN 0070382166

Easy reading. Brief collection of phrases and associations often based on answers to assorted multiple-choice questions. Expensive for the amount of material. New edition features new photomicrographs (gross and microscopic) and improved editing.

Medical Exam Review: Pathology

$19.95 Test/600 q

A&L/MEPC, Fayemi

Appleton & Lange, 1994, 317 pages, ISBN 0838584411

Good-quality questions with explanations. Good case-study chapter. Use as a supplement to other review books.

Pathology: Examination and Board Review

$29.95 Review/Few q

Newland

Appleton & Lange, 1995, 314 pages, ISBN 0838577199

Short, to-the-point text review with some high-quality charts and photomicrographs. Non-boards-style questions at the end of each chapter with letter answers only.

Pathology Notes

$26.95 Review only

Chandrasoma

Appleton & Lange, 1992, 788 pages, ISBN 0838551645

Lengthy but well organized and easy to read. Requires considerable time commitment. Good tables. No photographs. Good line drawings. Compare the format with *Pocket Companion to Robbins'* as to which best suits your style. Companion to *Concise Pathology* by same authors.

Pocket Companion to Robbins' Pathologic Basis of Diseases

$25.00 Review only

Robbins

Saunders, 1995, 620 pages, ISBN 0721657427

Good for reviewing associations between keywords and specific diseases. Very condensed, easy to understand. Explains most important diseases and pathologic processes. No photographs or illustrations. Useful as a quick reference.

B | Essentials of Pathophysiology

EBS, Kaufman

$39.95 Review/69 q

Little, Brown, 1996, 650 pages, ISBN 0316484059

Review book with few questions. Features clinical descriptions of important diseases, but too detailed for high-yield review. Good diagrams, tables, and black-and-white photographs. More appropriate as a course text and reference. For the highly motivated student. Limited student feedback.

B | Pathology

Oklahoma Notes, Holliman

$17.95 Review/140 q

Springer-Verlag, 1994, 279 pages, ISBN 0387943900

Dense text. Few diagrams and tables. No illustrations. Questions with letter answers only. Good when you have no time for comprehensive review books.

B | Pathology Illustrated

Govan

$54.95 Review only

Churchill-Livingstone, 1995, 843 pages, ISBN 0443050686

Lengthy, but fast reading. Well illustrated with many line drawings. User-friendly format. Worth considering despite price. New edition not reviewed.

B⁻ | Pathologic Basis of Disease Self-Assessment and Review

Compton

$21.75 Test/1600+ q

Saunders, 1995, 239 pages, ISBN 0721640419

Features a huge number of practice questions, some very difficult and detailed. A good buy for the number of questions. Time-consuming. Only for the dedicated student.

B⁻ | Pathology

NMS, LiVolsi

$27.00 Review/500 q

Williams & Wilkins, 1994, 508 pages, ISBN 0683062433

Outline form. Comprehensive review of large amount of material. Sometimes too detailed. Slow reading.

B⁻ | Pathology

PreTest, Brown

$17.95 Test/500 q

McGraw-Hill, 1996, 299 pages, ISBN 0070520860

Picky, difficult questions with detailed, complete answers. Often obscure or esoteric questions. Good-quality black-and-white photographs; no color photographs. Can be used as a supplement to other review books. For the motivated student who desires challenging exposure to lots of photographs.

Pathology Facts

$19.95   Review only

Harruff

Lippincott, 1994, 424 pages, ISBN 0397512589

A handbook-sized text database, organized by disease. Limited topic coverage. Worth considering.

Pathology QuizBank Vol. 2

$99.00   Software/1000+ q

Faculty UC Davis

Keyboard Publishing, 1995, ISBN 1573493295 (Mac), ISBN 1573493317 (Windows)

Expensive software database of board-style questions with good, detailed explanations. Some repetitive questions. Requires time commitment. Electronically referenced to Robbins' *Pathology Text Stack*. Quizzer has no timer or ability to custom-generate tests. Good product, but expensive. Best for library acquisition.

The Keyboard Pathology Series Personal Edition

$199.00   Software/1300+ q

Cotran

Keyboard Publishing, 1995, ISBN 1573492116 (Mac), ISBN 1573492124 (Windows)

Includes electronic edition of the 5th edition of Robbins' *Pathologic Basis of Disease* on CD-ROM and *Pathology QuizBank*. Very good if used as reference or with course. Beyond the student budget. More appropriate as a library purchase.

PreTest Pathology Study Disk

$28.00   Software/500 q

Brown

McGraw-Hill, 1995, ISBN 0078641594 (Mac); ISBN 0078641586 (Windows)

Subset of exactly the same questions found in *PreTest Pathology*. Picky, difficult questions with detailed answers. Program can vary the length of time allotted per question. Score report (of questionable value) gives breakdown of questions by type answered correctly (matching versus positive and negatively phrased questions). More expensive than the book, with mixed-quality pictures. Limited student feedback.

Wheater's Basic Histopathology

$49.00   Review only

Burkitt

Churchill-Livingstone, 1996, 252 pages, ISBN 0443050880

Color atlas with text. Contains pictures of pathologic histology. Not directed to boards-type review. May be more useful for photomicrograph-based questions. New edition not yet reviewed.

N | **Colour Atlas of Anatomical Pathology** | **$56.00** | Review
Cooke
Churchill-Livingstone, 1995, 261 pages, ISBN 0443050627
Beautifully photographed atlas of gross pathology. Expensive, but definitely
worth browsing.

N | **Essential Pathology** | **$49.95** | Review
Rubin
Lippincott, 1995, ISBN 0397514875
Thin book with good color illustrations that are useful for second year and
beyond. Limited feedback.

N | **Review Questions for Pathology** | **$19.95** | Test/
Jones
Parthenon, 1997, 180 pages, ISBN 1850705992
Not yet reviewed.

N | **Basic Concepts in Pathology** | **$24.95** | Review
Brown
McGraw-Hill, 1998, 312 pages
Expected in December 1997.

A⁻

Lippincott's Illustrated Reviews: Pharmacology $29.95   Review/230+ q

Harvey

Lippincott, 1997, 475 pages, ISBN 0397515677

Outline format with practice questions and many excellent and memorable illustrations and tables. Cross-referenced to Lippincott's *Biochemistry*. Good for the "big picture." Good pathophysiologic approach. Detailed, so must start early. For the motivated student. Ten illustrated case studies with questions and answers in the appendix.

A⁻

Pharm Cards: A Review for Medical Students $25.95   Review only

Johannsen

Little, Brown, 1995, 195 cards, ISBN 0316465496

Review in compact index-card format; very popular with students. High-lights important features of major drugs/drug classes. Perfect for class review; also offers a quick, focused review for the USMLE. Lacks pharmacokinetics. Good charts and diagrams. Highly rated by students who enjoy flash-card-based review. Follow instructions on "sample pharmcard" regarding use of the cards for USMLE review.

A⁻

Pharmacology: Examination and Board Review $29.95   Review/650+ q

Katzung

Appleton & Lange, 1995, 509 pages, ISBN 083858067X

Text is well organized in a narrative format. Good charts and tables. Large number of relevant and challenging questions with concise explanations. Good for drug interactions and toxicities. Text is quite detailed and requires substantial time commitment. Includes some low-yield/obscure drugs. The 40-page (417–457) crammable list of "top boards drugs" is especially high yield. Compare closely with *Lippincott's Illustrated Reviews: Pharmacology*.

B⁺

Digging Up the Bones: Pharmacology $17.95   Review/Cards

Linardakis

McGraw-Hill/Michaelis, 1996, 99 pages and 100+ flash cards, ISBN 007038214X

Easy reading. Brief collection of phrases and drug associations. Expensive for the amount of material. Contains 100+ flash cards of top drugs with clinical use, mechanisms, and side effects.

B⁺

Mosby Ace Pharmacology $29.95   Review/462 q

Ace, Enna

Mosby-Year Book, 1996, 394 pages, ISBN 0815131127 (Windows), ISBN 0815131526 (Mac)

Concise content review with some boards-style questions. Very thorough explanations. Test software included with text. Money-back guarantee if you fail.

B⁺ **Pharmacology: An Illustrated Review with Questions and Explanations** $29.95   Review/400+ q

Ebadi

Little, Brown, 1996, 336 pages, ISBN 0316199575

New edition with many more illustrations and tables. Comprehensive review of pharmacology, but the content and emphasis do not always reflect high-yield topics. Some emphasis on neuropharmacology. Good for the student who likes comprehensive chart/illustration–based review. Requires time commitment. Includes clinical case-based questions.

B⁺ **Pharmacology: Review for New National Boards** $25.00   Test/539 q

Billingsley

J & S, 1995, 186 pages, ISBN 0963287370

Question-and-answer book, typical for this series. Includes clinical vignettes. Good explanations cover many high-yield pharmacology topics. Easy, fast reading. Questions about drug structures probably low yield. Useful adjunct to a review book. Limited student feedback.

B **Blond's Pharmacology** $19.99   Review only

Kostrzewa

Sulzburger & Graham, 1995, 398 pages, ISBN 094581948X

Concise review of pharmacology. Many good diagrams. Some key topics inadequately covered.

B **Clinical Pharmacology Made Ridiculously Simple** $18.95   Review only

Olson

MedMaster, 1997, 162 pages, ISBN 0940780178

Includes general principles and many drug summary charts. Particularly strong in cardiovascular drugs and antimicrobials; incomplete in other areas. Mostly tables; lacks the humorous illustrations and mnemonics typical of this series. Well organized, but occasionally too detailed. Effective as a chart-based review book but not as a sole study source. Must supplement with a more detailed text.

B **Essentials of Pharmacology** $29.95   Review/250+ q

EBS, Theoharides

Little, Brown, 1996, 444 pages, ISBN 0316839361

Review text with some boards-style questions and letter answers. May be more appropriate as a course text than as a review book. New edition has many good tables that summarize important drug mechanisms and toxicities. Too much boldface is distracting. Limited student feedback.

B **MEPC Pharmacology** $19.95 Test/700 q

Krzanowski

Appleton & Lange, 1995, 267 pages, ISBN 0838562272

Questions with brief, direct explanations. Well referenced answers.

B **Medical Pharmacology at a Glance** $24.95 Review only

Neal

Blackwell Science, 1997, 92 pages, ISBN 0865427194

Contains sophisticated, well-thought-out figures followed by explanations. Visual synthesis of sites and mechanisms of drug actions. Occasionally, British terminology may be confusing. High yield for those with limited study time. Not designed for USMLE review, but worth considering for the diagrammatic approach. Useful only as a supplement to a review text. May be hard to find.

B **Pharmacology** $22.95 Review/450 q

BRS, Rosenfeld

Williams & Wilkins, 1993, 357 pages, ISBN 0683073613

Outline format. Good use of boldface, although few tables. Questions are of moderate difficulty with short answers. Worse than average for this series. New edition expected in October 1997 (ISBN 0683180509).

B **Pharmacology** $27.00 Review/450+ q

NMS, Jacob

Williams & Wilkins, 1996, 373 pages, ISBN 0683062514

Outline format. More tables and diagrams in new edition. Often too detailed. Lacks emphasis on high-yield material. Has a lengthy USMLE-type exam. Requires time commitment. Typical for this series.

B **Pharmacology** $17.95 Review/560+ q

Oklahoma Notes, Moore

Springer-Verlag, 1995, 235 pages, ISBN 0387943943

Conceptual approach. Features USMLE-type questions with brief explanations. A concise and readable review book.

B **Pharmacology** $17.95 Test/500 q

PreTest, DiPalma

McGraw-Hill, 1996, 253 pages, ISBN 0070520879

Typical for this series. Questions are picky and challenging with detailed answers. Lacks clinical vignettes. For the motivated student.

B⁻ **Med Charts, Pharmacology** $14.95 Review only
Rosenbach
ILOC, 1993, 171 pages, ISBN 1882531000
Contains tables and summaries. Good for quick review, but requires previous reading from other sources. May be helpful for students who prefer studying charts.

B⁻ **PreTest Pharmacology Study Disk** $28.00 Software/500 q
DiPalma
McGraw-Hill, 1995, ISBN 0078641616 (Mac), ISBN 0078641608 (Windows)
Subset of exactly the same questions found in *PreTest Pharmacology*. Picky, difficult questions with detailed answers. Program can vary the length of time allotted per question. Score report of questionable value gives breakdown of questions by type answered correctly (matching versus positive and negatively phrased questions). More expensive than the book. Limited student feedback.

NEW BOOKS—PHARMACOLOGY

N **Basic Concepts in Pharmacology** $24.95 Review only
Stringer
McGraw-Hill, 1996, 288 pages, ISBN 0070631654
Presents summaries of "elusive" concepts in pharmacology, from simple to complex. Not yet reviewed.

N **The Phunny Pharm** $18.95 Review only
Reidhead
Hanley & Belfus, 1997, 207 pages, ISBN 1560531142
Pharmacology review based on memory devices and illustrations. Sometimes too intricate. For the student who likes this approach; somewhat similar to the *Ridiculously Simple* series. Examine carefully.

N **Medical PharmFile** — Cards
Feinstein
Medfiles, 1998, ISBN 0965537315
Not yet reviewed. High-yield pharmacology in flash-card format similar to *Medical MicroCards*.

N **The Pharmacology Companion** $27.95 Review/Cards
Gallia
Alert and Oriented, 1997, 300 pages, ISBN 096401243X
Not yet reviewed. Chart format. Spiral bound with high-yield flash cards.

A

Physiology

$22.95 Review/400 q

BRS, Costanzo

Williams & Wilkins, 1995, 288 pages, ISBN 0683021346

Clear, concise review of physiology. Fast, easy reading. Comprehensive and efficient. Great charts and tables. Good practice questions with explanations with a clinically oriented final exam. Excellent review book, but may not be enough for in-depth coursework. Comparatively weak respiratory and acid–base sections.

B+

Ace Physiology

$29.95 Review/250 q

Ace, Ackermann

Mosby-Year Book, 1996, 285 pages, ISBN 081510054X (Windows), ISBN 0815109334 (Mac)

Concise yet thorough content review with some boards-style questions. Outline format is easy to read. Good illustrations. Test software included with text. Money-back guarantee if you fail.

B+

Clinical Physiology Made Ridiculously Simple

$18.95 Review only

Goldberg

MedMaster, 1995, 152 pages, ISBN 0940780216

Easy reading with many "ridiculous" associations. Style does not work for everyone. Not as well illustrated as the rest of series. Short length allows for quick review.

B+

Physiology: An Illustrated Review with Questions & Explanations

$29.95 Review/320 q

Tadlock

Little, Brown, 1995, 333 pages, ISBN 0316827649

New edition features updated text with superb illustrations and tables. Format and organization improved. Quite detailed. Best used with the course. Some questions include complex calculations not typical for the USMLE. Requires time commitment.

B

Blond's Physiology

$20.00 Review only

Grossman

Sulzburger & Graham, 1995, 439 pages, ISBN 0945819420

Comprehensive but easy-to-read review text of physiology. Clear and simple classic diagrams and charts. Better than average for this series. Strong endocrine chapter. Good hormone list.

B Color Atlas of Physiology

$29.00   Review only

Despopoulos

Georg Thieme Verlag, 1991, 369 pages, ISBN 0865773823

Compact, with more than 156 colorful but complicated diagrams on the right and dense explanatory text on the left. Some translation problems. A unique, highly visual approach worthy of consideration. Useful as an adjunct to other review books.

B MEPC Physiology

$19.95   Test/700 q

Penney

Appleton & Lange, 1996, 257 pages, ISBN 0838562221

Questions with brief, direct answers. Reflects USMLE Step 1 format. Compare with *PreTest Physiology*. Good as an adjunct to other review texts. Limited student feedback.

B Physiology

$27.00   Review/300 q

NMS, Bullock

Williams & Wilkins, 1995, 641 pages, ISBN 068306259X

Very complete text in outline form. Often too detailed, but some good diagrams. Moderately difficult questions with detailed answers. Provides some pathophysiology and clinical correlations. More useful if used as a course text and reference; too long as a review text. Inexpensive for the amount of material. For the motivated student.

B Physiology

$17.95   Test/500 q

PreTest, Ryan

McGraw-Hill, 1996, 228 pages, ISBN 0070520852

Questions with detailed, well-written explanations. Some questions too difficult or picky. May be useful for the motivated student following extensive review from other sources.

B Physiology: A Review for the New National Boards

$25.00   Test/506 q

Jakoi

J & S, 1994, 214 pages, ISBN 0963287346

Good review book, but inadequate as sole source of review. Quick reading. Below-average question quality for this series. Answer discussions cover many important topics.

B⁻ Essentials of Physiology

$35.95   Review/100 q

EBS, Sperelakis

Little, Brown, 1996, 680 pages, ISBN 0316806285

Dense review text with some boards-style questions and letter answers. Numerous diagrams, including some that are not particularly helpful. May be more appropriate as a course text than as a review book. Significant time commitment.

B⁻ **Physiology**   **$17.95**   Review/345 q
Oklahoma Notes, Thies
Springer-Verlag, 1995, 280 pages, ISBN 0387943978
Dense text. Inconsistent quality of sections. Emphasizes general concepts,
but incomplete. Boards-type questions with short answers. Some errors.

B⁻ **PreTest Physiology Study Disk**   **$28.00**   Software/500 q
Ryan
McGraw-Hill, 1995, ISBN 0078641578 (Mac), ISBN 007864156X (Windows)
Subset of exactly the same questions found in *PreTest Physiology*. Many
questions are picky and difficult. Program can vary the length of time allotted per question. Score report of questionable value gives breakdown of
questions by type answered correctly (matching versus positive and negatively phrased questions). More expensive than the book with mixed-quality
pictures. Limited student feedback.

NEW BOOKS—PHYSIOLOGY

N **Appleton & Lange's Review of Physiology**   **$29.95**   Test/700+ q
Penney
Appleton & Lange, 1998, ISBN 0838502741
Boards-style questions with letter answers and explanations. Not yet re-
viewed.

N **Concepts in Physiology**   **$17.95**   Review/100+ q
Gupta
Parthenon, 1996, 135 pages, ISBN 1850707308
System-based review in paragraph form. Some sections have clinical
questions at the end of the chapter with explanations. Format may not ap-
peal to all students. Limited student feedback.

N **Linardakis' Illustrated Review of Physiology** **$37.95**   Review/200+ q
Linardakis
Michaelis Medical, 1998, 340 pages, ISBN 1884084176
Expected in early 1998. Comprehensive, illustration-based review of medi-
cal physiology. Integrated text and color illustrations.

N **Review Questions for Physiology**   **$19.95**   Test/600 q
Pasley
Parthenon, 1997, 180 pages, ISBN 1850706018
Not yet reviewed.

Commercial Review Courses

Compass Medical Education
    Network
FMSG/IMP Step 1 Review Course
Kaplan Educational Centers
National Medical School Review
Northwestern Learning Center
Postgraduate Medical Review
    Education
The Princeton Review
Youel's Prep, Inc.

Commercial preparation courses can be helpful for some students, but these courses are expensive and require significant time commitment. They are usually effective in organizing study material for students who feel overwhelmed by the volume of material. Note that the multiweek courses may be quite intense and thus leave limited time for independent study. Also note that some commercial courses are designed for first-time test takers while others focus on students who are repeating the examination. Some courses focus on foreign medical graduates who want to take all three Steps in a limited amount of time. Student experience and satisfaction with review courses are highly variable. We suggest that you discuss options with recent graduates of review courses you are considering. Course content and structure can evolve rapidly. Some student opinions can be found in discussion groups on the World Wide Web.

Compass Medical Education Network

Compass Medical Education Network, formerly known as ArcVentures Medical Education Services, offers a series of live-lecture preparation courses for USMLE Step 1. Compass is an affiliate of Rush Presbyterian–St. Luke's Medical Center in Chicago, Illinois, and has been providing live-lecture review courses for the USMLE since 1988.

Courses are taught by faculty members who are recognized not only for their medical expertise but also for their teaching abilities. For Step 1 courses, faculty consist of medical school professors and experts in the basic sciences.

All of Compass' courses are live-lecture and feature Compass' comprehensive notes. These notes, which are updated annually, are written by the faculty, correspond to the lectures, and feature high-yield USMLE information. Compass courses also provide hundreds of practice questions as well as test-taking strategies. All Compass courses (excluding the PrePrep course) are covered by a guarantee: if a Compass student doesn't pass the USMLE, he or she can take the course again for half the price.

Compass' 1998 schedule includes PrePrep, IntensePrep, AcceleratedPrep, and ExtendedPrep courses. Courses in the US are offered in Chicago; Detroit; Houston; Los Angeles; Miami; Clifton, New Jersey; New York City; and Washington, DC. International locations include San Juan, Puerto Rico; Guadalajara, Mexico; and India. In addition, Compass IntensePrep Step 1 courses will be offered at more than 20 US medical school campuses in 1998.

The four-week Compass Step 1 IntensePrep course is designed specifically for second-year medical students who are first-time takers of the exam. This course reviews the seven basic sciences, with emphasis on materials most likely to be found on the exam. Through live lectures, course notes, and hundreds of practice questions, students receive a structured review of the basic sciences. In addition, this course offers students a full-length (720-question) simulated USMLE exam. A Step 1 AcceleratedPrep course will also be offered in 1998. This course is similar to Compass' Step 1 IntensePrep course but is six weeks in length and will be held in Cherry Hill, New Jersey.

The Compass Step 1 Prep (seven weeks in length) and ExtendedPrep (15 weeks in length) courses offer more in-depth coverage of the basic sciences. These courses include small group sessions that are specifically designed to reinforce the lectures and to help students retain more information through discussion of USMLE-type practice questions. Both courses also include a comprehensive diagnostic exam and practice tests for each subject area. A PrePrep course can also be taken prior to either the Prep or the ExtendedPrep course to provide an initial review of the material.

Tuition for Compass courses ranges from $975 for the IntensePrep course to $5000 for the ExtendedPrep course. For more information, including course schedules, complete descriptions, and an application, please contact Compass at 1-800-818-9128 or write to:

Compass Medical Education Network
820 W. Jackson Boulevard
Chicago, IL 60607

E-mail should be sent to: csimek@arcventures.com

Compass can also be found online at http://www.compass-meded.com

FMSG/IMP Step 1 Review Course

FMSG Publishing, in conjunction with IMP, Ltd., conducts two-day "live-lecture" courses for the USMLE Step 1. Typically held on weekends in New York City one to two months prior to the exam, each course includes 12 hours of lecture with accompanying study notes plus a simulated three-hour practice exam and review. Courses are designed specifically to help domestic and IMG candidates assess their aptitude, determine their weaknesses, and maximize their study time while reviewing high-yield topics, repeat concepts, and the most pertinent facts related to the Step 1 exam. Lectures are given by Dr. Stanley Zaslau and/or other US-trained physicians. Courses are also available in Europe. For further information, call 1-800-443-4194 or 1-716-689-6000, fax 1-716-689-6187, or write to:

IMP, Ltd. (International Medical Placement)
100 Sylvan Parkway, Suite 200
Amherst, NY 14228

E-mail should be sent to: impltd@worldnet.att.net

FMSG Publishing can also be found online at: http://www.cyberdeas.com/imp

Kaplan Educational Centers

Kaplan's 1988 Step 1 review course is organized by organ system. The course is designed to allow medical students to focus on the most exam-worthy material using a variety of review tools, including a set of seven books, video lectures, and over 1000 USMLE-style questions (with comprehensive written explanations). All of the materials in Kaplan's Step 1 course are newly updated for 1998.

The Kaplan course includes diagnostic testing and an individual study plan. Students begin their preparation with a three-hour diagnostic test and comprehensive questionnaire. This data is computer-analyzed, and each student receives a customized study plan that assesses strengths and weaknesses and suggests a study timeline. All enrolled students also receive a copy of the new *USMLE Step 1 Starter Kit* (Appleton & Lange) featuring two 180-question diagnostic tests with comprehensive explanations and on-line computer feedback.

Kaplan's Step 1 course also includes a set of seven organ-system-based review books. Each page includes an outline written by faculty experts along with numerous student-suggested "margin notes" with high-yield tips, clinical correlates, and mnemonics. There is also ample space for students to add their own margin notes.

All Kaplan course lectures are on video. This allows a student to watch only the lecture he or she needs at a convenient time. (Comprehensive live-lecture programs are also offered in selected locations, including some medical school campuses.) The video lecture modules can be reviewed by organ system or by discipline. Instructors are all faculty at US medical schools and are selected on the basis of their teaching ability and their familiarity with the USMLE Step 1. Many instructors are noted review-book authors.

Kaplan's course includes USMLE-style practice questions with detailed explanations of correct and incorrect answer choices. In 1998, Kaplan will be introducing over 1000 new practice questions into the course. Most of these questions will feature clinical vignettes, and all will also include comprehensive written explanations. The course concludes with four simulated exams that emulate the USMLE in booklet length, style, and content.

Kaplan's USMLE Step 1 course is offered at over 120 locations worldwide. Course price varies with length of study and ranges from $595 (30-day option offered for second-year medical students) to $2700 and up (three-month Step 1 and Step 2 combination course geared to medical graduates). In 1998, Kaplan is also offering a "books only" option for $325 plus tax and shipping. For information about any Kaplan USMLE course, call 1-800-KAP-TEST or write to:

Kaplan Medical
888 Seventh Avenue, 22nd Floor
New York, NY 10106

For information about arranging a live Step 1 course on your campus, call 1-800-950-0350 x5939.

Kaplan can also be found online at: http:www.kaplan.com/usmle

National Medical School Review

National Medical School Review (NMSR) programs provide an interactive, integrated review for the USMLE Step 1. They utilize a variety of learning modes, including 100% live lectures by faculty; diagnostic testing that helps students identify their content strengths; and weaknesses; multiple-choice question practice; and study skills instruction.

NMSR faculty members are chosen for their expertise in teaching USMLE content material, and many have authored or contributed to highly acclaimed review books for the USMLE. All programs emphasize the current high-yield information tested on Step 1 while also focusing on methods that are intended to maximize understanding and retention of material at test time. Faculty members use an integrated instructional approach that includes audiovisual techniques.

Each program includes study skills instruction that is given by learning skills specialists and that includes lectures on study methods, test taking, and other study skills designed to help students prioritize, consolidate, understand, retain, and apply the information taught. Students also receive an extensive set of review materials, including notes, faculty-authored review textbooks, and practice questions that are continually updated to reflect the content tested on Step 1. Material is given to students on the first day of the program and is theirs to keep and study. Audio taping of lectures is permitted.

NMSR offers three live-lecture Step 1 review programs. The 105+ hour Preview Program is designed primarily for US medical students taking Step 1 for the first time; the 240+ hour Review Program covers material in greater depth for students who need more time for review or who have had an initial failure; and the 450+ hour Supplemental Instruction Program (250+ lecture hours and 200+ facilitated small group hours) is designed for students who have been away from the content for an extended period of time, scored less than 156, or have had multiple failures.

NMSR also offers a "startup study kit" that includes special "pre-review" materials and is sent to all students when they enroll. Step 1 students receive the five-volume *Board Simulator Series* (Williams & Wilkins), which features more than 3850 questions with extensive answer explanations.

Fees for the Step 1 programs are: 105+ hour Preview Program, $1000; 240+ hour Review Program, $2700; 450+ hour Supplemental Instruction Program, $5000. Substantial discounts are available for enrollment in multiple programs, and NMSR's guarantee allows a student to repeat a program at a significantly reduced rate. The programs are available at several sites in the United States. A staff of medical education specialists are available to answer questions concerning the USMLE, licensing, and other points of interest to the physician-in-training. To receive an application and/or more information, call 1-800-533-8850 or 1-714-476-6282, fax 1-714-476-6286, or write:

National Medical School Review
4500 Campus Drive, Suite 201
Newport Beach, CA 92660

E-mail should be sent to: nmsr@nmsr.com

NMSR can also be found online at: http://www.nmsr.com

Northwestern Learning Center

Northwestern Learning Center offers live-lecture review courses for both the USMLE Step 1 and the COMLEX Level 1 examinations. Two types of courses are available for each exam: NBI 100—Primary Care for the Boards[98] and NBI 300—Intensive Care for the Boards[98]. NBI 100 is an on-site, 15-hour live-lecture review that is offered in two- or three-day formats and utilizes Northwestern Learning Center's TALLP[98] techniques in conjunction with a systematic review of high-yield boards facts and concepts. This course is designed to organize students and to help them focus on the most essential aspects of their boards preparation. NBI 300 is a comprehensive, live boards preparation review conducted by a team of university faculty and/or authors of top boards review texts. It also includes over 1800 pages of lecture notes and a large pool of simulated exams. NBI 300 is offered each year in 15- or 18-day formats both across the country and overseas. It is also available in a customized, on-site format for groups of second-year students.

Tuition for NBI 100 ranges from $130 to $250 and for NBI 300 from $390 to $880 per student, depending on group size and early enrollment discounts. NBI 100 home-study materials are also available for $110. The Center also offers a tuition refund guarantee and a liberal cancellation policy. For more information, call 800-837-7737 or 517-332-0777, or write to:

Northwestern Learning Center
4700 S. Hagadorn
East Lansing, MI 48823

E-mail should be sent to: testbuster@aol.com or northwestern@voyager.net

The Center may also be found online at: http://www.northwesternlearning.com/nw

Postgraduate Medical Review Education

Postgraduate Medical Review Education (PMRE) has over 22 years of experience with medical licensing exam preparation.

PMRE offers a complete home-study course for USMLE Step 1 in the form of audio cassettes and concise books beginning at $350. PMRE has packages of 9000 questions and answers for both basic and clinical sciences.

Every month, PMRE offers videotaped reviews for the USMLE and SPEX exams at their offices in Miami Beach, Florida, at a cost beginning at $1000. PMRE also guarantees that if a student does not pass the USMLE, he or she will receive a full refund for their reviews.

For more information, call 1-800-ECFMG-30 or write to:

PMRE
407 Lincoln Road, Suite 12E
Miami Beach, FL 33139

E-mail should be sent to: PMRE@aol.com

PMRE can also be found online: http://www.PMRE.com

The Princeton Review

The Princeton Review offers several programs of varying length to prepare students and graduates for the USMLE Step 1. Class time is broken into three sessions: proctored assessment exams, exam reviews, and workshops. All Princeton Review programs are taught live by medical students and graduates whose Step 1 scores exceed the 80th percentile and who have completed formal training.

Students in all courses sit for a battery of proctored, timed exams that span the basic sciences and that emphasize the increasingly clinical nature of the Step 1. Two of these exams are three hours long and are conducted without a break to simulate one of the exams given on the two days of the USMLE. Students also receive a computer-analyzed diagnostic score report that pinpoints any remaining areas of weakness while also tracking progress made during the course. Instructors review all exams with students. In addition to the practice examinations, students in all courses receive *Rapid Preparation for the USMLE Step 1* (J&S Publishing).

Some courses also include workshops wherein instructors teach the content tested on the Step 1 in a small group setting. No more than 15 students are ever placed in any workshop with a teacher. Princeton Review students who enroll in a workshop course also receive a complete set of basic science course manuals that review the highest-yield content found on the boards. The manuals contain text, tables, and diagrams; medical images such as CTs, MRIs, and gross and microscopic images; clinical cases; and over 1000 practice items. Manuals are revised each year to reflect Step 1 topics, formats, and cognitive approaches.

Live Princeton Review programs for the Step 1 are offered in more than 35 cities across the United States and Canada as well as throughout Europe, the Caribbean, and Asia. Second-year students of US medical schools are also encouraged to contact The Princeton Review to find out about programs that are run directly on medical school campuses.

To contact the Princeton Review office nearest you, call 1-800-USMLE84 or write to:

The Princeton Review of the Mid-Atlantic
St. Leonard's Court
39th and Chestnut, Suite 317
Philadelphia, PA 19107

The Princeton Review can also be found online: http://www.review.com

Youel's Prep, Inc.

David Bruce Youel, MD, has been presenting medical board preparation programs for 21 years. Youel's Prep provides comprehensive sets of preparation books and offers live-lecture and preparation programs for the USMLE Step 1 and for the NBOME COMLEX Level 1.

The Prepper's Manual (1998 edition) describes what to study, how to remember it, and how to use it at test time and is relevant for all steps/levels. This 350-page book is available for $69.

The Home Study Program (1998 edition) covers all steps and levels. Step- and level-specific facts are labeled with relevant numbers. The program includes nine books: Prepper's Manual; Multi-Systems I: Cardiovascular, Pulmonary, Hematology; Multi-Systems II: Immunology, Infections, Neoplasms; Multi-Systems III: Neurology, Behavior, Psychiatry; Multi-Systems IV: Endocrinology and Metabolism; Multi-Systems V: Reproduction and Renal; Multi-Systems VI: Gastroenterology and Dermatology; Multi-Systems VII: Musculoskeletal; and Q&A for The Home Study Program. This nine-volume, 3200-page series is available for $600 per set or $69 per book.

The FUNdaMENTALS (1998 edition) is written specifically for the USMLE Step 1 and the COMLEX Level 1. It consists of five books: Disease Book I: Heart, Lung, Blood, Gastroenterology, Renal; Disease Book II: Reproduction, Immunology, Microbiology; Molecular Medicine Book: Biochemistry, Physiology, Endocrinology, Pharmacology; Big and Little Parts Book: Anatomy; and Q&A for The FUNdaMENTALS. This 1825-page volume is available for $300 per set or $69 per book.

All Youel's Prep books are written by Dr. Youel and are formatted in a style that is designed to encourage active learning. Facts are clustered together in question-focused boxes that include language links, mnemonic links, logic locks, and carefully planned repetition.

All-live lectures and discussions are conducted by Dr. Youel and are designed as active learning sessions. The programs provide seven eight-hour sessions that are held mostly at US medical schools. Scheduling is customized to each school. The programs discuss the relevant books and provide practice examinations. Day 1 teaches what to study, how to remember it, and how to use high-yield facts at test time. These techniques are then applied throughout the week.

Program tuition for medical students of schools hosting a Youel's Prep program are $600 with The Home Study Program; $500 with The FUNdaMENTALS or The Clinical Book; and $375 for lectures only. Program tuition for programs held at hotels and for registrants not from a host school are $775 with The Home Study Program; $675 with The FUNdaMENTALS or The Clinical Book; and $375 for lectures only.

The purchase price of book sets is applied to tuition regardless of how much later the live program is taken. Once fully paid for any program, the same step/level program may be repeated as many times as desired, before or after the boards. First-year students are encouraged to attend. Both the books and the programs are also designed to improve scores on regular medical school examinations.

Contact Youel's Prep, Inc., at 1-800-645-3985 or 1-561-795-1555, fax 1-561-795-0169, or write to:

Youel's Prep, Inc.
701 Cypress Green Circle
Wellington, FL 33414.

E-mail should be sent to YouelsPrep@aol.com

Publisher Contacts

If you do not have convenient access to a medical bookstore, consider ordering directly from the publisher.

Alert & Oriented
7850 El Paseo Grande #5
La Jolla, CA 92037
(888) 253-7844
(619) 551-7667
joel@alertandonline.com
www.alertandonline.com

Appleton & Lange
P.O. Box 120041
Stamford, CT 06912
(800) 423-1359
(203) 406-4690
Fax: (203) 406-4602
www.appletonlange.com

Blackwell Science
350 Main Street
Malden, MA 02148
(800) 759-6102
(781) 388-8255
Fax: (781) 388-8250
www.blacksci.co.uk

Churchill Livingstone
300 Lighting Way
Secaucus, NJ 07094
(800) 553-5426
(973) 319-9800
Fax: (201) 319-9659

FMSG c/o IMP
100 Sylvan Pkwy
Amherst, NY 14228
(800) 443-4194
(716) 689-6000
Fax: (716) 689-6187
impltd@worldnet.att.net
www.cyberdeas.com/imp

ILOC Inc.
P.O. Box 232
Granville, OH 43023
(800) 495-4562
(614) 587-2658
Fax: (614) 587-2679

J&S Publishing
1300 Bishop Lane
Alexandria, VA 22302
(703) 823-9833
Fax: (703) 823-9834
Jandspub@ix.netcom.com
www.jandspub.com

Lippincott-Raven/Little, Brown
P.O. Box 1580
Hagerstown, MD 21741
(800) 777-2295
Fax: (301) 824-7390

McGraw-Hill Customer Service
P.O. Box 545
Blacklick, OH 43004
(800) 262-4729
Fax: (614) 755-5645
www.mghmedical.com

MedMaster, Inc.
P.O. Box 640028
Miami, FL 33164
(800) 335-3480
(305) 653-3480
Fax: (305) 653-9678
stgoldberg@aol.com

Mosby-Year Book
11830 Westline Industrial Drive
St. Louis, MO 63146
(800) 325-4177 ext. 5017
Fax: (800) 535-9935
www.mosby.com

National Learning Corporation
212 Michael Drive
Syosset, NY 11791
(800) 645-6337
Fax: (516) 921-8743

Springer-Verlag, NY Inc.
Attention: Service Center
333 Meadowlands Parkway
Secaucus, NJ 07094
(800) 777-4643
Fax: (201) 348-5405
www.Springer-NY.com
orders@Springer-NY.com

W.B. Saunders
6277 Sea Harbor Drive
Orlando, FL 32887
(800) 545-2522
Fax: (800) 874-6418

Williams & Wilkins
P.O. Box 1496
Baltimore, MD 21298-9724
(800) 638-0672
Fax: (800) 477-8438
www.wwilkins.com

Data in Section III were verified by Discount Medical Books & Supplies and Reiter's Professional Books—independent bookstores that are able to ship books from multiple publishers at list price both domestically and internationally.

Discount Medical Books & Supplies
345 Judah Street
San Francisco, CA 94122
(415) 664-5555
Fax: (415) 664-7810
medical@discmedbooks.com

Reiter's Scientific & Professional Books
2021 K Street, N.W.
Washington, DC 20006-1003
(800) 537-4314
(202) 223-3327
Fax: (202) 296-9103
books@reiters.com

Abbreviations and Symbols

Abbreviation	Meaning
AA	amino acid
AAV	adeno-assisted virus
Ab	antibody
ACE	angiotensin-converting enzyme
ACh	acetylcholine
AChE	acetylcholinesterase
ACL	anterior cruciate ligament
ACTH	adrenocorticotropic hormone
AD	autosomal dominant
ADA	adenosine deaminase
ADH	antidiuretic hormone (vasopressin)
ADHD	attention-deficit hyperactivity disorder
Ag	antigen
AIDS	acquired immunodeficiency syndrome
ALA	aminolevulinate synthase
ALL	acute lymphocytic leukemia
ALS	amyotrophic lateral sclerosis
ALT	alanine transaminase
AML	acute myelogenous leukemia
ANA	antinuclear antibody
ANOVA	analysis of variance
ANP	atrial natriuretic peptide
ANS	autonomic nervous system
AOA	American Osteopathic Association
AP	arterial pressure
APC	antigen-presenting cell
aPTT	activated partial thromboplastin time
ARDS	acute respiratory distress syndrome
ASD	atrial septal defect
ASO	antistreptolysin O
AST	aspartate transaminase
ATP	adenosine triphosphate
ATPase	adenosine triphosphatase
AV	atrioventricular
AVM	arteriovenous malformation
AZT	azidothymidine
BAL	British anti-Lewisite (dimercaprol)
BM	basement membrane
BP	blood pressure
BPG	bis phosphoglycerate
BPH	benign prostatic hyperplasia
CAD	coronary artery disease
cAMP	cyclic adenosine monophosphate
CCK	cholecystokinin
CCT	cortical collecting tubule
CD	cluster of differentiation
CDC	Centers for Disease Control
CDP	cytidine diphosphate
CE	cholesterol ester
CETP	cholesteryl-ester transfer protein
CF	cystic fibrosis
CFTR	cystic fibrosis transmembrane regulator
CFX	circumflex (artery)
cGMP	cyclic guanosine monophosphate

Abbreviation	Meaning
ChAT	choline acetyltransferase
CHF	congestive heart failure
CJD	Creutzfeldt–Jakob disease
CL	clearance
CLL	chronic lymphocytic leukemia
CM	chylomicron
CML	chronic myelogenous leukemia
CMT	Computerized Mastery Test
CMV	cytomegalovirus
CN	cranial nerve
CNS	central nervous system
CO	cardiac output
CoA	coenzyme A
COMLEX	Comprehensive Osteopathic Medical Licensing Examination
COMT	catechol-O-methyltransferase
COPD	chronic obstructive pulmonary disease
COX	cyclooxygenase
C_p	concentration in plasma
CPK-MB	creatine phosphokinase, MB fraction
CRH	corticotropin-releasing hormone
CSA	Clinical Skills Assessment (exam)
CSF	cerebrospinal fluid
CT	computed tomography
CV	cardiovascular
CXR	chest x-ray
D	dopamine
DAG	diacylglycerol
DEA	Drug Enforcement Agency
DES	diethylstilbestrol
DIC	disseminated intravascular coagulation
DIMS	disorder in initiating and maintaining sleep
DKA	diabetic ketoacidosis
DMD	Duchenne muscular dystrophy
DMN	dorsal motor nucleus
2,4-DNP	2,4-dinitrophenol
DOES	disorder of excessive somnolence
DOPA	dihydroxyphenylalanine (methyldopa)
DPG	diffuse proliferative glomerulonephritis; diphosphoglycerate
DPM	Doctor of Podiatric Medicine
DPPC	dipalmitoyl phosphatidylcholine
ds	double stranded
dTMP	deoxythymidine monophosphate
DTR	deep tendon reflex
DTs	delirium tremens
EBV	Epstein–Barr virus
ECF	extracellular fluid
ECFMG	Educational Commission for Foreign Medical Graduates
ECT	electroconvulsive therapy
EDRF	endothelium-derived relaxing factor
EDTA	ethylenediamine tetraacetic acid
EDV	end-diastolic volume

Abbreviation	Meaning	Abbreviation	Meaning
EEG	electroencephalogram	HNPCC	hereditary nonpolyposis colorectal cancer
EF-2	elongation factor 2	HPV	human papillomavirus
EGF	epidermal growth factor	HSV	herpes simplex virus
ELISA	enzyme-linked immunosorbent assay	HTLV	human T-cell lymphotropic virus
EM	electron microscopy	HTN	hypertension
EMB	eosin–methylene blue	IC	inspiratory capacity
EOM	extraocular muscle	ICF	intracellular fluid
EPS	extrapyramidal symptoms	ICU	intensive care unit
ER	endoplasmic reticulum; emergency room	IDDM	insulin-dependent diabetes mellitus
ERP	effective refractory period	IDL	intermediate-density lipoprotein
ERV	expiratory reserve volume	I/E	inspiratory/expiratory
ESR	erythrocyte sedimentation rate	IF	intrinsic factor; immunofluorescence
ESV	end-systolic volume	IFN	interferon
EtOH	ethyl alcohol	Ig	immunoglobulin
FAD	oxidized flavin adenine dinucleotide	IHSS	idiopathic hypertrophic subaortic stenosis
FADH$_2$	reduced flavin adenine dinucleotide	IL-1, -2, -3, -4, -5	interleukin-1, 2, 3, 4, 5
FAP	familial adenomatous polyposis	IM	intramuscular
FDA	Food and Drug Administration	IMG	international medical graduate
FEV	forced expiratory volume	IMP	inosine monophosphate
FF	filtration fraction	IND	investigational new drug
FFA	free fatty acid	INH	isonicotine hydrazine (isoniazid)
FFP	fresh frozen plasma	IP$_3$	inositol triphosphate
FH$_x$	family history	IPV	inactivated polio vaccine
FLEX	Federal Licensing Examination	IRV	inspiratory reserve volume
FMG	foreign medical graduate	IVC	inferior vena cava
FMN	flavin mononucleotide	JCV	JC virus
FSH	follicle-stimulating hormone	JGA	juxtaglomerular apparatus
FSMB	Federation of State Medical Boards	KSHV	Kaposi's sarcoma–associated herpesvirus
FTA-ABS	fluorescent treponemal antibody— absorbed	LA	left atrium
FVC	forced vital capacity	LAD	left anterior descending; left atrial defect
G3P	glucose-3-phosphate	LAF	left anterior fascicle
G6PD	glucose-6-phosphate dehydrogenase	LCA	left coronary artery
GABA	γ-aminobutyric acid	LCAT	lecithin-cholesterol acyltransferase
GBM	glomerular basement membrane	LCL	lateral collateral ligament
GFAP	glial fibrillary acidic protein	LCME	Liaison Committee on Medical Education
GFR	glomerular filtration rate	LCV	lymphocytic choriomeningitis virus
GH	growth hormone	LDH	lactate dehydrogenase
GI	gastrointestinal	LDL	low-density lipoprotein
G$_i$	G protein, inhibitory	LES	lower esophageal sphincter
GM-CSF	granulocyte-macrophage colony- stimulating factor	LFT	liver function test
GMP	guanosine monophosphate	LH	luteinizing hormone
GN	glomerulonephritis	LLQ	left lower quadrant
GnRH	gonadotropin-releasing hormone	LM	light microscopy
GRP	gastrin-releasing peptide	LMN	lower motor neuron (signs)
G$_s$	G protein, stimulatory	LPS	lipopolysaccharide
GTP	guanosine triphosphate	LT	leukotriene; long thoracic
HAV	hepatitis A virus	LV	left ventricle; left ventricular
Hb	hemoglobin	MAC	*Mycobacterium avium–intracellulare* complex; membrane attack complex
HBsAG	hepatitis B surface antigen	MAO	monoamine oxidase
HBV	hepatitis B virus	MC	musculocutaneous
hCG	human chorionic gonadotropin	MCL	medial collateral ligament
HCV	hepatitis C virus	M-CSF	macrophage colony stimulating factor
HDL	high-density lipoprotein	MEN	multiple endocrine neoplasia
HDV	hepatitis D virus	MEOS	microsomal ethanol oxidizing system
HEV	hepatitis E virus	MHC	major histocompatibility complex
HGPRT	hypoxanthine-guanine phosphoribosyltransferase	MI	myocardial infarction
HHV	human herpesvirus	MLF	medial longitudinal fasciculus
HIV	human immunodeficiency virus	MMR	measles, mumps, rubella
HLA	human leukocyte antigen	MPTP	1-methyl-4-phenyl-1, 2, 3, 6-tetrahydro- pyridine
HMG	human menopausal gonadotropin	MRI	magnetic resonance imaging
HMG-CoA	hydroxymethylglutaryl-CoA	MTP	metatarsal–phalangeal
HMP	hexose monophosphate		

Abbreviation	Meaning	Abbreviation	Meaning
NAD	oxidized nicotinamide adenine dinucleotide	RDS	respiratory distress syndrome
NADH	reduced nicotinamide adenine dinucleotide	REM	rapid eye movement
NADP	oxidized nicotinamide adenine dinucleotide phosphate	RER	rough endoplasmic reticulum
		RES	reticuloendothelial system
NADPH	reduced nicotinamide adenine dinucleotide phosphate	RPF	renal plasma flow
		RPR	rapid plasma reagin
NBME	National Board of Medical Examiners	RSV	respiratory syncytial virus
NBOME	National Board of Osteopathic Medicine Examination	RUQ	right upper quadrant
		RV	residual volume; right ventricle; right ventricular
NBPME	National Board of Podiatric Medical Examiners		
		RVH	right ventricular hypertrophy
NE	norepinephrine	SA	sino-atrial
NIDA	National Institute on Drug Abuse	SAM	S-adenosylmethionine
NIDDM	non-insulin-dependent diabetes mellitus	SC	sickle cell, subcutaneous
NREM	non–rapid eye movement	SCID	severe combined immunodeficiency disease
NSAID	nonsteroidal anti-inflammatory drug		
OAA	oxaloacetic acid	SD	standard deviation
OBS	organic brain syndrome	SEM	standard error of the mean
OMT	osteopathic manipulative technique	SER	smooth endoplasmic reticulum
OPV	oral polio vaccine	SES	socioeconomic status
PABA	para-aminobenzoic acid	SGOT	serum glutamic oxaloacetic transaminase
PAH	para-aminohippuric acid		
PALS	periarterial lymphoid sheath	SGPT	serum glutamic pyruvate transaminase
PAN	polyarteritis nodosa	SLE	systemic lupus erythematosus
P-ANCA	perinuclear pattern of antineutrophil cytoplasmic antibodies	SMA	superior mesenteric artery
		SOMA	Student Osteopathic Medical Association
PAS	periodic acid–Schiff (stain)	SRS-A	slow-reacting substance of anaphylaxis
PCAT	phosphatidylcholine-cholesterol acyltransferase	ss	single stranded
		SSPE	subacute sclerosing panencephalitis
PCI_2	prostacyclin I_2	STD	sexually transmitted disease
PCL	posterior cruciate ligament	SV	stroke volume
PCP	*Pneumocystis carinii* pneumonia; phencyclidine hydrochloride	SVC	superior vena cava
		SVT	supraventricular tachycardia
PCR	polymerase chain reaction	$t_{1/2}$	half-life
PCWP	pulmonary capillary wedge pressure	TAT	thematic apperception test
PD	posterior descending	TB	tuberculosis
PDA	patent ductus arteriosus	TBW	total body water
PDE	phosphodiesterase	TCA	tricarboxylic acid
PDGF	platelet-derived growth factor	TCR	T-cell receptor
PEP	phosphoenolpyruvate	TG	triglyceride
PFK	phosphofructokinase	TGF	transforming growth factor
PFT	pulmonary function tests	TGV	transposition of great vessels
PG	prostaglandin	TIBC	total iron binding capacity
PID	pelvic inflammatory disease	TLC	total lung capacity
PIP_2	phosphatidylinositol 4,5-bisphosphate	TMP-SMX	trimethoprim-sulfamethoxazole
PK	pyruvate kinase	TNF	tissue necrosis factor
PKU	phenylketonuria	TNM	tumor, node, metastasis
PML	progressive multifocal leukoencephalopathy	ToRCH	toxoplasmosis, rubella, CMV, herpes
		tPA	tissue plasminogen factor
PMN	polymorphonuclear	TPP	thiamine pyrophosphate
PNH	paroxysmal nocturnal hemoglobinuria	TSH	thyroid-stimulating hormone
PNS	peripheral nervous system	TSS	toxic shock syndrome
POMC	pro-opiomelanocortin	TSST	toxic shock syndrome toxin
PP	pyrophosphate	TV	tidal volume
PPRF	parapontine reticular formation	TXA	thromboxane
PR	pulmonic regurgitation	UDP	uridine diphosphate
PRPP	phosphoribosylpyrophosphate	UMN	upper motor neuron (signs)
PSA	prostate-specific antigen	URI	upper respiratory infection
PSS	progressive systemic sclerosis	USMLE	United States Medical Licensing Examination
PT	prothrombin time		
PTH	parathyroid hormone	UTI	urinary tract infection
PTT	partial thromboplastin time	VC	vital capacity
RA	right atrium	V_d	volume of distribution
RBC	red blood cell	VDRL	Venereal Disease Research Laboratory
RCA	right coronary artery	VF	ventricular fibrillation

Abbreviation	Meaning	Symbol	Meaning
VLDL	very low-density lipoprotein	↑	increase(s)
VMA	vanillylmandelic acid	↓	decrease(s)
V/Q	ratio of ventilation to perfusion	→	leads to
VSD	ventricular septal defect	1°	primary
VWF	Von Willebrand factor	2°	secondary
VZV	varicella-zoster virus	3°	tertiary
WBC	white blood cell	≈	approximately; homologous
X̄	statistical mean	≡	defined as
		⊖	negative effect
		⊕	positive effect

Index of Mnemonics

Index

Polyarteritis nodosa, 218
Polycyclic aromatic hydrocarbons, 266
Polymerase chain reaction (PCR), 124
Polymerases: DNA, 123
Polymerases: RNA, 125
Polymyxins, 238, 243
Portal-systemic anastomoses, 76
Postgraduate Medical Review Education (PMRE), 363
Post-traumatic stress disorder, 113
Potter's syndrome, 72
Power, 100
Practice tests, 24–25
    See also practice *under* Review books/materials
Praziquantel, 245
Prazosin, 250, 255
Precipitin curve, 182
Precision vs. accuracy, 99
Predictive value, 98
Prednisone, 264, 274
Pregnancy
    hormones during, 302
    hypertension, 213
Prescriptions. *See* Antimicrobial drugs; Cancer drugs; Central nervous system (pharmacology); Pharmacology; pharmacology *under* Cardiovascular system; Toxicology; *specific drugs*
Prevalence vs. incidence, 98
Primaquine, 266
Primidone, 253
Princeton Review, 364
Prions, 173
Probucol, 262
Procainamide, 260, 266
Procaine, 254
Procarbazine, 266
Progesterone, 303
Projection, 116
Projective tests, 118
Propafenone, 260
Propofol, 253
Propylthiouracil, 273
Prostatic adenocarcinoma, 200
Protein/cell
    cell cycle phases, 142
    cholesterol lipoproteins, 143
    collagen synthesis/structure, 143
    CO_2 transport in blood, 144
    enzyme kinetics, 141
    enzyme regulation methods, 144
    Hb structure regulation, 144
    hemoglobin, 143
    hormonal effects on cAMP, 144
    keratin composition and function, 142
    microtubule, 142
    phosphatidylcholine function, 142
    PIP_2 second messenger system, 144
    plasma membrane composition, 142
    sodium pump, 144
Protein synthesis, 139, 240
Protozoa, medically important, 171
Psammoma bodies, 226
Pseudogout, 211
Pseudohermaphroditism, 192
Pseudomonas aeruginosa, 161

Psychiatry, 120
    amnesia types, 109
    antipsychotic mechanism, 115
    bipolar disorder, 111
    compulsion, 113
    cultural/ethnic, 108
    cyclothymic disorder, 111
    delirium, 111
    delirium tremens, 110
    delusion vs. loose association, 114
    dementia, 111
    depressive episode, major, 111
    electroconvulsive therapy, 115
    factitious disorder, 112
    forensic, 108
    gain: 1°, 2°, 3°, 112
    hallucination vs. illusion vs. delusion, 114
    hypomanic episode, 111
    malingering, 112
    manic episode, 111
    obsession, 113
    orientation as to person/place, 108
    panic disorder, 112
    personality, 113–114
    phobias, specific/social, 112
    post-traumatic stress disorder, 113
    schizophrenia, 114
    somatoform disorders, 112
    substance abuse/dependence, 109–110
Psychoanalysis, 117
Psychology, 120
    classical conditioning, 117
    dyad, 117
    ego defenses, 115
    elderly, changes in the, 118
    existential psychotherapy, 118
    fear: conditioners, 117
    Gestalt therapy, 117
    hopelessness, factors in, 117
    intelligence testing, 118
    mind, structural theory of the, 115
    Oedipus complex, 117
    operant conditioning, 117
    projective tests, 118
    psychoanalysis, 117
    reinforcement schedules, 117
    sexual dysfunction, 118
    sick role, 117
PTH, 298, 300
Publications, NBME/USMLE, 8–10
    See also Database of basic science review resources; Review books/materials, Resources, informational
Pulmonary circulation, 290
Pulmonary flow volume loops, 289
Pyridostigmine, 248
Pyruvate dehydrogenase complex, 135
Pyruvate dehydrogenase deficiency, 127

Q

Questions
    difficult, 29–30
    experimental, 30
    matching sets, 4
    multiple-choice, 29
    one-best-answer items, 4
Quinidine, 260, 266
Quinine, 245, 266
Quinolones, 238

R

Rabies, 178
Radial nerve, 91
Radiology, 96
Rationalization, 116
Reaction formation, 116
Recurrent laryngeal nerve, 73
Red blood cells, 136, 226
Reed–Sternberg cells, 227
Regression, 105, 116
Reinforcement schedules, 117
Reiter's syndrome, 212
Reliability and validity, 99
REM sleep/rebound, 107
Renal system
    amino acid clearance, 297
    electrolyte clearance, 297
    failure to make urine and excrete nitrogenous wastes, 297
    filtration fraction, 296
    glomerular filtration barrier, 297
    glucose clearance, 296
    hormones acting on, 298
    hyperaldosteronism, 299
    kidney endocrine functions, 297
    measuring fluid compartments, 297
    nephron physiology, 299
    PAH, 296
    plasma flow, 296
    renal clearance, 296
    renin–angiotensin system, 298
Renin–angiotensin system, 298
Replication
    DNA, 123
    viral, 172
Reportable diseases, 101
Repression, 116
Reserpine, 247, 255
Residencies and international medical graduates, 44
Resistance/pressure/flow, 282
Resources, informational
    international medical graduates, 45–47
    publications, NBME/USMLE, 8–10
    United States Medical Licensing Examination, Step 1 (USMLE Step 1), 35–37
    See also Commercial review courses; Database of basic science review resources; Review books/materials
Respiratory system
    acid-base physiology, 290
    altitude, response to high, 288
    CO_2 transport, 291
    hypoxemia, 291
    important lung products, 288
    lung volumes, 288
    neonatal respiratory distress syndrome, 222
    obstructive lung disease, 291
    oxygen dissociation curve, 290
    particle size and lung entrapment, 288
    pulmonary circulation, 290
    pulmonary flow volume loops, 289
    restrictive lung disease, 292
    V/Q mismatch, 290
Retroperitoneal structures, 77

New from the authors of *First Aid for the USMLE Step 1*

First Aid for the Wards

Le, Bhushan, & Amin

This brand-new high-yield student-to-student guide is designed to help students make the transition from the basic sciences to the hospital wards and succeed on their clinical rotations. The book features an orientation to the hospital environment, tips on being an effective and efficient junior medical student, student-proven advice tailored to each core rotation, a database of high-yield clinical facts, and recommendations for clinical pocket books, texts, and references. ISBN 0-8385-2595-4, A2595-5.

First Aid for the Match

Le, Bhushan, & Amin

This top-rated (5 stars, *Doody Review*) student-to-student guide helps medical students effectively and efficiently navigate the residency application process, helping them make the most of their limited time, money, and energy. The book draws on the advice and experiences of successful student applicants as well as residency directors. Also featured are application and interview tips tailored to each specialty, successful personal statements and CVs with analyses, current trends, and common interview questions with suggested strategies for responding. ISBN 0-8385-2596-2, A2596-3.

About the Authors

Vikas Bhushan, MD, completed residency training in diagnostic radiology at the University of California at Los Angeles. He is currently working part-time *locum tenens* in radiology while taking time off to travel and write. His interest in medical education led to the development and publication of the original *First Aid for the USMLE Step 1* in 1992. He is active in medical informatics and digital radiology. Vikas earned his MD with Thesis from the University of California at San Francisco. Vikas is single and resides in Los Angeles. He can be reached at vbhushan@aol.com

Tao Le, MD, earned his medical degree from the University of California at San Francisco. He has been involved in major writing and editing projects over the past six years. As a medical student he was editor-in-chief of *Synapse,* a campus-wide student-run newspaper with a weekly circulation of 5000. He is a resident in internal medicine at Yale–New Haven Hospital. He is married and lives in New Haven with his wife, Thao, a resident in pediatrics. Tao can be reached at taotle@aol.com

Chirag Amin, MD, graduated from medical school at the University of Miami and has begun residency training in orthopedic surgery at Orlando Regional Medical Center. Chirag has been involved extensively in teaching and in writing books. He led the completion of *Jump Start MCAT: A High-Yield Student-to-Student Guide* (Williams & Wilkins). Chirag is single and lives in Orlando, Florida. He can be reached at chiragamin@aol.com

Vipal Soni is a third-year medical student at the UCLA School of Medicine. He helped coordinate the 1998 revision of *First Aid for the USMLE Step 1* and was a contributor to *Jump Start MCAT: A High-Yield Student-to-Student Guide.* He has been involved in medical research, and his interests include music and tennis. Vipal is single and lives in Los Angeles. He can be reached at vsoni@ucla.edu

Hoang (Henry) Nguyen is a third-year MD/PhD student at Northwestern University Medical School and is currently pursuing research in neuroscience and development. He has previously worked on other books, including *Underground MCAT Answers* and *JumpStart MCAT* as well as *Let's Go: Southeast Asia.* Although his first love is the classics, he hopes to pursue a career in academic medicine and research. Henry is single and lives in the Bucktown area of Chicago, where he spends his free time writing, reading, and enjoying music. He can be reached at hbnguyen@nwu.edu

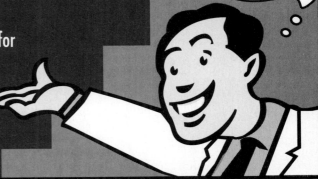
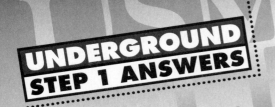
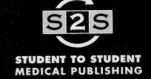

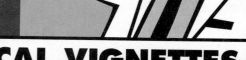
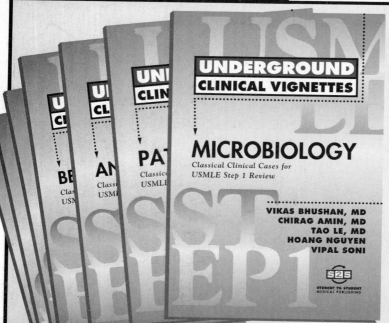